CASE REVIEW

Nuclear
Medicine

Series Editor

David M. Yousem, MD
Professor, Department of Radiology
Director of Neuroradiology
Johns Hopkins Hospital
Baltimore, Maryland

Other Volumes in the CASE REVIEW Series

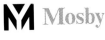
Mosby

An Imprint of Elsevier Science

St. Louis London Philadelphia Sydney Toronto

Harvey A. Ziessman, MD
Director of Nuclear Medicine
Professor of Radiology
Division of Nuclear Medicine
Georgetown University Hospital
Washington, DC

Patrice K. Rehm, MD
Associate Professor of Radiology
Director of Nuclear Medicine
University of Virginia Health Science Center
Charlottesville, Virginia

WITH 362 ILLUSTRATIONS

CASE REVIEW

Nuclear Medicine

CASE REVIEW SERIES

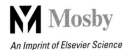

Acquisitions Editor: Stephanie Donley
Publication Services Manager: Pat Joiner
Designer: Mark A. Oberkrom

Mosby, Inc.
11830 Westline Industrial Drive
St. Louis, Missouri 63146

Printed in the United States of America

International Standard Book Number 0-323-00658-2

02   03   04   05   06   TG/MVY   9   8   7   6   5   4   3   2   1

To Karen and Bob

Nuclear medicine combines anatomic and functional imaging in a clinical and research setting. Its role in diagnosing disease and monitoring treatment has expanded with time, just as its research applications have also grown. Since the diseases evaluated by nuclear medicine span all organ systems, if you truly understand this subspecialty, you will know a great deal about medicine in general.

Drs. Ziessman and Rehm have provided the reader with an excellent contribution to the Case Review series. They have emphasized the latest advances in nuclear medicine but teach the reader in a user-friendly, case-at-a-time format. This is not a dry text laboring under the weight of descriptions of quality assurance techniques and decay curves. Instead, this is a brilliant teaching instrument that demonstrates this marvelous specialty in action using relevant clinical cases. I wish I had this book when I was cramming for the boards 14 years ago—I was stumped by superscans and hepatic regenerating nodules when I was in Louisville.

The philosophy of the Case Review series is to review each specialty in a challenging interactive way. Each book in the series has gradations of difficulty so that the reader can assess his or her proficiency and can use this self-evaluation to guide continued education. Since each case in the book is distinct, this is the kind of text that can be picked up and read at any time in your day, in your career.

I am very pleased to welcome Dr. Ziessman's and Dr. Rehm's *Nuclear Medicine* edition to the very popular Case Review series that includes *General and Vascular Ultrasound* by William D. Middleton; *Musculoskeletal Imaging* by Joseph Yu; *Obstetric and Gynecologic Ultrasound* by Al Kurtz and Pam Johnson; *Spine Imaging* by Brian Bowen; *Thoracic Imaging* by Phil Boiselle and Theresa McLoud; *Genitourinary Imaging* by Ron Zagoria, William Mayo-Smith, and Glenn Tung; *Gastrointestinal Imaging* by Peter Feczko and Robert Halpert; *Brain Imaging* by Laurie Loevner; and *Head and Neck Imaging* by me.

David M. Yousem, MD
Case Review Series Editor

Case Review: Nuclear Medicine is similar in format to *Case Reviews* previously published on other subjects. This volume contains 200 cases that cover all the major areas of nuclear medicine clinical practice. Cases are categorized as Opening Round, Fair Game, and Challenge, according to our estimated difficulty; understanding that difficulty will vary with the reader's experience and training. Each image-based case includes questions, answers, comments, and references to the medical literature and to specific pages in *Nuclear Medicine: The Requisites*. The two textbooks complement each other, enhancing the learning opportunity.

The format is intended to provide the reader more than merely a test of image recognition. The text serves as a means of review of basic concepts of physiology and pathophysiology, radiopharmaceutical biodistribution and kinetics, and mechanisms of radiopharmaceutical uptake and clearance. Image recognition combined with an understanding of the physiologic basis of the scintigraphic images is necessary to derive the appropriate differential diagnosis. The game-like format offers a relaxed and enjoyable method to learn and review nuclear medicine.

In recent years, the field of nuclear radiology/nuclear medicine has made many major advances in radiopharmaceuticals and instrumentation. Positron emission tomography (PET) is a prime example. What many considered not long ago a mere research tool has rapidly become a clinical study in rapidly increasing demand. Fluorodeoxyglucose (FDG) PET revolutionized tumor imaging and is required for state-of-the-art oncology imaging. This volume contains many pertinent examples of how FDG-PET is being used clinically on a daily basis. Other recently developed radiopharmaceuticals, such as monoclonal antibodies and peptides, and up-to-date methods for using established radiopharmaceuticals are presented.

Most imaging aspects of nuclear medicine are included in this book, with case representation roughly in proportion to the clinical demand. Nuclear cardiology or cardiac nuclear medicine, which represents a large portion of a typical nuclear medicine practice, is the focus of many examples in the *Case Review.*

Harvey A. Ziessman, MD
Patrice K. Rehm, MD

We would like to thank and acknowledge the contributions to this book by Suhny Abbara, MD; Anup Agarwal, CNMT; Sherry S. Deane; Asaf Durakovic, MD; Douglas Eggli, MD; Edward Kotylarov, MD, PhD; Kenneth Levin, MD; Michael Oberhofer, MD; Janice O'Malley, MD; Lalitha Shankar MD, PhD; and Denny D. Watson, PhD. Special thanks goes to Daniel C.E. Lane with Educational Media at Georgetown University Medical Center for the many hours spent on digital processing and printing images for this text.

Color Plates

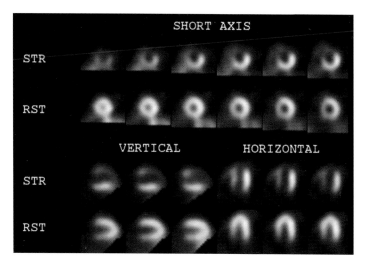

Case 17

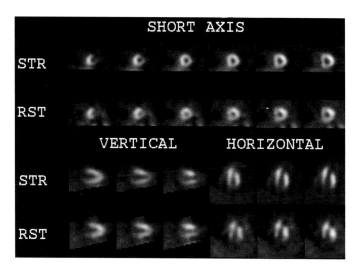

Case 18

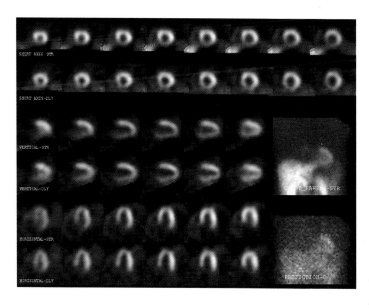

Case 19

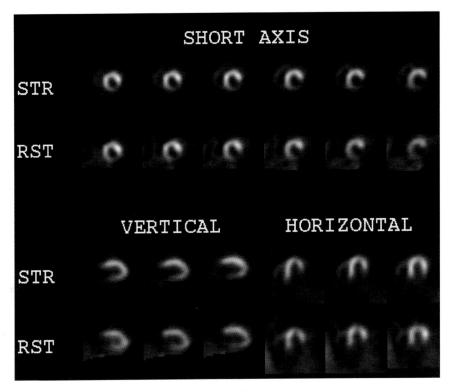

Case 83

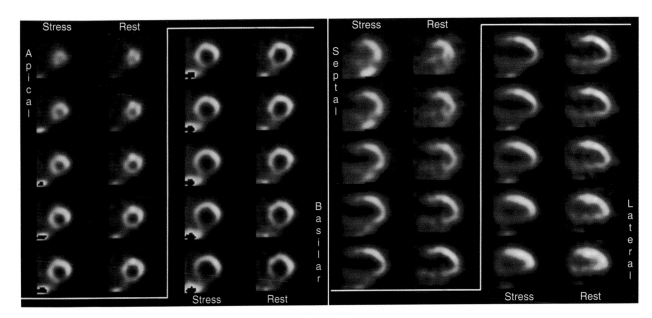

Case 84

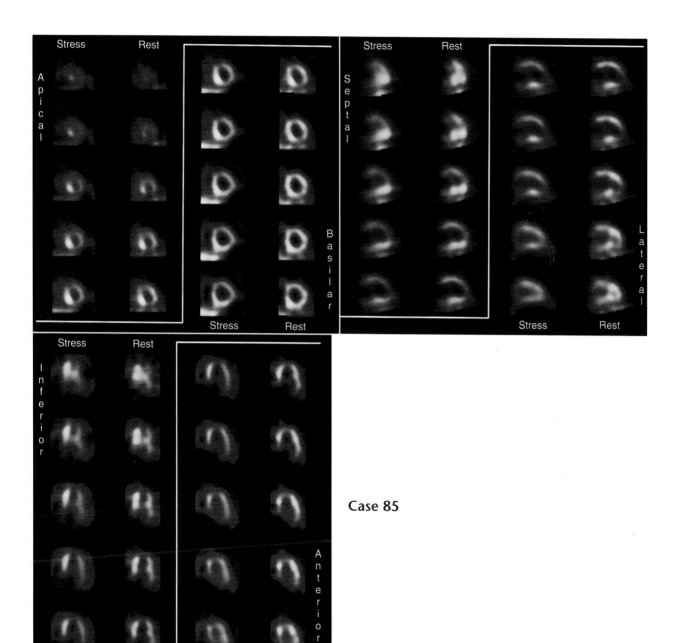

Case 85

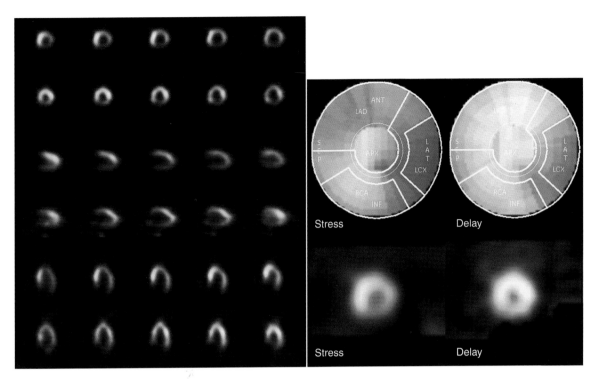

Case 87

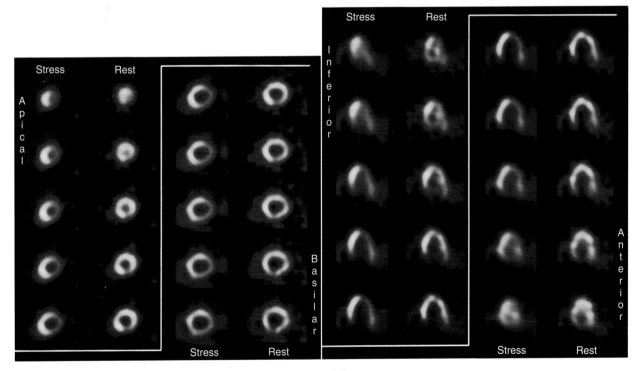

Case 89

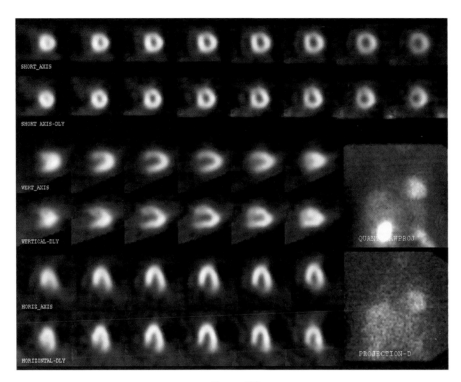

Case 90

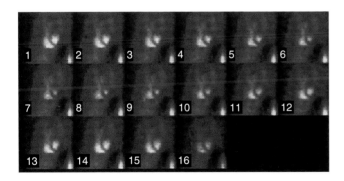

Case 91

Case 93

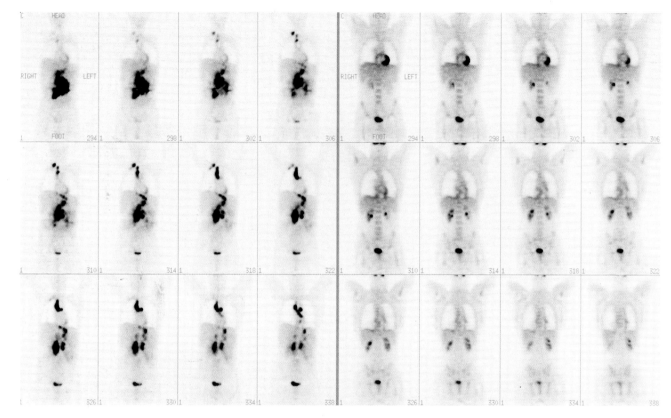

Case 104

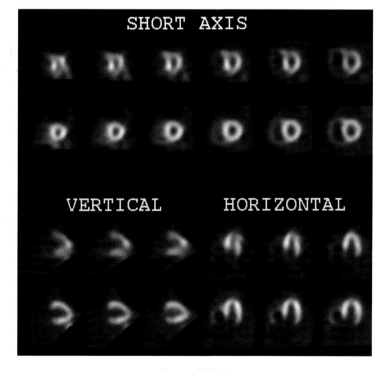

Case 150*A*

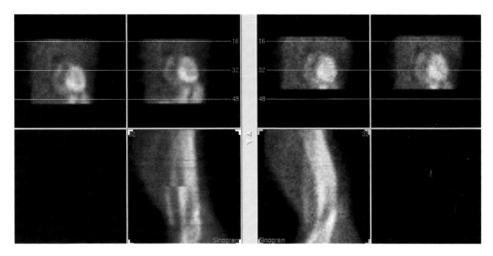

Case 150*B*

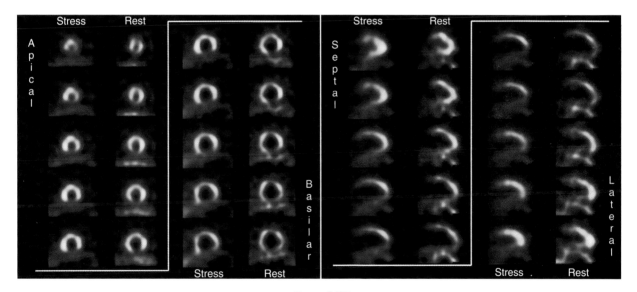

Case 152

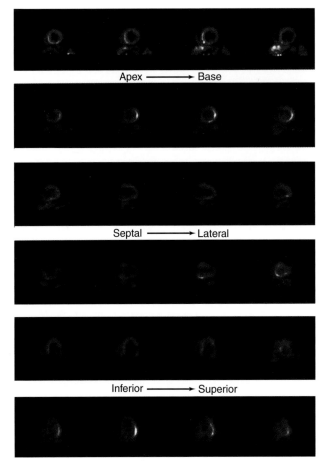

Apex ⟶ Base

Septal ⟶ Lateral

Inferior ⟶ Superior

Case 156

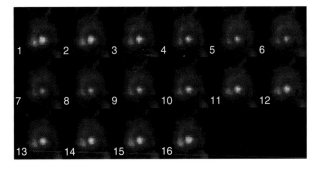

Case 157A

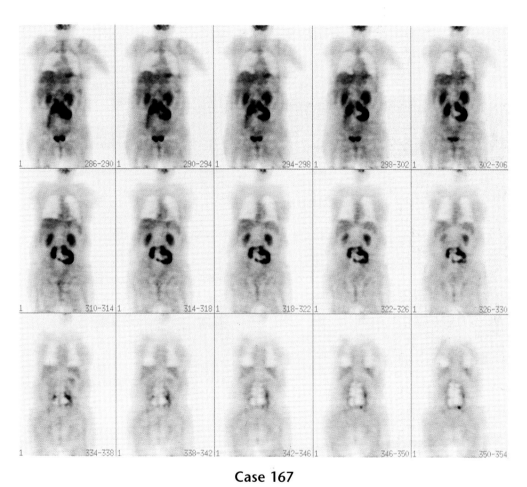

Case 167

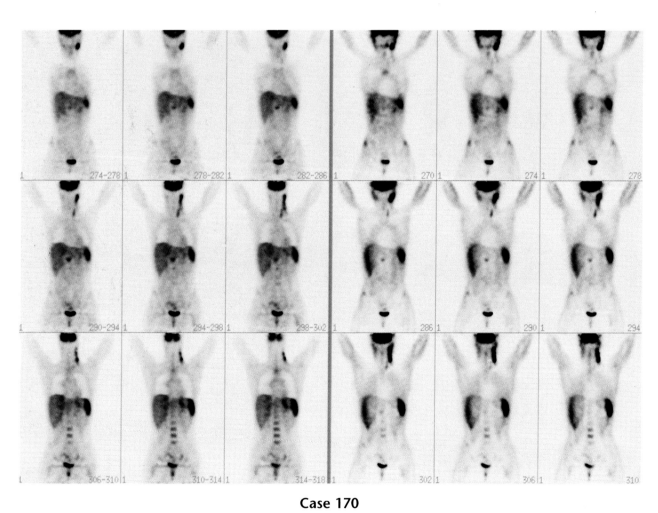

Case 170

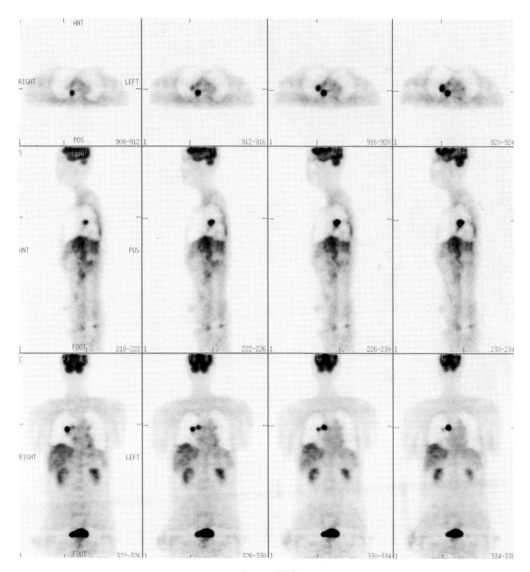

Case 198

Opening Round Cases

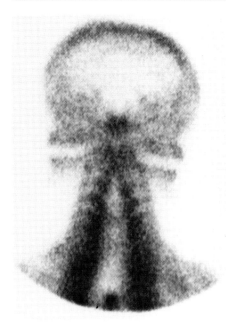

1. What is the radiopharmaceutical used for this study?
2. Describe the image findings. Interpret this limited study.
3. Name the mythological Roman god with two heads.
4. What is a radioisotope, a radionuclide, a radionucleotide, and a radiotracer?

Skeletal System: Janus—Two-Headed Roman God

1. ^{99m}Tc methylene diphosphonate.

2. Bone scan in patient with apparently two heads looking in opposite directions. The patient moved his head; the technologist did not move his/hers.

3. Janus.

4. If you do not know, you cannot proceed until you read the comments below.

Reference
Roman mythology.

Cross-Reference
Nuclear Medicine: THE REQUISITES, ed 2, pp 110-116.

Comment
Janus is the two-faced Roman god of beginnings and endings, the god of gates and doors, from which the month of January gets its name. He is depicted with two faces gazing in opposite directions. Looking back at the short history of nuclear medicine, many advances in the field, in both instrumentation and radiopharmaceuticals, and most importantly in their clinical use, are evident. An exciting advance is the adoption of fluorodeoxyglucose (FDG) positron emission tomography (PET) as a clinical reality and its transformation of the practice of oncologic medicine. Like Janus, we should not only look back to know where we have come from, but we must then look forward to the many opportunities ahead.

Nucleotides are basic structural building blocks of DNA and RNA, i.e., ribose or deoxyribose sugar joined to a purine or pyrimidine base and a phosphate group. Clinical nuclear medicine uses radionuclides, not radionucleotides. As different types of atoms are called elements, different types of nuclei are termed *nuclides*. Nuclides with the same number of protons are isotopes, e.g., ^{131}I, ^{123}I. An element is characterized by its atomic number (Z) alone, whereas a nuclide is characterized by its mass number (A) and its atomic number (Z). Radionuclides refer to radioactive elements of all types, whether natural or manmade. Technetium was the first manmade radionuclide. Radiopharmaceuticals are radionuclides attached to chemicals or drugs used to investigate physiological and biochemical processes, e.g., ^{99m}Tc labeled to methylene diphosphonate (MDP). Radiopharmaceuticals often are referred to as *radiotracers,* because only trace amounts of the drugs are used, indicating that they are markers of physiological processes, e.g., bone metabolism, but without pharmacological effect.

A   B

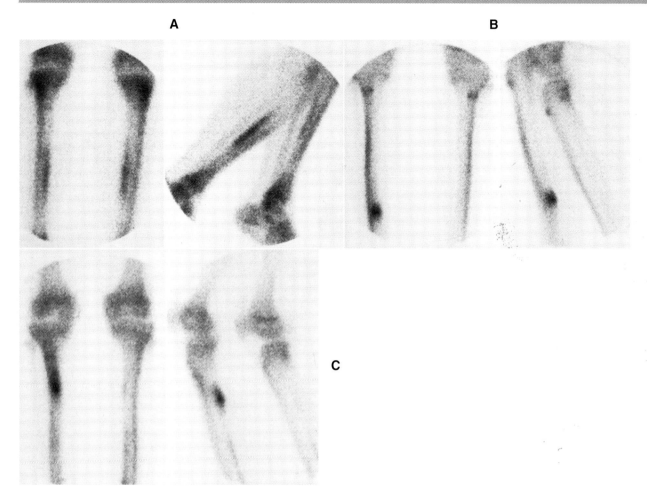

C

Lower extremity pain in three different patients *(A, B, C)*, all members of the track team.

1. Describe the findings in Patient *A*.
2. What is the most likely diagnosis?
3. Describe the findings in Patients *B* and *C*.
4. Provide the most likely diagnosis for Patients *B* and *C*.

Skeletal System: Stress Fractures

1. Increased activity in a linear pattern along the posterior and medial aspect of both mid-tibias.

2. Shin splints.

3. Patient *B:* focal ovoid activity posteromedial right tibia at the junction of the proximal two thirds and distal one third. Patient *C:* focal fusiform activity posteromedially in the right proximal tibia and linear activity along the posteromedial left tibia proximally and more prominently distally.

4. Patient *B:* stress fracture. Patient *C:* stress fracture and shin splints.

Reference

Thrall JH, section editor: *Nuclear radiology* (fourth series) *test and syllabus,* Reston, Va, 1990, American College of Radiology, pp 121-129.

Cross-Reference

Nuclear Medicine: THE REQUISITES, ed 2, pp 130-131.

Comment

Bone is a dynamic tissue in which intermittent forces stimulate remodeling of the bone architecture to withstand applied stresses. Stress leads to remodeling initiated by osteoclasts that produce small areas of resorption and microfractures that are remodeled with lamellar bone. If bone formation cannot keep up with bone resorption, bone weakening results. In response to the temporarily weakened bone, periosteal reaction, endosteal proliferation, or both may occur at the site of stress. If the stress is not reduced, the repair mechanisms may become overwhelmed, resulting in fracture.

Stress fractures on bone scan appear as focal oval or fusiform activity based at the cortex with the axis of the abnormality parallel to that of the bone, or they may appear as a transverse band of increased activity. The scan abnormality often precedes radiographic changes by 1 to 2 weeks. Tibial stress fractures most commonly occur posteromedially at the junction of the middle and distal thirds of the tibia, as in Patient *B.* Shin splints or tibial stress syndrome are terms used to describe anterior leg pain and tenderness. Often there is no identifiable inciting event, but pain occurs after athletic activity and is relieved by rest. Scan findings vary, but generally bilateral linear tibial uptake involves the cortex in multiple areas or diffusely; the uptake may be symmetrical or asymmetrical. The pattern differs from the pattern of stress fracture. However, because of the nature of the inciting stresses, stress fractures commonly coexist with shin splints.

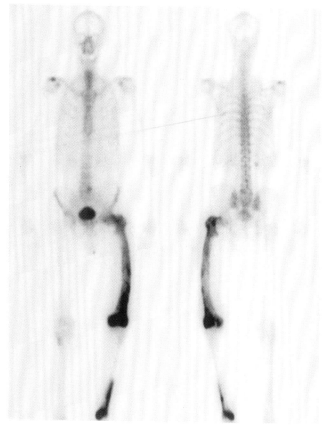

1. Describe the bone scan abnormality.
2. Provide descriptive terms that could be used to describe the pattern in the tibia.
3. Provide the differential diagnosis.
4. The patient may experience clinical symptoms related to another organ system. Discuss the mechanism.

Skeletal System: Paget's Disease

1. Abnormal highly increased uptake in the entire left femur, which appears bowed and widened, and the distal third of the left tibia, which tapers proximally.

2. A sharp leading edge, referred to as "flame-shaped" or "blade of grass," may be demonstrated on the lytic phase on radiograph and on bone scintigraphy.

3. Paget's disease, fibrous dysplasia, chronic osteomyelitis, primary bone tumors, but principally osteosarcoma.

4. High-output congestive heart failure may occur. Once believed to be the result of arteriovenous shunting within the bone lesion, now hyperemia and increased blood flow through the lesion, and not shunting, are likely causes.

References

Brown ML: Bone scintigraphy in benign and malignant tumors, *Radiol Clin North Am* 31:731-738, 1993.

Sartoris DJ: *Musculoskeletal imaging: the requisites,* St Louis, 1996, Mosby, pp 303-307.

Cross-Reference

Nuclear Medicine: THE REQUISITES, ed 2, pp 119, 139-140.

Comment

Paget's disease is a benign disorder characterized by excessive and abnormal bone remodeling. Common after the age of 40, Paget's disease may be recognized because of bone pain, tenderness, or increase in bone size, but frequently is identified incidentally by an elevated serum alkaline phosphatase level or on radiographs or bone scans ordered for other reasons. The x-ray appearance has three phases: lytic, sclerotic, and mixed lytic-sclerotic. The classic appearance is one of bone enlargement, increased density, and coarsened trabecular pattern. Lesions typically start at the end of a long bone; 20% are monostotic. The disease is characterized by an initial phase of excess bone resorption with a lytic front, followed by an intense osteoblastic reaction with deposition of woven bone. Skeletal architecture becomes disorganized with a mixed pattern of lytic and sclerotic disease. This imbalance of bone remodeling in favor of formation leads to cortical thickening and bone expansion. Bone scintigraphy demonstrates abnormal intense radiotracer uptake extending from the subcortical region for the length of the lesion, which may be most or all the bone. The lesion may be three-phase positive in the active phase of the disease, although Paget's disease is most commonly identified on the delayed or bone phase. A three-phase study is not necessary for diagnosis. Bone scans can be used to evaluate therapy with calcitonin or new-generation biphosphonates. Response to therapy is indicated by a uniform or nonuniform decrease in radiotracer uptake.

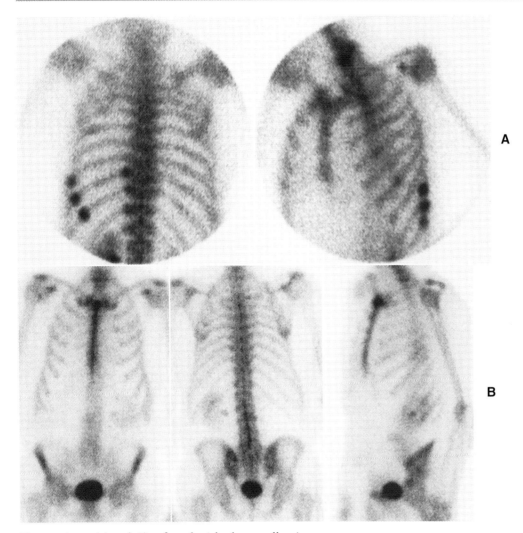

A

B

Two patients (*A* and *B*) referred with chest wall pain.

1. Describe the bone scan findings.
2. Is there a pattern to the abnormalities?
3. What causes should be considered?
4. Based on the scan findings, provide the most likely diagnoses.

Skeletal System: Rib Fractures and Sternotomy

1. Patient *A:* focal increased uptake in multiple ribs postero-laterally and at the costovertebral junctions. Patient *B:* increased vertical linear uptake in the sternum from the manubrium to the xiphoid.

2. The uptake in adjacent ribs (Patient *A*) and the vertical uptake in the sternum both have a geometric and characteristic pattern.

3. Trauma or surgery.

4. Patient *A:* multiple rib fractures. Patient *B:* median sternotomy for coronary artery bypass grafting (CABG) 6 months ago.

Reference

Holder L, Brown ML: Orthopedic imaging in trauma and sports medicine. In Collier BD Jr, Fogelman I, Rosenthall L: *Skeletal nuclear medicine,* St Louis, 1996, Mosby, pp 225-239.

Cross-Reference

Nuclear Medicine: THE REQUISITES, ed 2, pp 138-139.

Comment

Increased uptake on bone scans is nonspecific. However, the pattern of uptake can be diagnostic. Common polyostotic processes such as metastases are unlikely in these cases. Metastases occur randomly and are unlikely to involve only contiguous bones. Occasionally, this can occur with a large pleural-based mass eroding into adjacent bones, but then the appearance is not likely to be linear. The pattern of rib uptake represents an "Aunt Minnie" that is pathognomonic for fractures. Depending on clinical circumstances, the clinician may desire further radiographic evaluation, but this is not necessary for diagnosis. Abnormalities often are depicted on bone scintigraphy before the development of radiographic changes.

Abnormalities of the sternum range from benign or malignant neoplasm to infection and trauma. The linear nature of the finding provides the indication that this is postoperative. Findings indicating previous median sternotomy are not an uncommon occurrence on bone scans given the prevalence of CABG surgery. In some patients the uptake may not be defined or perfectly linear. Infection superimposed on median sternotomy would be a less likely consideration; osteomyelitis would be expected to extend beyond the sharp linear pattern to nonuniformly involve the remainder of the sternum. At times the standard anterior and posterior views of the sternum may not adequately depict the finding because of overlay of the sternum with the thoracic spine. Shallow anterior oblique views may be helpful.

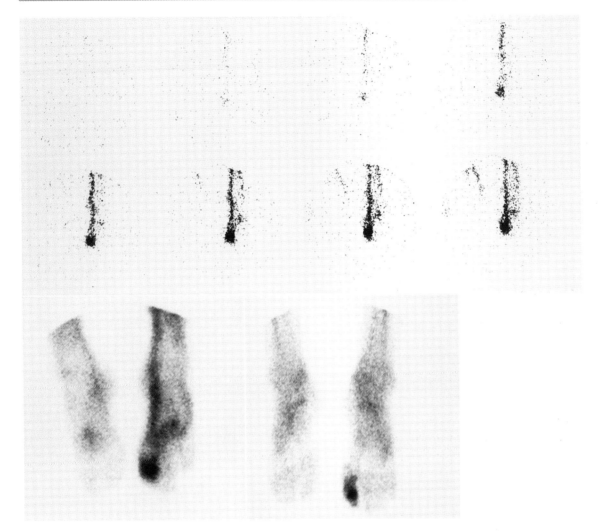

A 60-year-old patient with diabetes with cellulitis of the distal foot, referred to rule out osteomyelitis of the left great toe.

1. Describe the physiology of each of the three phases.

2. Describe the scintigraphic findings in this case.

3. Interpret the study.

4. What is the sensitivity and specificity of the three-phase bone scan for osteomyelitis?

Skeletal System: Pedal Osteomyelitis— Three-Phase Positive

1. First phase: arterial blood flow to the bone. Second phase: blood pool or interstitial space distribution immediately following the flow. Third phase: bone uptake phase at 3 hours after injection. All three phases are typically focally increased with osteomyelitis. With cellulitis, only the first two phases are positive.

2. Increased flow, blood pool, and delayed uptake to the left first digit distal phalanx.

3. Consistent with osteomyelitis of the digit. Recent fracture must be excluded with radiography.

4. Sensitivity and specificity of approximately 95% if the radiograph is normal or has only suggestive changes of osteomyelitis.

Reference
Palestro CJ, Thomas MB: Scintigraphic evaluation of the diabetic foot. In Freeman LM: *Nuclear medicine annual 2000,* Philadelphia, 2000, Lippincott Williams & Wilkins, pp 143-172.

Cross-Reference
Nuclear Medicine: THE REQUISITES, ed 2, pp 134-136, 185-188.

Comment
Foot ulcers frequently serve as the portal of entry for infection and osteomyelitis in patients with diabetes. Radiographic findings may be negative or show only suggestive changes in early phases. A negative three-phase bone scan rules out osteomyelitis with a high degree of certainty. Although three-phase positive studies are characteristic of osteomyelitis, patients with vascular insufficiency may have decreased flow and blood pool. Checking for foot warmth and pedal pulses can aid in interpretation. A cold region in the distal extremity in the setting of infection suggests gangrene and nonviability.

The specificity of the three-phase scan can be problematic. Differentiating joint infection from bone infection is important. With synovitis, uptake is seen in bone on both sides of the joint. Good resolution and proper intensity setting is necessary. Any cause for bone remodeling, e.g., healing fracture, orthopedic implants, and neuropathic osteoarthropathy, may result in a three-phase positive scan. Radiographs often demonstrate these potential problems. In these cases, radiolabeled leukocytes can be helpful. Differentiating bone from overlying soft tissue infection can sometimes be difficult with ^{111}In oxine leukocytes because of its limited resolution. [99m]Tc hexamethyl-propyleneamine-oxime (HM-PAO) offers an advantage in such situations, and soft tissue uptake usually can be distinguished from bone uptake.

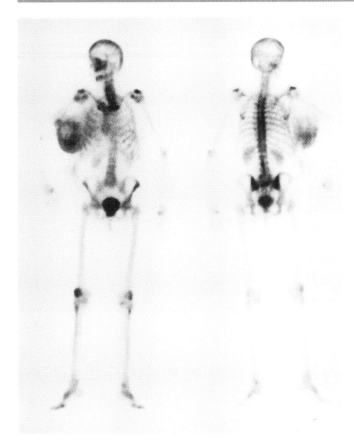

Patient referred for bone scan because of right-sided chest pain.

1. Describe scintigraphic findings.
2. Provide a differential diagnosis.
3. What other examinations may be helpful in this setting?
4. What is the likely reason for ordering the bone scan?

CASE 6

Skeletal System: Abnormal Breast Uptake

1. Nonuniform abnormal soft tissue uptake exists in the soft tissue overlying the chest, likely in the right breast.

2. Breast cancer, aseptic or septic mastitis, primary skin disease, such as psoriasis, vascular or lymphatic obstruction, radiation therapy.

3. Breast examination, mammography, and possible biopsy.

4. To determine whether breast cancer bone metastases are present.

References

Kopans DB: Breast imaging, ed 2, Philadelphia, 1998, Lippincott-Raven, pp 340-341, 591.

Jacobson AF, Fogelman I: Skeletal scintigraphy in breast and prostate cancer: past, present, and future. In Freeman LM, editor: *Nuclear medicine annual 1999,* Philadelphia, 1999, Lippincott Williams & Wilkins.

Cross-Reference

Nuclear Medicine: THE REQUISITES, ed 2, pp 124-125.

Comment

Breast uptake on bone scans can be a normal finding. The greater the amount of uptake and degree of asymmetry, the more likely a pathological condition exists, as in this case. The majority of benign lesions caused by fibroadenomas, mammary dysplasia, and cystic mastitis have bilateral uptake. Malignant uptake usually is unilateral. On further questioning, this patient reported that the breast had been inflamed for weeks and a biopsy had recently been performed. The combination of the bone scan findings and clinical history limit the diagnosis to inflammatory carcinoma or mastitis. Inflammatory carcinoma (shown by biopsy) consists of diffuse early invasion of the dermal lymphatics by an aggressive form of infiltrating carcinoma. An underlying primary lesion may not be evident. Inflammatory carcinoma is uncommon, comprising less than 1% of invasive breast cancers. Its prognosis is worse than infiltrating ductal carcinoma that has secondarily invaded the skin. Soft tissue involvement by malignant neoplasms, either primary or metastatic, may demonstrate abnormal uptake of bone radiotracer. The lesions most commonly seen because of the frequency of the tumor and its avidity for tracer are primary or metastatic breast, lung, metastatic colon cancer, and neuroblastoma.

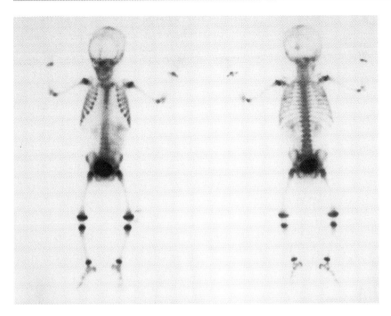

A 2-year-old child has an abdominal mass.

1. Describe the scintigraphic bone scan findings.
2. Name a likely organ of origin.
3. What is the most likely diagnosis?
4. Is the current examination adequate for staging of the patient's illness?

A

B

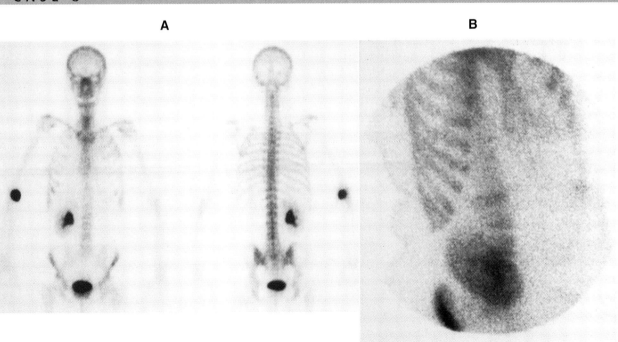

1. Describe the abnormal bone scan findings in scan *A*.
2. Provide a differential diagnosis.
3. Describe the findings in scan *B*, a delayed spot image.
4. Explain the change and provide the most likely diagnosis.

CASE 7

Skeletal System: Neuroblastoma

1. Large region of nonuniform abnormal soft tissue uptake predominantly in the left side of the abdomen that appears to cross the midline. Its boundaries cannot be distinguished from the two kidneys.

2. Adrenal gland.

3. Neuroblastoma.

4. No.

Reference

Bissett GS III, Strife JL, Kirks DR: Genitourinary tract. In Kirks DR, editor: *Practical pediatric imaging,* ed 2, Boston, 1991, Little, Brown, pp 1110-1125.

Cross-Reference

Nuclear Medicine: THE REQUISITES, ed 2, p 124.

Comment

Neuroblastoma is a malignant tumor of the sympathetic nervous system and occurs most frequently in early childhood. More than 85% of the tumors secrete variable amounts of catecholamines and their metabolites. Staging requires determination of the extent of disease, necessitating anatomical imaging with CT, MRI, and histological evaluation of the bone marrow. The Evans staging system is used most commonly. Stage I disease is confined to the structure of origin. Stage II disease involves tumor extension in continuity but not across the midline, or tumors arising in the midline. Stage III disease extends in continuity across the midline. Stage IV disease is disseminated disease with metastases involving the skeleton, soft tissues, distant lymph nodes or organs. Stage IV-S disease occurs in patients whose primary tumor would be stage I or II but for metastatic disease to liver, skin, or bone marrow but not the skeleton.

Most neuroblastomas take up bone radiopharmaceuticals with varying degrees. The intensity of uptake does not correlate with the degree of malignancy or prognosis. Even primary tumors without radiographic evidence of calcification often have increased bone radiopharmaceutical uptake. The bone scan is also a sensitive detector of metastatic neuroblastoma to bone and is abnormal weeks before radiographic changes are present. The combination of bone scan and ^{131}I metaiodobenzylguanidine (MIBG) has the highest sensitivity for detection of bone involvement, and both are used in evaluating response to therapy.

Notes

CASE 8

Skeletal System: Extrarenal Pelvis and Mobile Solitary Right Kidney

1. Solitary right kidney with a prominent renal pelvis. Incidental uptake at antecubital injection site.

2. Ureteropelvic junction obstruction or obstruction secondary to other processes, extrarenal pelvis.

3. The renal pelvis has drained and the kidney is now seen inferomedial to its prior location.

4. Image *B* was taken with the patient erect, leading to gravity drainage of an extrarenal pelvis. The kidney is mobile (ptotic).

Reference

Dunnick NR, Sandler CM, Newhouse JH, et al: *Textbook of uroradiology,* ed 3, Philadelphia, 2001, Lippincott Williams & Wilkins.

Cross-Reference

Nuclear Medicine: THE REQUISITES, ed 2, pp 115-116.

Comment

This case demonstrates how a simple maneuver can clarify scintigraphic findings and eliminate the need for further evaluation. If imaging had stopped with the full renal pelvis, the differential diagnosis would have included obstruction and likely prompted further diagnostic evaluation, probably ultrasonography and a diuretic renal scan. Review of the completed scan by the physician before the patient leaves the department allows for tailoring of the scan protocol, which can lead to a more definitive interpretation and avoidance of further unnecessary testing. In this case the anterior oblique view with the patient erect demonstrates emptying of the renal pelvis. A postvoid supine image after the patient returned from the restroom also would have shown emptying but would not have revealed the renal mobility.

The kidneys usually are paired retroperitoneal organs that are oriented parallel with the psoas muscles on either side of the lumbar spine. The top of the kidney is located more medial than the lower portion. However, the kidney can be mobile, and their positions may vary with inspiration or patient position. This case is a good example of renal mobility, demonstrated because the image was obtained with the patient in the supine and then erect position.

Notes

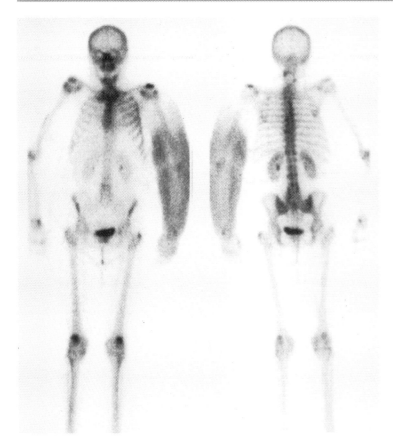

Pain in the left shoulder; rule out metastasis.

1. Describe the findings.
2. Name three general processes that could account for the findings.
3. What is the likely primary tumor for which metastases are being excluded?
4. What is the most likely diagnosis?

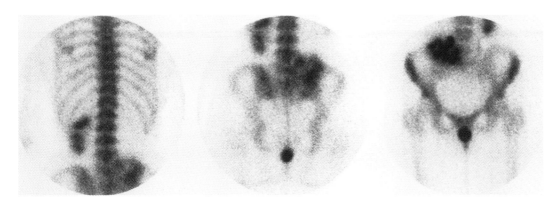

1. Describe the bone scan findings.
2. Provide the general classification for this finding and the likely diagnosis.
3. Name other conditions that fall into the same spectrum of abnormalities.
4. Are increased risks associated with this condition?

Skeletal System: Lymphedema

1. The soft tissues of the left arm are enlarged and show abnormal increased soft tissue activity; the left anterior ribs are uniformly more intense than the right.

2. Venous or lymphatic obstruction, soft tissue neoplasm, soft tissue injury.

3. Breast cancer.

4. Lymphedema secondary to axillary lymph node dissection and left mastectomy.

Reference
Gray HW, Krasnow AZ: Soft tissue uptake of bone agents. In Collier BD Jr, Fogelman I, Rosenthall L, editors: *Skeletal nuclear medicine,* St Louis, 1996, Mosby, pp 386-389.

Cross-Reference
Nuclear Medicine: THE REQUISITES, ed 2, pp 122-123.

Comment
The combination of findings of increased visualization of the anterior ribs and soft tissue uptake in an enlarged upper extremity is essentially an "Aunt Minnie" for lymphedema as a result of axillary lymph node dissection and mastectomy. Other causes of lymphatic or venous obstruction should be considered, such as prior lymphadenectomy for melanoma, tumor replacement of lymph nodes causing obstruction to lymph flow, or venous obstruction from idiopathic thrombus or prior indwelling catheter. Processes primarily related to the arm that could cause this appearance, such as sarcoma or electrical, frostbite, or crush injuries, are considerations but are seen much less frequently.

In patients with breast cancer, the axillary lymph node dissection generally is considered to be primarily diagnostic. It is controversial whether surgical excision of involved nodes also provides a therapeutic benefit. However, associated morbidity is associated with excision, which increases with the extent of lymphadenectomy. The patient may experience transient or lifelong discomfort, abnormal sensation, or lymphedema as in this patient. Lymphedema in the ipsilateral arm develops in 15% of women with breast cancer after therapy. This complication may be slightly higher in women treated with lumpectomy and radiation than in patients whose disease is staged with sentinel lymph node procedures

Notes

Skeletal System: Bone Abnormalities of Renal Position

1. The right kidney is not seen in the renal fossa. Nonuniform activity is noted in the right sacroiliac region, which extends beyond the expected superior margin of the bone.

2. Congenital renal anomaly, pelvic kidney.

3. Anomalies of number (supernumerary kidney), position (malrotation), or fusion (horseshoe).

4. Yes. Ureteropelvic junction obstruction, vesicoureteral reflux, decreased function, increased risk of trauma. Urine stasis resulting from distorted anatomy increases the risk of stone formation.

Reference
Tung GA, Zagoria RJ, Mayo-Smith WW: *Genitourinary radiology: the requisites,* St Louis, 2000, Mosby, pp 55-58.

Cross-Reference
Nuclear Medicine: THE REQUISITES, ed 2, pp 142-143.

Comment
Renal anomalies involve the following factors: (1) number, which includes agenesis or the extremely rare condition of supernumerary kidney; (2) position, which includes nonrotation, malrotation, and ectopia; and (3) fusion, which includes horseshoe kidney and cross-fused ectopia. Renal ectopia is an anomaly that arises from alteration of the normal caudal to cranial movement of the kidneys during development. Underascent is much more common than overascent (which gives rise to the thoracic kidney). In these cases, adjacent vessels usually provide the blood supply to the ectopic kidney. Renal ectopia may be associated with anomalies of fusion and contralateral renal anomalies. Underascent of the kidney ranges from pelvic kidneys that lie in the true pelvis, in the iliac fossa opposite the iliac crest, to location in the lower abdomen but not at the expected level adjacent to L2. Normal pelvic kidneys do not have the same appearance as normally located kidneys because of variable degrees of rotation and alteration in the calices. Pelvic kidneys usually are asymptomatic, although there are increased risks as noted.

Cross-fused ectopia is an uncommon congenital anomaly in which one kidney crosses the midline and fuses with the opposite kidney, so that both kidneys lie on one side of the spine. However, its ureter inserts in the normal position, but extends across the midline to enter the bladder on the side opposite to the kidney. Fused kidneys usually produce no symptoms but are susceptible to the complications seen in other ectopic kidneys.

Notes

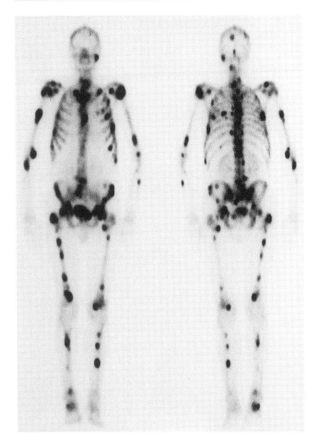

A 67-year-old man has an elevated serum prostate-specific antigen (PSA) level.

1. Describe the findings on this bone scan and interpret the study.

2. What would you predict the serum PSA level to be?

3. Which metastatic cancers have predominantly lytic lesions in bone and thus lower sensitivity for their detection by bone scanning?

4. If a patient with prostate cancer has a significantly elevated serum PSA level postoperatively but negative bone scan findings, what other imaging options are indicated?

Skeletal System: Metastatic Prostate Cancer

1. Abnormal focal uptake throughout the axial and appendicular skeleton strongly suggestive of metastatic disease. The many distal appendicular lesions usually are seen with late-stage disease.

2. Considerably greater than 20 ng/ml. The prevalence of bone scan–evident metastases is less than 1% below this level.

3. Multiple myeloma, followed by thyroid cancer, renal cell carcinoma, lymphoma.

4. CT and MRI have a poor sensitivity for detection of prostate cancer soft tissue/nodal metastases, less than 20%. An [111]In ProstaScint study is indicated.

Reference

Jacobson AF, Fogelman I: Skeletal scintigraphy in breast and prostate cancer: past, present, and future. In Freeman LM, editor: *Nuclear medicine annual 1999,* Philadelphia, 1999, Lippincott Williams & Wilkins.

Cross-Reference

Nuclear Medicine: THE REQUISITES, ed 2, p 122.

Comment

Bone scans are very sensitive for detection of bone metastases in most cancers, 50% to 80% more sensitive than radiographs. Fifty percent of the bone mineral content must be lost before a metastasis is detectable on x-ray films. Although bone scans are not routinely indicated in patients with PSA levels less than 20 ng/ml, baseline scans are appropriate in patients with high Gleason scores, skeletal symptoms, abnormal radiographic findings, and patients with preexisting skeletal conditions that might render interpretation of scans difficult. Patients with PSA levels greater than 100 ng/ml invariably have wide spread skeletal involvement. Eighty percent of metastatic lesions are in the axial skeleton. In patients with known metastases the incidence of extremity or skull involvement rises to 50%.

The sensitivity of the bone scan for detection of bone lesions caused by multiple myeloma is considerably lower (~50%) because these lesions are often lytic, i.e., predominantly osteoclastic. Bone scans are used to determine the effectiveness of therapy, although serum PSA levels are increasingly used for this purpose. Nonetheless, the bone scan still is useful for the evaluation of symptomatic patients or when a change in management is contemplated. The serum PSA level may not be as useful in patients who have had hormonal therapy. One study found that 35% of patients receiving antiandrogen therapy with definite metastatic disease had normal levels of PSA.

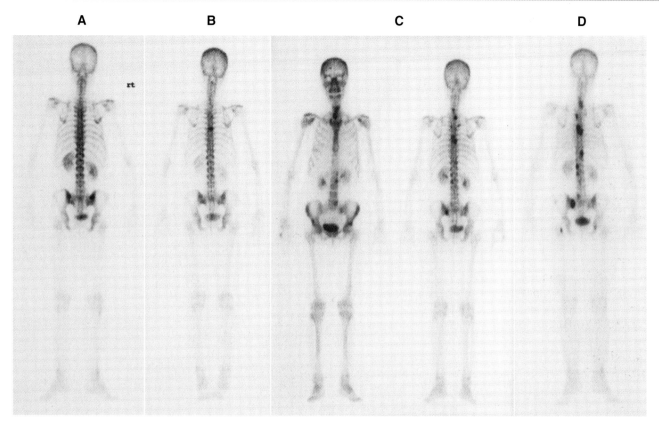

A   B   C   D

Patient with breast cancer. The serial bone scans are dated as follows: *A, 4/97; B, 5/99; C, 8/99; D, 4/00.*

1. Describe the bone scan findings and changes over time. The 4/97 scan was completely normal.

2. What is the likelihood of tumor with new focal uptake in a single rib in a patient with known cancer? What is the likelihood with new solitary spine lesions?

3. What are different general scan patterns in metastatic disease?

4. What is the cause of the relatively cold defect in the left hemithorax?

Skeletal System: Breast Cancer

1. *B,* New increased uptake at T7 suspicious for tumor; *C,* multiple new lesions in the thoracic spine, fourth right rib, left sacrum, and single focus in the anterior skull all strongly suspicious for tumor; *D,* continued progression with new tumor sites in the spine and left sacrum and new focal uptake in left iliac crest, right intertrochanteric femur, and right acetabulum.

2. Less than 20%; greater than 40%.

3. Solitary focal lesion, multiple focal lesions, diffuse involvement (superscan), cold lesion, soft tissue uptake, flare phenomenon.

4. Breast prosthesis.

Reference

Jacobson AF, Fogelman I: Skeletal scintigraphy in breast and prostate cancer: past, present and future. In Freeman LM, editor: *Nuclear medicine annual 1999,* Philadelphia, 2000, Lippincott Williams & Wilkins, pp 121-156.

Cross-Reference

Nuclear Medicine: THE REQUISITES, ed 2, pp 117-123.

Comment

Bone scans in stage I and II breast cancer have a low yield and generally are not justified, except for patients with poor prognosis stage II disease (tumor >3 cm or with aggressive histological findings). With later stage III and IV disease, bone scans usually are obtained. Because routine follow-up bone scans have no demonstrated effect on survival, bone scans usually are reserved for patients with specific bone symptoms and those with radiologic findings suggestive of metastatic disease. Bone scanning is also used for evaluation of patients with symptoms, worrisome physical findings, abnormal laboratory test results or radiographs, because evidence of new or progressive metastatic disease is likely to result in institution of new or additional therapy.

The flare phenomenon is seen in patients who have had a good response to chemotherapy. The scan paradoxically appears worse, with prior lesions more prominent; occasionally lesions are seen that were not present on prior scans. The reason for this finding is that the bone is demonstrating an osteoblastic reparative response. Patients may have increased pain with the onset of chemotherapy, but typically the pain resolves before the scan is obtained. The increased scan uptake may be seen for 2 to 3 months after chemotherapy and may also be seen with radiation therapy.

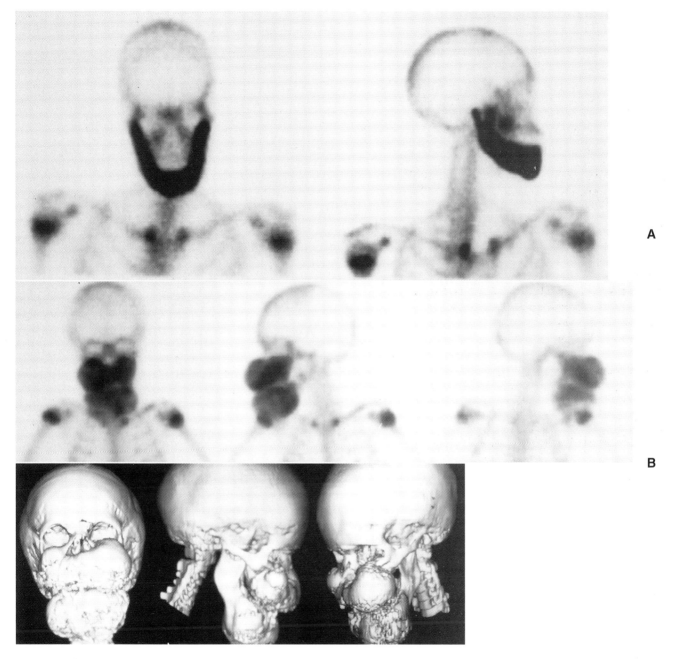

Because of a "jaw problem," a bone scan *(A)* and a bone scan and CT-30 reconstruction *(B)* were obtained in two children.

1. Describe the bone scan findings.

2. What additional information would be helpful?

3. Provide a short differential diagnosis.

4. The mother says there is no known disease in the child *(B)* or family. What is the most likely diagnosis?

CASE 13

Skeletal System: Fibrous Dysplasia

1. *A* shows increased uptake in the entire mandible. *B* shows intense increased uptake in the mandible and maxilla, which appear deformed and overgrown.

2. Check the rest of the bone scan for other sites; obtain a history of known underlying or familial disease.

3. Fibrous dysplasia, cherubism.

4. Fibrous dysplasia.

References

Blickman H: *Pediatric radiology: the requisites,* ed 2, St Louis, 1998, Mosby, pp 220-221.
Sartoris DJ: *Musculoskeletal imaging: the requisites,* St Louis, 1996, Mosby, pp 216-217.

Cross-Reference

Nuclear Medicine: THE REQUISITES, ed 2, pp 139-141.

Comment

Fibrous dysplasia is a common congenital, nonhereditary skeletal disorder of unknown origin. It is characterized by a developmental anomaly of bone formation in which the marrow is replaced by fibrous tissue. Fibrous dysplasia occurs during periods of bone growth in older children and adolescents and slowly enlarges for life. Seventy-five percent of cases are monostotic. Other frequently affected sites include the proximal femur (35%), tibia (20%), and facial bones and ribs (15%).

Sclerotic thickening caused by involvement of the facial bones is called leontiasis ossea ("resembling a lion's face"). Cherubism is a rare but different entity and results in bilateral swelling in the jaw with multilobular expansile bone lesions, which may simulate fibrous dysplasia. However, in contrast to fibrous dysplasia, cherubism is a familiar disorder. Skeletal deformities also can occur as a result of repeated pathological fractures.

CT is most useful to determine the extent of involvement in a particular skeletal region. Identification of polyostotic involvement is one of the main indications for skeletal scintigraphy because many of these sites are asymptomatic. Hypertrophy of soft tissues and bones can be seen in several other conditions, including neurofibromatosis, macrodystrophia lipomatosa, hemangiomas as in Kippel-Trénaunay-Weber disease, and lymphangiomatosis.

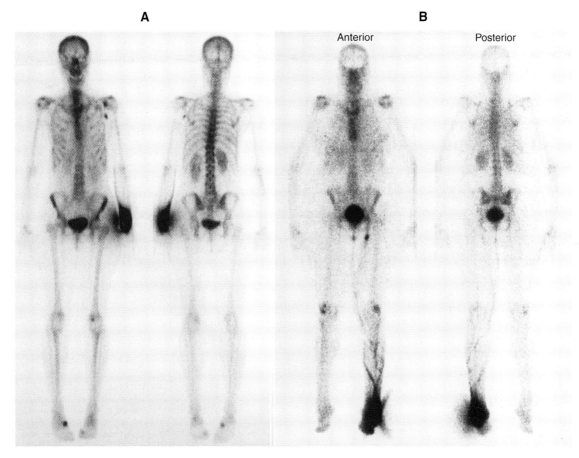

A

B

Anterior   Posterior

1. Describe the findings in patient *A*.
2. Describe the findings in patient *B*.
3. Provide the most likely reason for this appearance.
4. Explain the mechanism for the scan appearance.

CASE 14

Skeletal System: Radiopharmaceutical Infiltration, Scatter, and Lymph Node Uptake

1. Intense uniform activity in the soft tissues of the distal left forearm and focal activity in the left axilla, nonuniform activity in the left lateral buttock.

2. Intense activity in the left foot, linear activity indicating lymphatic channels, and left inguinal lymph node. Scatter is seen lateral to the left foot.

3. Partial extravasation of the bone radiotracer at the site of intravenous injection in the left forearm.

4. Demonstration of an axillary lymph node because of lymphatic clearance of the extravasated radiopharmaceutical. Scatter from the arm infiltrate results in apparent (but unreal) increased activity in the buttock.

Reference

McAfee JG, Reba RC, Majd M: The musculoskeletal system. In Wagner HN, Szabo Z, Buchanan JW, editors: *Principles of nuclear medicine,* ed 2, Philadelphia, 1995, WB Saunders, p 991.

Cross-Reference

Nuclear Medicine: THE REQUISITES, ed 2, p 20.

Comment

Abnormalities related to injection technique are not uncommon and vary from faintly visible activity at the site of injection to the appearance in this case. If an even larger portion of the administered radiopharmaceutical was infiltrated, the demonstration of bone structures could be reduced at the time of routine imaging (3 to 4 hours after injection). The infiltration serves as a radiopharmaceutical reservoir with slow absorption through the lymphatics ultimately to the central circulation, such that renal clearance also is delayed. A mixed arterial-venous injection or solely arterial injection occasionally occurs and is shown by the arterial distribution of radiotracer distal to the injection site, which is not evident in this case. Local skin contamination at the site of injection (perhaps a leaky hub on the syringe) could result in intense activity on the forearm and scatter artifact, but demonstration of a lymph node would not occur in that setting.

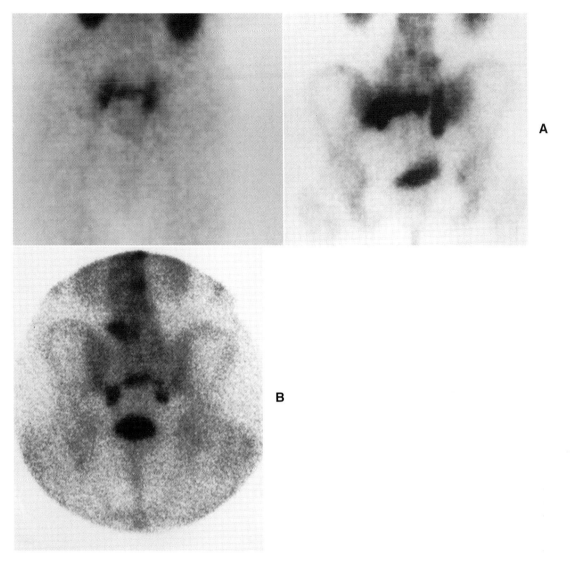

A

B

Two patients have low back pain. Patient *A* has blood pool (left) and delayed images (right) available; for Patient *B*, only delayed images are shown.

1. Describe the bone scan abnormalities.

2. Provide the differential diagnoses.

3. List three other sites that are at increased risk for the same process.

4. What is the most likely underlying process in both patients?

Skeletal System: Sacral Insufficiency Fracture

1. Patient *A* has increased blood pooling and delayed uptake bilaterally in the region of the sacroiliac joints and across the sacrum (**H** pattern). The bone scan for Patient *B* demonstrates abnormal increased radiotracer in a curvilinear linear pattern across the lower sacrum.

2. Both of these are diagnostic of sacral insufficiency fractures.

3. Proximal femur, wrist, and proximal humerus.

4. Osteoporosis.

References

Sartoris DJ: *Musculoskeletal imaging: the requisites,* St Louis, 1996, Mosby, p 14.

Balseiro J, Brower AC, Ziessman HA: Scintigraphic diagnosis of sacral fractures, *AJR Am J Roentgenol* 148:111, 1987.

Cross-Reference

Nuclear Medicine: THE REQUISITES, ed 2, pp 138-139.

Comment

Insufficiency fractures are an important and common complication of osteoporosis, a condition resulting from diminished bone quantity that is seen most commonly in postmenopausal women, but also in patients with hyperparathyroidism and those receiving steroid therapy. In many cases, fractures occur with minimal or no trauma. Common sites of osteoporosis-related fractures outside the pelvis are the vertebral bodies, femoral neck and intertrochanteric region, distal radius, humeral neck, proximal and distal tibia, and sternum. Bone density studies are used increasingly to predict fracture risk in postmenopausal women or patients at increased risk of osteoporosis.

Because of the increased radiolucency of affected bone, fractures may be difficult to identify on radiographs. However, usually they are easily detectable on bone scintigraphy because of the high sensitivity of bone scanning for identification of sites of increased bone turnover and osteoblastic activity. Insufficiency fractures in the pelvis typically involve the sacrum, symphysis pubis, or pubic rami. Sacral fractures are associated with characteristic bone scan appearances, such as the **H** or "Honda sign" indicating vertical involvement of sacral ala and horizontal involvement of the sacrum (an "Aunt Minnie"). Portions of the **H** may only be seen at times. Another common pattern is that of linear, curvilinear, a "dot and dash" appearance as seen in case *B*. After pelvic radiation, radiation-induced fractures can have a similar appearance.

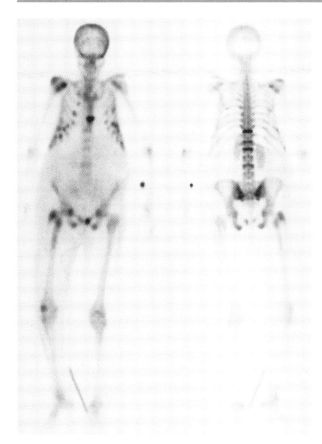

An elderly woman with a history of prior right hip fracture comes to the emergency department because of pelvic pain and inability to walk. A bone scan was obtained.

1. Describe the scintigraphic findings.
2. What is the differential diagnosis?
3. What is the most likely diagnosis?
4. Name three medical conditions that predispose patients to this underlying disease process.

Skeletal System: Multiple Insufficiency Fractures

1. Multiple focal areas of increased radiotracer uptake are noted in several ribs, multiple sites in both pubic rami, lower sternum, and multiple vertebra.

2. Multifocal involvement by benign or malignant tumor, multifocal osteomyelitis, fractures.

3. Multiple insufficiency fractures. Degenerative change is present in the right shoulder and postoperative change related to previous right hip orthopedic fixation.

4. Hypercortisolism, hyperparathyroidism, hyperthyroidism.

Reference

Fernandez-Ulloa M, Klostermeier TT, Lancaster KT: Orthopaedic nuclear medicine: the pelvis and hip, *Semin Nucl Med* 28:25-40, 1998.

Cross-Reference

Nuclear Medicine: THE REQUISITES, ed 2, pp 138-139.

Comment

Osteoporotic insufficiency fractures commonly occur in the pelvis, vertebra, hip, wrist, proximal humerus, proximal and distal tibia, ribs, and sternum. Although multiple bone abnormalities may suggest tumor metastases, close review of the character and location of the findings usually leads to the correct diagnosis. The spine abnormalities have a linear appearance that suggests fracture (either wedge compression fracture or vertebral end-plate deformity). The rib abnormalities occur in adjacent ribs in a linear pattern that strongly suggests fractures. None of the sites of increased uptake have a pattern to suggest other causes, such as a suspicious segmental or regional abnormality in one of the long bones or flat bones. Osteoporosis risk factors include female gender, family history of osteoporosis, estrogen deficiency, calcium deficiency, low body weight, sedentary lifestyle, amenorrhea, and smoking.

Insufficiency fractures usually are not seen on routine radiographs. Bone scanning allows localization of these fracture sites because of its high sensitivity for sites of increased bone turnover. CT can be used to confirm that these foci of uptake are indeed fractures. However, the pattern usually is quite characteristic on bone scans. Fractures of the pelvis invariably result in at least three fracture sites. This patient has at least six. Sacral insufficiency fractures typically have intense uptake in sacroiliac joint areas and sacrum (H pattern). Careful analysis of this patient also suggests sacral fractures.

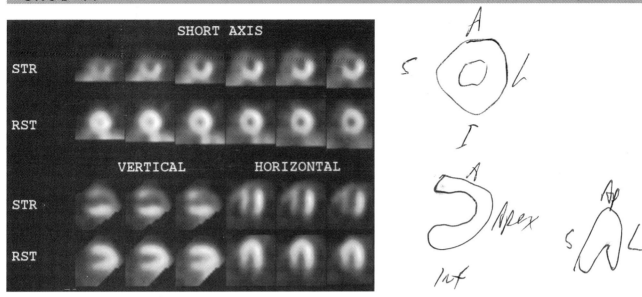

A 55-year-old man with exertional chest pain had a stress single photon emission computed tomography (SPECT) myocardial perfusion study.

1. Describe the perfusion abnormalities and give your interpretation.
2. Name the culprit vessel or vessels.
3. List any ancillary scan findings.
4. List clinical findings related to the stress test relevant to interpretation of the scan.

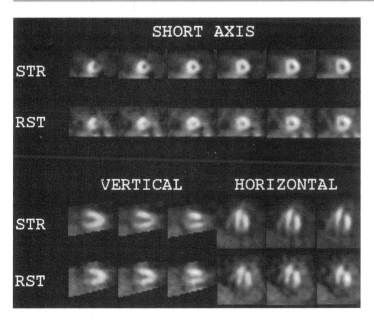

A 60-year-old man with a history of remote myocardial infarct and CABG surgery. Echocardiography results were normal.

1. Describe the SPECT findings.
2. Provide the differential diagnosis.
3. Give the most likely diagnosis.
4. Explain the discrepancy between the cardiac echocardiogram and the SPECT scan.

Cardiovascular System: Left Anterior Descending Artery Ischemia

1. Severe decreased perfusion in the majority of the anterior wall, apex, and septum, which normalizes on the rest image indicating extensive severe ischemia.

2. Left anterior descending (LAD) coronary artery.

3. Transient cavity dilation.

4. Ventricular tachyarrhythmias, angina-related ST-segment abnormalities, decrease in systolic blood pressure, level of exercise achieved.

Reference
Yao SS, Rozanski A: Myocardial perfusion scintigraphy in conjunction with exercise and pharmacologic stress: prognostic applications in the clinical management of patients with coronary artery disease. In DePuey EG, Garcia EV, Berman DS, editors: *Cardiac SPECT imaging,* ed 2, Philadelphia, 2001, Lippincott Williams & Wilkins, pp 263-296.

Cross-Reference
Nuclear Medicine: THE REQUISITES, ed 2, pp 78-79.

Comment
Although stress myocardial perfusion studies are sensitive for detection of coronary artery disease (CAD; 85% to 90%), the sensitivity for diagnosis of multivessel disease is less. Ischemia in multiple vascular distributions may not be evident on the perfusion study because the most severe lesion produces symptomatic ischemia and exercise is discontinued before producing ischemia in myocardial regions of less diseased vessels.

Both transient ischemic dilation and stress-induced ^{201}Tl uptake are important indicators of multivessel disease. Stress-induced left ventricular cavity dilation is apparent by comparison of stress *(str)* and rest *(rst)* images. This finding is often the result of an actual increase in the left ventricular volume, indicating stress-induced ventricular dysfunction. However, particularly when ^{99m}Tc-labeled myocardial perfusion agents are used, this finding may represent diffuse subendocardial ischemia rather than actual increased cavity size. Transient cavity dilation sometimes is called transient ischemic dilatation and correlates with significant and usually multivessel CAD.

Anginal-type chest pain and depression of the ST-T segment on ECG evaluation during stress are suggestive of ischemia. Indicators of severe ischemia include a decrease in the patient's systolic blood pressure, 2-mm or more ST-T wave segment depression, and ventricular arrhythmia (frequent premature ventricular contractions, ventricular tachycardia). These findings are reasons to stop the exercise, if possible, preferably 1 minute after the stress injection to allow time for radiopharmaceutical uptake so that diagnostic images can still be obtained.

Cardiovascular System: Apical Infarct

1. Fixed stress *(str)* and rest *(rst)* severe apical lateral perfusion defect of small size. Heart and cavity size appear normal.

2. Myocardial infarction, apical thinning, attenuation.

3. Small apical lateral scar.

4. Technical factors, operator error, interpretation error.

Reference
Yao SS, Rozanski A: Myocardial perfusion scintigraphy in conjunction with exercise and pharmacologic stress: prognostic applications in the clinical management of patients with coronary artery disease. In DePuey EG, Garcia EV, Berman DS, editors: *Cardiac SPECT imaging,* ed 2, Philadelphia, 2001, Lippincott Williams & Wilkins, pp 263-296.

Cross-Reference
Nuclear Medicine: THE REQUISITES, ed 2, pp 76-79.

Comment
This apical perfusion defect in a man is unlikely to be caused by attenuation, even with gynecomastia, because of its severity and sharp demarcation. The appearance of apical thinning is related to the normal lesser myocardial mass at the apex. In a normal-sized heart, apical thinning may be seen on the horizontal long-axis view but rarely is evident on the vertical long-axis and short-axis views, as in this case. With ventricular dilation, apical thinning becomes more prominent and may be seen on more than the horizontal long-axis slices. However, this ventricle is not dilated. A gated wall motion study would be helpful. Apical akinesis is seen with an infarct. A septal wall motion abnormality (hypokinesis or dyskinesis) might be expected in this patient because of his previous CABG surgery. The subdiaphragmatic liver activity just inferior to the heart suggests that the patient had either pharmacological stress or inadequate exercise. Exercise shifts blood flow away from abdominal viscera to the exercising muscles.

Echocardiography is operator dependent, and stress echocardiography even more so. Operator skills and effort on a given case can affect the results. In some patients, particularly those with chronic obstructive pulmonary disease, the acoustic window may be suboptimal and limit the examination. Normal wall motion or hyperkinesis of the adjacent myocardial regions can obscure a small hypokinetic segment of myocardium. In this case in which the perfusion abnormality is small, it is not surprising that it was missed by echocardiography.

Notes

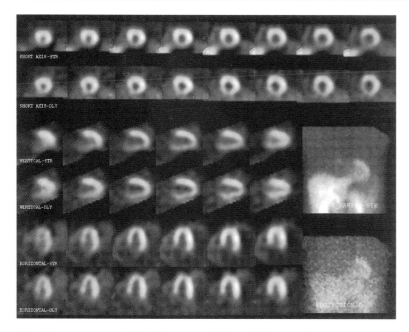

Dual-isotope stress SPECT myocardial perfusion study.

1. Describe the various imaging protocols used for ^{99m}Tc myocardial perfusion tracers.

2. What radionuclides are used for a dual-isotope study?

3. List the advantages of the dual-isotope technique compared with a single-isotope study.

4. Describe the SPECT findings and interpret the study.

Cardiovascular System: Dual-Isotope Study— Mild Inferior Ischemia

1. Two-day stress/rest; same-day rest/stress; same-day stress/rest.

2. [201]Tl chloride for rest; ^{99m}Tc sestamibi or tetrofosmin for stress.

3. The dual-isotope technique requires a shorter time to complete the examination. Wall-motion assessment and gated SPECT are available from ^{99m}Tc perfusion study. [201]Tl can be used to assess viability.

4. Mild decreased inferior wall perfusion at stress with mild improvement at rest. Mild inferior wall ischemia (right coronary artery). (Liver activity on the stress images suggests pharmacological stress. Normal biliary clearance is present on projection images.)

Reference

Berman DS, Hayes SW, Germano G: Assessment of myocardial perfusion and viability with ^{99m}Tc perfusion agents. In DePuey EG, Garcia EV, Berman DS, editors: *Cardiac SPECT imaging,* ed 2, Philadelphia, 2001, Lippincott Williams & Wilkins, pp 179-210.

Cross-Reference

Nuclear Medicine: THE REQUISITES, ed 2, pp 66-72, 85, 390, 392-393.

Comment

Various imaging protocols are used for ^{99m}Tc myocardial perfusion scans. Defect contrast and image quality are superior with the 2-day protocol because both scans are obtained after the injection of high doses of tracer (20 to 30 mCi). However, this study requires a 2-day patient visit. A same-day low-dose rest/high-dose stress protocol frequently is used. Its disadvantage is reduction in stress defect contrast caused by persistent radioactivity from the rest study at the time of the stress scan. Same-day low-dose stress/high-dose rest protocols require a scan interval similar to that for ^{201}Tl scans; thus it is practical in laboratories when both types of studies are being performed routinely. However, it has less than ideal count rates from the stress images because of the low administered dose.

Two separate, rather than simultaneous, acquisitions are recommended for dual-isotope studies because of ^{99m}Tc downscatter into the ^{201}Tl window. Because ^{201}Tl imaging is performed before injection of the ^{99m}Tc agent, downscatter is not a problem. [201]Tl does not contribute significantly to the ^{99m}Tc window because of the lower ^{201}Tl photopeak and the much higher dose of [99m]Tc. Because imaging begins by 10 minutes after ^{201}Tl injection, the rest/stress study can be completed in 90 minutes, quicker than protocols using a single radiotracer. Other advantages are the functional information from the ^{99m}Tc agent and potential viability information from delayed ^{201}Tl imaging.

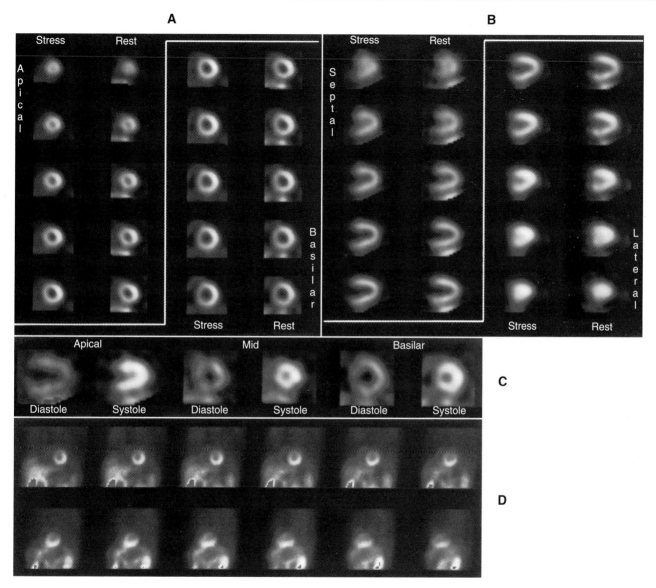

A 50-year-old woman has atypical chest pain. The exercise treadmill test result with adequate exercise was interpreted as negative. SPECT perfusion images (*A*, gated short-axis; *B*, vertical long-axis; *C*, SPECT wall thickening; *D*, sequential raw data projection acquisition images) are provided.

1. Describe the SPECT myocardial perfusion image findings and gated SPECT.

2. What information is available from the raw data sequential projection images?

3. What is the most likely diagnosis?

4. List the advantages of electrocardiograph-synchronization (gating) to SPECT.

Cardiovascular System: Breast Attenuation, Wall Thickening

1. Mild fixed anteroseptal hypoperfusion that demonstrates uniform brightening on gated SPECT, indicating normal myocardial wall thickening on gated images.

2. Apparent decreased radiotracer in the upper portions of the heart is most obvious on the left anterior oblique and lateral frames. No obvious patient motion.

3. Normal perfusion study with normal wall thickening and breast attenuation.

4. Assessment of regional wall motion/wall thickening and left ventricular ejection fraction (LVEF).

References

Hachamovich R, Berman DS, Kiat H, et al: Exercise myocardial perfusion SPECT in patients without known coronary artery disease: incremental prognostic value and use in risk stratification, *Circulation* 93:905-914, 1996.

DePuey EG, Heller G, Taillefer RL: Clinical applications of gated myocardial perfusion SPECT. In DePuey EG, Garcia EV, Berman DS, editors: *Cardiac SPECT imaging,* ed 2, Philadelphia, 2001, Lippincott Williams & Wilkins, pp 211-230.

Cross-Reference

Nuclear Medicine: THE REQUISITES, ed 2, pp 67-68, 71-79.

Comment

Gated SPECT analysis allows for assessment of regional wall motion, wall thickening, and calculated regional LVEF. For gated SPECT the cardiac cycle is usually divided into 8 frames, in contrast to 16 or more frames for planar equilibrium ^{99m}Tc red blood cell ventriculography. The fewer number of frames has somewhat poorer accuracy because of limited temporal resolution. For example, true end-systole and end-diastole may not be detected because of summation of counts in the longer time frames. The higher count rates available with ^{99m}Tc agents compared with ^{201}Tl and the use of multiheaded cameras are advantageous in maximizing the count rate for gated SPECT.

Stress myocardial perfusion imaging is considerably more accurate for assessment of CAD than stress electrocardiograms. Stress electrocardiography has a sensitivity of only 70% for detection of CAD and a false-positive rate as high as 40%. False-positive results are a particular problem in female patients. In contrast, stress myocardial perfusion studies have an overall accuracy rate of approximately 85%. Individuals with normal scan results and nonanginal symptoms have less than a 1% incidence of major cardiac events in the subsequent 2 years.

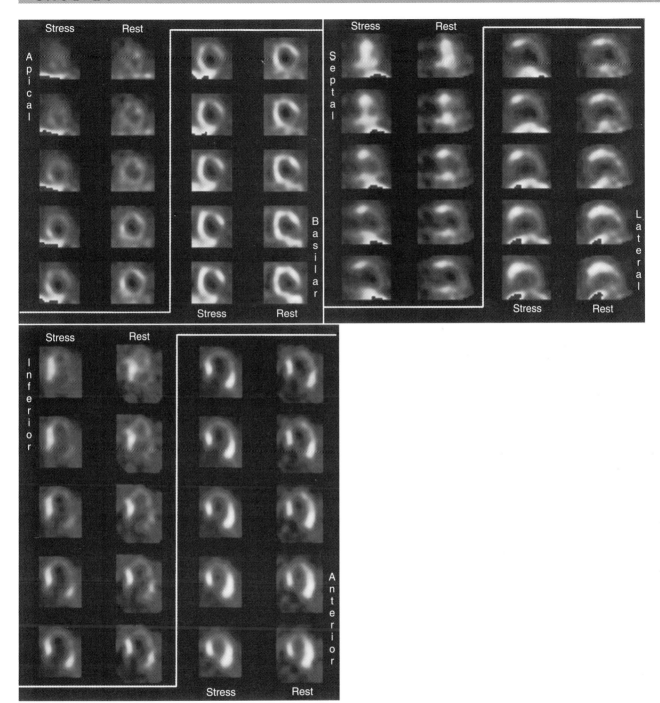

After the rest scan the patient said he could not stay for the stress study but would reschedule. However, the patient came to the emergency department the next morning with chest pain. ⁹⁹ᵐTc sestamibi was injected during the pain, and the images were labeled "stress."

1. Describe the SPECT findings.

2. Name the most likely culprit coronary artery or arteries.

3. Which radiopharmaceuticals are preferred in this setting?

4. Provide the reason for your choice of radionuclide.

Cardiovascular System: Emergency Department Chest Pain

1. Moderately severe perfusion defect of the entire anterior wall extending to the apex that partially reverses on rest images, severe perfusion defect of the defect involving the lateral and inferolateral wall that partially reverses.

2. LAD and left circumflex coronary arteries or left main coronary artery.

3. ^{99m}Tc sestamibi or ^{99m}Tc tetrofosmin.

4. The exact image timing of ^{99m}Tc-labeled agents is not crucial because no significant redistribution occur. In an emergency setting, matters of patient management and logistics may take priority over immediate scanning.

Reference

Heller GV, Stowers SA, Hendel RC, et al: Clinical value of acute rest technetium-99m tetrofosmin tomographic myocardial perfusion imaging in patients with acute chest pain and nondiagnostic electrocardiograms, *J Am Coll Cardiol* 31:1011-1017, 1998.

Cross-Reference

Nuclear Medicine: THE REQUISITES, ed 2, pp 72-80, 88-89.

Comment

Studies have shown that performing perfusion imaging in the emergency department in patients with unexplained chest pain is cost-effective. Abnormal findings on SPECT perfusion imaging accurately predict acute myocardial infarction in patients with symptoms, a nondiagnostic electrocardiogram, and no history of myocardial infarction. A normal study is associated with a very low cardiac event rate. The use of acute rest SPECT for patients in the emergency department can substantially and safely reduce the number of unnecessary hospital admissions. However, this practice requires cooperation and coordination by a number of clinical services and hospital personnel.

In an emergency setting, matters of patient management and logistics may take priority over scanning. Although ^{201}Tl can be used in a similar fashion to evaluate acute chest pain, the need to image without delay after injection is a significant disadvantage. After initial uptake, ^{201}Tl undergoes "redistribution," i.e., an ongoing dynamic equilibrium of ^{201}Tl between the myocardium and the blood pool exists. ^{99m}Tc-labeled agents offer the flexibility of injection early in the evaluation process, but delay of the scan until "things are under control." This feature has increased the utilization of myocardial perfusion SPECT in the acute care setting.

A

B

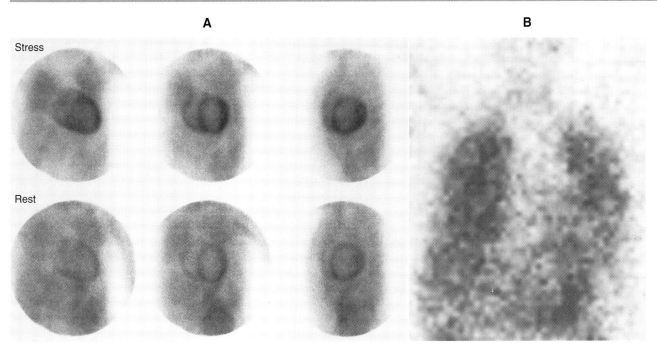

Stress

Rest

Scans for two patients are provided. *A,* Stress and 4-hour delayed planar thallium scan. *B,* Poststress SPECT anterior raw data projection image. Stress/rest SPECT showed single-vessel ischemia.

1. Describe the planar scintigraphic findings in patient *A* and the abnormal finding in patient *B.*

2. What other information is necessary for interpretation of these examinations?

3. Name ancillary findings of CAD other than perfusion defects that are relevant in interpreting myocardial perfusion scans.

4. What is the most appropriate diagnosis in patients *A* and *B?*

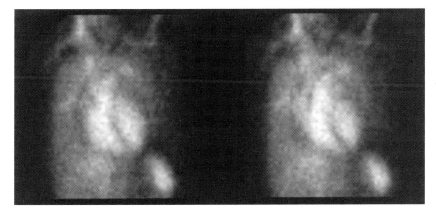

A 45-year-old man has dyspnea on exertion. Cardiac catheterization found no coronary disease. Images at end-diastole *(left)* and end-systole *(right)* are shown.

1. Name the radiopharmaceutical, the examination being performed, and describe the findings.

2. Which view is shown, and why was it selected to calculate LVEF? Name other views often obtained.

3. List the terms used to describe myocardial wall motion.

4. Provide a classification for cardiomyopathies.

Cardiovascular: Planar Thallium with Increased Lung Activity

1. *A,* Both ventricles are dilated with prominent right ventricular uptake. No evidence of ischemia or scar. Increased lung activity on the stress images.

2. The level of exercise achieved. At a low level of stress, the scan can provide false-negative indication of CAD.

3. Poststress lung uptake and transient ischemic dilation.

4. *A,* Dilated cardiomyopathy with right ventricular hypertrophy. *B,* Multivessel CAD.

Reference

Gerson MC, editor: *Cardiac nuclear medicine,* ed 3, New York, 1997, McGraw-Hill.

Cross-Reference

Nuclear Medicine: THE REQUISITES, ed 2, pp 66-68, 76-79, 82.

Comment

^{201}Tl has been used as a myocardial radiotracer for more than two decades. Myocardium distribution is proportional to blood flow over the physiological range. When ^{201}Tl is injected at peak stress, it redistributes according to initial blood flow. Imaging is performed within 10 minutes of injection. So-called redistribution represents the combination of differential washout and secondary tracer uptake from circulating ^{201}Tl.

Lung activity on stress ^{201}Tl studies should always be assessed. In normal subjects the lung background activity is low. However, it is increased at rest in patients with left ventricular failure. Stress-induced uptake is correlated with left ventricular end-diastolic pressure and pulmonary capillary wedge pressure. Increased lung activity uptake on stress images indicates left ventricular decompensation and often is a sign of multivessel CAD. However, uptake can also be the result of other causes of poorly compensated heart disease. A quantitative ratio of lung/myocardial activity (L/M) is often used to confirm the imaging abnormality. The L/M ratio should be less than 0.5; ratios above this value are abnormal. Lung uptake does not have the same significance when ^{99m}Tc myocardial perfusion agents are used because these tracers are normally taken up by the lung to a higher degree than ^{201}Tl.

Notes

Cardiovascular System: Cardiomyopathy on Equilibrium-Gated Blood Pool Ventriculography or Multigated Acquisition

1. ^{99m}Tc-labeled erythrocytes. Equilibrium-gated blood pool ventriculography (RVG) or MUGA (multigated acquisition). Frames at end-diastole and end-systole show globally decreased wall motion. Visual estimate shows very decreased LVEF.

2. The left anterior oblique view provides the best septal separation of the two ventricles. Occasionally anterior and left lateral posterior oblique views also are obtained.

3. Global or regional—akinesis, hypokinesis, dyskinesis, tardokinesis.

4. Classification according to the functional status of the ventricle: restrictive, dilated, or hypertrophic; or according to cause: alcoholic, infectious, metabolic, toxic, drug-induced, or ischemia/CAD, idiopathic.

References

Borer JS: Measurement of ventricular function and volume. In Zaret BL, Beller GA, editors: *Nuclear cardiology,* St Louis, 1999, Mosby.

Dilsizian V, Rocco TP, Bonow RO, et al: Cardiac blood-pool imaging. II: Applications in noncoronary heart disease, *J Nucl Med* 31:10-22, 1990.

Cross-Reference

Nuclear Medicine: THE REQUISITES, ed 2, pp 91-93, 98-99, 103-104.

Comment

Wall motion abnormalities may be global, as in this patient, or regional. Regional abnormalities are usually caused by CAD, primarily infarction, or less commonly, acute ischemia. Definitions of the terms used to describe cardiac wall motion are:

- Normal
- Akinesis: complete absence of wall motion
- Hypokinetic: residual but diminished contraction
- Dyskinesis: paradoxic wall motion, opposite to the direction of expected motion. Dyskinesia is seen in the septum of patients after coronary bypass grafting as a result of disruption of the pericardium and in patients after myocardial infarctions with aneurysmal wall motion
- Tardokinesis: motion present but delayed compared with adjacent segments

Cardiomyopathies can be classified functionally: restrictive, dilated, or hypertrophic, according to the cause, or as primary or secondary. When the cause is known, cardiomyopathy is labeled as alcoholic, infectious, metabolic, toxic, drug-induced, or ischemic; otherwise it is idiopathic. Dilated cardiomyopathies usually are associated with a dilated LV and a depressed LVEF. In contrast, hypertrophic and restrictive cardiomyopathies usually are associated with small or normal LV.

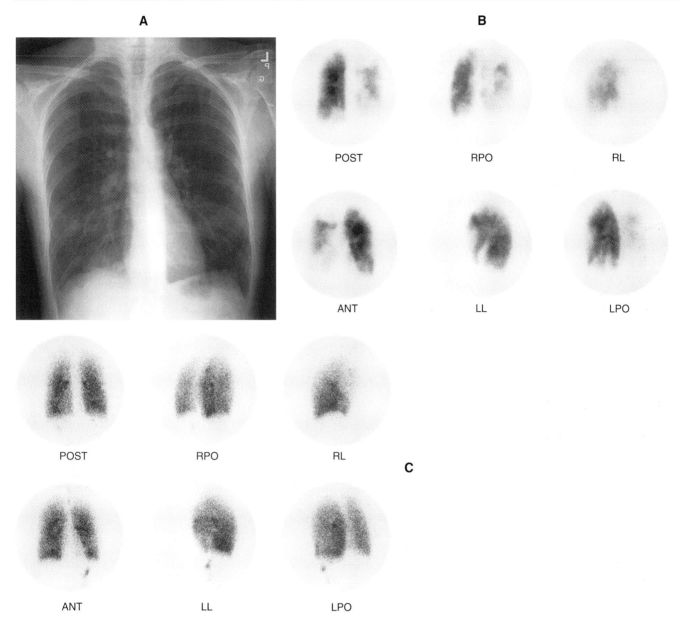

A 62-year-old patient has right-sided chest discomfort and shortness of breath. *A,* Posteroanterior chest radiograph; *B,* perfusion; *C,* ventilation.

1. Describe the ventilation-perfusion image findings.

2. Interpret the study. Give your reasoning.

3. What is the likelihood of pulmonary embolus in this patient?

4. What are the most common chest x-ray findings in patients with pulmonary emboli?

Pulmonary System: High Probability of Pulmonary Embolus

1. Perfusion is decreased in the right lower lobe except for the superior segment. Ventilation is truncated in the right lower lobe consistent with subpulmonic effusion.

2. High probability for pulmonary embolus. Mismatch between perfusion and ventilation is evident in the basal segments. The perfusion defect is considerably larger than the effusion on the radiograph.

3. Greater than 80%.

4. Most common: normal. Next most common: atelectasis; these also are the most common chest x-ray findings in patients determined by angiography not to have emboli.

References

Freitas JE, Sarosi MG, Nagle CC, et al: Modified PIOPED criteria used in clinical practice, *J Nucl Med* 36:1573-1578, 1995.

Juni J, Alavi A: Lung scanning in the diagnosis of pulmonary embolism: the emperor redressed, *Semin Nucl Med* 21:281-296, 1991.

Cross-Reference

Nuclear Medicine: THE REQUISITES, ed 2, pp 152-160.

Comment

The PIOPED criterion that a perfusion defect larger than the radiographic abnormality indicates a high probability of pulmonary embolism should be used cautiously. The chest radiograph is obtained with maximal inspiration. The lung scan image is acquired during tidal breathing. Thus the heart is more horizontal on the lung scan than on the radiograph, and the lung fields appear larger on the lung scan than on the radiograph. However, in this case perfusion defect undoubtedly is larger than the defect on the radiographic finding. No ventilatory defects are apparent, only a truncated lower lung field.

A patient with a high-probability scan has a greater than 80% probability of pulmonary embolus. However, fewer than half of patients determined to have pulmonary embolus by angiography have a high-probability scan. Thus a high-probability scan is not sensitive for the diagnosis of pulmonary embolus, but it is fairly specific. Conversely, this means that 20% of patients have another diagnosis. The most common cause is lung cancer. The mediastinal tumor preferentially occludes the pulmonary artery, which is easily compressible in contrast to the more rigid bronchi. Old emboli are another common cause of a false-positive study for pulmonary embolus. Vasculitis or sickle cell disease are other causes.

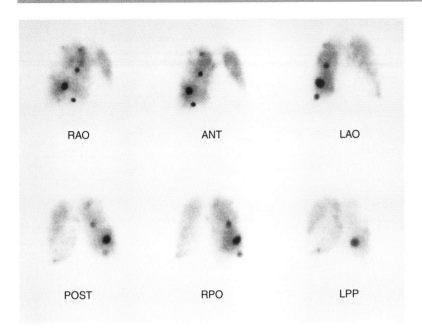

RAO   ANT   LAO

POST   RPO   LPP

A 45-year-old woman was referred for a ventilation-perfusion study. The perfusion scan only is shown.

1. Describe the abnormal scintigraphic findings.

2. What is the most likely cause for the findings?

3. What is the radiation dose to the patient from a perfusion study? From a ^{133}Xe ventilation study?

4. Given the longer physical half-life and larger administered dose of ^{133}Xe, compared with ^{99m}Tc macro-aggregated albumin (MAA), explain the lower resulting radiation dose to the lungs.

Pulmonary System: "Hot Spots" on Lung Scan

1. Multiple "hot spots" are present in the upper and lower lobes, predominately in the right lung field.

2. Radioactive emboli as a result of poor technique caused by drawing back blood into the syringe containing the ^{99m}Tc MAA before injection of the radiotracer, causing clumping.

3. The lungs, the target organs, receive approximately 1 rad/5 mCi from ^{99m}Tc MAA. Approximately 0.2 rads to the lung from a 20-mCi xenon study.

4. The biological half-life is brief. The patient breathes ^{133}Xe gas to equilibrium, then expels it into a trap. Only ^{133}Xe absorbed as a result of fat solubility has any appreciable biological half-life.

References

Preston DF, Greenlaw RH: "Hot spots" on lung scans, *J Nucl Med* 11:422-425, 1970.

Conca DM, Brill DR, Shoop JD: Pulmonary radioactive microemboli following radionuclide venography, *J Nucl Med* 18:1140-1141, 1977.

Cross-Reference

Nuclear Medicine: THE REQUISITES, ed 2, pp 119-150.

Comment

The cause of this abnormal hot spot scan pattern is poor technique. Technologists are taught that blood should *not* be drawn back into the syringe to prove it is in the vein before infusion of ^{99m}Tc MAA, in contrast to other injections. The blood causes the MAA to aggregate, and when it is reinfused, it forms a pattern indicating hot pulmonary microemboli. ^{99m}Tc MAA particles should be agitated before injection to avoid settling and aggregation of the particles, which also can cause hot spots. This hot spot pattern has been reported in patients with thrombophlebitis when the injection is given distally in an extremity with proximal thrombophlebitis, e.g., if radionuclide venography is combined with the perfusion study. Injection of the radiopharmaceutical can dislodge part of the labeled thrombus.

Other important technical aspects of MAA injection include ensuring that the patient breathes deeply and is in the supine position to ensure uniform particle distribution. Gravity produces a lower lobe predominance if the patient is upright. The MAA should be injected through a 23-gauge or larger needle to prevent particle fragmentation. Six to eight views should be acquired. The anterior, posterior, and posterior oblique views are the most important. Lateral views should be interpreted cautiously because of shine-through from the opposite side. Anterior oblique views sometimes are helpful.

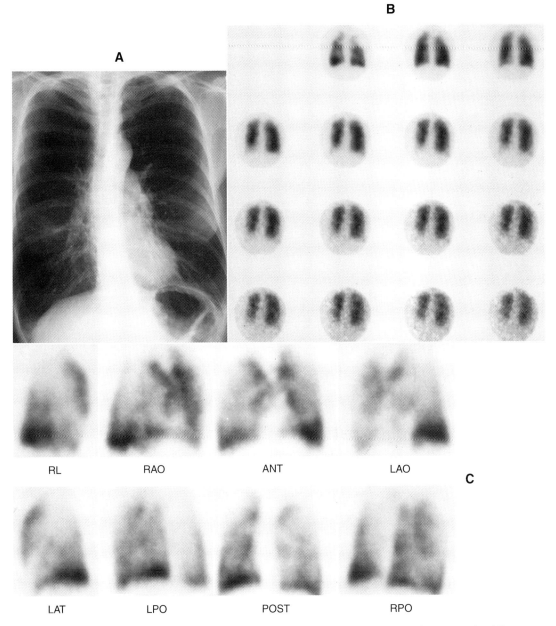

A chest radiograph *(A)*, posterior ¹³³Xe ventilation *(B)*, and eight-view perfusion study *(C)* were performed for shortness of breath.

1. Describe the findings on the ventilation study.

2. Describe the findings on the perfusion study.

3. Provide an interpretation regarding the presence or absence of pulmonary embolism.

4. What term could be applied to this perfusion pattern?

Pulmonary System: Ventilation-Perfusion— Stripe Sign, Emphysema

1. Decreased upper lobe ventilation is seen on the single breath with air trapping in both upper lobes and the right lower lobe on washout images.

2. Decreased perfusion to the majority of both lungs, with preserved perfusion in the subpleural lung, most evident at the lung bases and medial aspect of both upper lobes.

3. Low probability.

4. Stripe sign.

References

Worsley DF, Alavi A: Radionuclide imaging of acute pulmonary embolism, *Radiol Clin North Am* 38:1035-1052, 2001.

Sostman HD, Gottschalk A: The stripe sign: a new sign for diagnosis of nonembolic defects on pulmonary perfusion scintigraphy, *Radiology* 142:737-741, 1982.

Cross-Reference

Nuclear Medicine: THE REQUISITES, ed 2, pp 160, 396.

Comment

The stripe sign refers to a subpleural margin of activity in a lung region with decreased perfusion. The perfusion defect is not pleural based because a rim or stripe of activity at the pleura is greater than the activity seen in the defect. This assessment should be made from the best tangential view of the area in question. The stripe sign is useful and reliable for discounting pulmonary embolus as the cause of the perfusion defect. The sign is approximately 90% reliable as an indication of nonembolic disease, and thus of low probability. However, the remainder of the lungs should be inspected because the sign is only a predictor for the area when it appears, and not for the patient overall. For example, if the scan demonstrates an area with a stripe sign and two or more segmental mismatches, the study would appropriately be characterized as high probability.

Emphysema is a major cause of chronic airflow obstruction, a diagnosis indicating pathological permanent abnormal enlargement of air spaces distal to the terminal bronchiole. The best radiographic indicator is hyperinflation, but vascular change, bullae, and increased lung markings also may be demonstrated. The ^{133}Xe study is a sensitive indicator of obstructive lung disease as shown in this case.

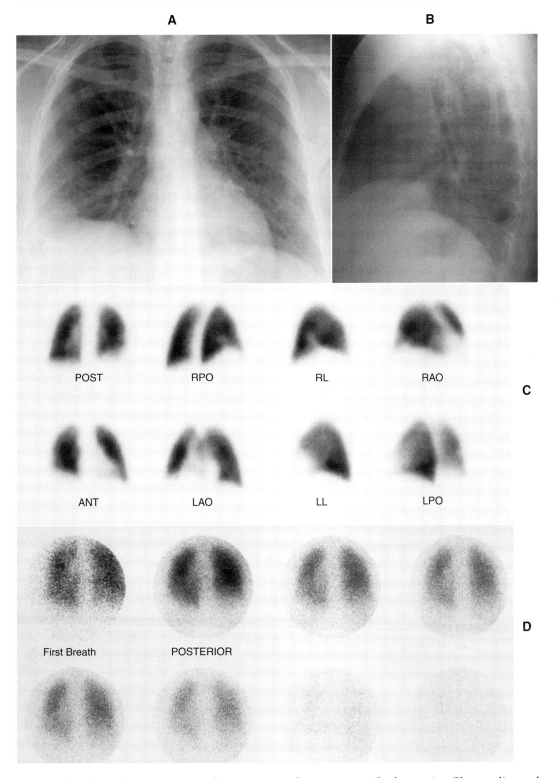

A young female patient presents at the emergency department with chest pain. Chest radiographs *(A, B)*, perfusion scan *(C)*, and ventilation study *(D)* are shown.

1. Describe the findings on the chest radiograph.

2. Describe the perfusion and ventilation scans.

3. Categorize the study regarding the presence or absence of pulmonary embolism using PIOPED criteria.

4. What is the most common finding on chest radiographs with thromboembolism?

Pulmonary System: Hampton's Hump—
Intermediate Probability

1. Posteroanterior and lateral chest radiographs demonstrate a pleural-based opacity in the lateral right lung base.

2. A single wedged-shaped, pleural-based defect in the same location as the radiographic abnormality, probably the anterobasal segment of the right lower lobe. Normal ^{133}Xe ventilation study.

3. Intermediate probability for pulmonary embolism.

4. Chest x-ray findings in pulmonary embolus without infarction are uncommon. When present, they are usually associated with a large, central embolus. Discoid atelectasis is the next most common finding.

Reference

Armstrong P, Wilson AG, Dee P, et al: *Images of diseases of the chest,* ed 3, pp 75, 407-408, St Louis, 2000, Mosby.

Cross-Reference

Nuclear Medicine: THE REQUISITES, ed 2, pp 152-159.

Comment

The radiographic signs of acute pulmonary embolism without infarction or hemorrhage include oligemia of the lung (Westermark's sign), increase in size of the main pulmonary artery, and elevation of the hemidiaphragm. All are nonspecific. Most emboli do not cause infarction. However, when present, infarction appears as lung consolidation and occurs predominantly in the lower lung fields. The radiographic finding described by Hampton and Castleman (1940) is known as Hampton's hump: "infarcts are always in contact with pleural surfaces and the shadows are rarely, if ever, triangular in shape." When pulmonary embolism is associated with consolidation because of hemorrhage and not true infarction, the infiltrate clears quickly, often within a week. In contrast, true infarction resolves over several months and may be associated with permanent linear scarring. Because cavitation is rare, it suggests secondary infection.

Because there is a single segmental mismatch, the study cannot be categorized as low probability. Two or more mismatched segmental defects are not present, so the study cannot be categorized as high probability. Therefore by default and definition, the study indicates intermediate probability for pulmonary embolism or is indeterminate from a diagnostic standpoint. Angiography findings were positive.

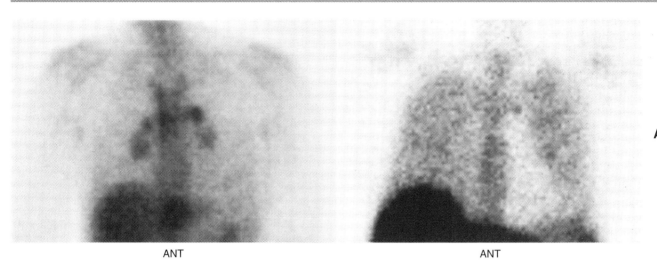

ANT   ANT

A

B

Two patients with the same disease (*A* and *B*) had ^{67}Ga scintigraphy.

1. Describe the lung patterns seen on the ^{67}Ga lung scans.

2. What is the finding on the head and neck scan?

3. Match the lung scan with the head and neck scan.

4. What is the disease, and how is ^{67}Ga scintigraphy used in these patients?

Infection and Inflammation: Sarcoidosis

1. Patient *A,* "lambda sign" (hilar and paratracheal nodal uptake); patient *B,* diffuse pulmonary uptake.

2. Classic "panda" sign.

3. Either *A* or *B.* The panda sign can be seen at any stage of disease.

4. Sarcoidosis. [67]Ga scintigraphy is used to confirm the clinical diagnosis and to differentiate active alveolitis from inactive fibrosis.

References

Kurdziel KA: The panda sign, *Radiology* 215:884-885, 2000.

Sulavik SB, Spencer RP, Weed DA, et al: Recognition of distinctive patterns of gallium-67 distribution in sarcoidosis, *J Nucl Med* 31:1909-1914, 1990.

Cross-Reference

Nuclear Medicine: THE REQUISITES, ed 2, pp 171-173.

Comment

The panda sign is highly suggestive of sarcoidosis. It is seen less frequently in other inflammatory diseases involving the lacrimal and salivary glands, e.g., Sjögren's syndrome and in patients who have had irradiation of the head and neck. The panda sign is not specific for sarcoidosis, but with the lambda sign or diffuse pulmonary uptake, or bilateral symmetrical hilar adenopathy on chest radiographs, the findings highly suggest sarcoidosis. The pattern of uptake in *B* can be seen in a variety of other inflammatory and infectious pulmonary diseases other than sarcoidosis, including *Pneumocystis carinii,* pneumoconioses, hypersensitivity pneumonitis, active idiopathic pulmonary fibrosis, and toxicity from therapeutic drugs, e.g., bleomycin.

More than 90% of patients with sarcoidosis have pulmonary manifestations; 25% have permanent loss of lung function, and 5% to 10% die of complications. [67]Ga is useful in the evaluation of patients in whom sarcoidosis is suspected and for evaluation of therapy effectiveness. [67]Ga is more sensitive than chest radiography for detection of early disease.

The chest radiograph has been used to stage sarcoidosis as follows: stage 0 (normal), stage 1 (bilateral symmetrical hilar adenopathy), stage 2 (bilateral hilar adenopathy with pulmonary infiltration), and stage 3 (diffuse symmetrical lung infiltration). The panda and lambda signs often are seen together, most commonly in stages 1 and 2, but also may be present in stage 0 and 3.

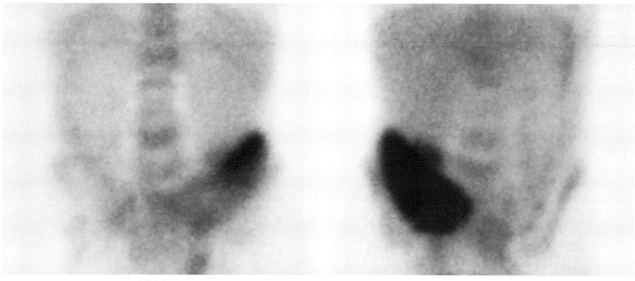

POST   ANT

A 57-year-old man has had abdominal discomfort and fever for 3 weeks.

1. Describe the findings on this ^{67}Ga study and give a likely diagnosis.
2. What is the mechanism of ^{67}Ga uptake in infection/inflammation?
3. List the photopeaks of ^{67}Ga. List the ones used for imaging. What collimator should be used to acquire the study?
4. What is the recommended administered dose of ^{67}Ga, its half-life, and imaging times?

C A S E   2 9

Infection and Inflammation: Intraabdominal Abscess

1. Very increased uptake in the right lower quadrant strongly suggests an intraabdominal abscess. Tumor cannot be excluded.

2. Increased vascular permeability, bacterial uptake, and binding to leukocytes play a role; however, binding to lactoferrin of degranulated neutrophils at the site of infection is probably the primary mechanism.

3. Photopeaks occur at 91 to 93, 185, 300, and 394 keV. The lower three photopeaks are used for imaging. A medium-energy collimator should be used.

4. The recommended adult dose of ^{67}Ga is 5 mCi; the half-life is 78 hours. Imaging at 48 hours is routine. However, if an abscess is suspected, imaging at 6 to 24 hours may provide an early diagnosis.

Reference

Rypins EB, Evans DG, Hinrichs W, et al: Tc-99m HMPAO white blood cell scan for diagnosis of acute appendicitis in patients with equivocal clinical presentation, *Ann Surg* 226:58-65, 1997.

Cross-Reference

Nuclear Medicine: THE REQUISITES, ed 2, pp 168-177.

Comment

The strict clinical definition of fever of unknown origin is (1) fever of at least 38.3° C on more than 3 occasions, (2) no diagnosis after 3 weeks of investigation, and (3) hospitalization of at least 7 days. A perforated appendix with intraabdominal abscess was found during surgery. ^{67}Ga has been used for infection imaging since the early 1970s. Today its role is limited because of the availability of radiolabeled leukocytes. ^{67}Ga occasionally is useful in patients with persistent fever but no localizing signs on examination and negative CT findings. In the setting of a fever of unknown origin, it may localize the site of infection, tumor, or both. Tumor occasionally is manifest as a cause of fever of unknown origin. However, if an intraabdominal source of infection is being sought, ^{67}Ga scanning is disadvantageous because of normal bowel clearance that may obscure pathological uptake.

Radiolabeled leukocytes, labeled with ^{99m}Tc hexamethyl-propyleneamine-oxime (HM-PAO) or ^{111}In oxine, are used more commonly for detection of infection, particularly intraabdominal infection. Disadvantages of labeled leukocytes are the requirement of up to 50 ml of the patient's blood for labeling, the time needed for cell labeling (minimum of 2 hours), and the serious problem of blood-borne diseases. A monoclonal antibody against granulocytes may be approved for clinical use soon.

A

B

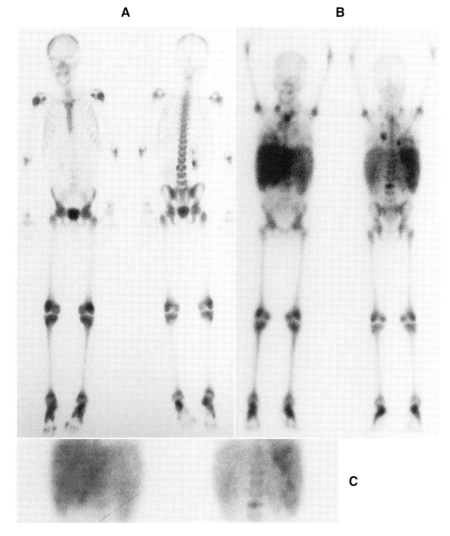

C

A 9-year-old patient had back pain and fever for 4 weeks. Bone *(A)*, gallium-67 whole-body *(B)* and abdominal spot views *(C)* are shown.

1. Describe the scintigraphic findings on the bone and gallium scans.

2. When both tests are ordered at the same time, which should be performed first?

3. Provide the differential diagnosis and the most likely diagnosis.

4. Based on the available information, characterize the stage of disease.

Oncology: Bone/Gallium—Stage IV Hodgkin's Disease

1. The bone scan shows mild increased uptake at L3. The ^{67}Ga scan shows abnormal uptake in the L3 vertebral body, as well as the neck bilaterally (right side greater than the left side), mediastinum, right paratracheal regions, posterior thorax, and right lung base; and multifocal uptake in the liver. The lower-intensity camera setting optimizes liver visualization *(C)*.

2. Bone scan.

3. Hodgkin's disease, tuberculosis, or atypical mycobacteria; Hodgkin's disease is likely.

4. Stage IV.

Reference
Rehm PK: Radionuclide evaluation of patients with lymphoma, *Radiol Clin North Am* 39:957-978, 2001.

Cross-Reference
Nuclear Medicine: THE REQUISITES, ed 2, pp 116-121, 199-202.

Comment
The findings indicate soft tissue and bone involvement; thus gallium-avid tumors and inflammatory and infectious conditions form the primary differential diagnosis. Given the distribution and age group, the gallium-avid tumor for primary consideration would be Hodgkin's disease. Infectious or inflammatory diseases would be considered. However, the involvement of a single vertebra on the bone scan, rather than two adjacent vertebral levels, would be atypical for vertebral osteomyelitis. Given the patient's age and distribution of findings, Hodgkin's disease is the most likely diagnosis. The presence of skeletal (independent of marrow) involvement indicates stage IV disease. ^{67}Ga is taken up both by the marrow and bone.

To avoid downscatter of higher-energy photons of ^{67}Ga (393, 300, and 185 keV) into the ^{99m}Tc window centered at 140 KeV, the bone scan should be completed before the gallium is injected. If gallium is injected first, because of its physical (78 hours) and biological half-lives (25 days) and the high energy of its photons compared with ^{99m}Tc, the bone scan should be delayed several days to avoid high background and downscatter degradation of the bone image. ^{67}Ga can be injected as soon as the bone scan is complete. Imaging of ^{67}Ga is initiated 48 to 72 hours after injection. Although 5 mCi of ^{67}Ga is administered for infection/inflammation imaging, 10 mCi of ^{67}Ga is recommended for adult tumor imaging to allow for higher-resolution images and SPECT. The higher dosimetry is considered acceptable for oncology patients.

A   B

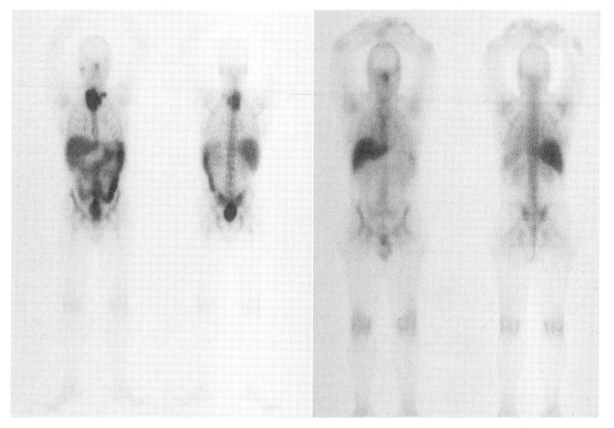

A 32-year-old man has non-Hodgkin's lymphoma. *A* shows the ^{67}Ga study at initial staging, and *B* was performed after a full course of chemotherapy. CT showed a residual chest mass after chemotherapy.

1. What is the adult dose of ^{67}Ga for tumor evaluation? When is imaging performed?

2. Compare the accuracy of ^{67}Ga and CT for initial staging and evaluating response to therapy.

3. Describe the findings of the two studies and interpret them.

4. How can the problem of bowel activity be minimized on ^{67}Ga scans?

Oncology: ^{67}Ga—Non-Hodgkin's Lymphoma Before and After Therapy

1. The adult dose is 10 mCi, which is twice the dose used for inflammatory and infectious evaluation. Imaging typically is performed 48 to 72 hours after injection.

2. CT scanning provides better sensitivity for initial staging. ^{67}Ga scanning is superior to CT in evaluation of the effectiveness of therapy and determination of whether residual masses after therapy represent residual tumor or merely necrosis and fibrosis.

3. *A,* A large mass in the anterior mediastinum extends to the supraclavicular regions. Considerable colonic/rectal activity is present. Because of the latter activity, tumor cannot be excluded in the mid-pelvis to the lower pelvis. *B,* Complete response to therapy has occurred. The residual chest mass on CT is caused by necrosis and fibrosis, not tumor.

4. Laxatives may be given, and imaging may be delayed as needed at 4 to 7 days after injection.

Reference
Rehm PK: Radionuclide evaluation of patients with lymphoma, *Radiol Clin North Am* 39:957-978, 2001.

Cross-Reference
Nuclear Medicine: THE REQUISITES, ed 2, pp 198-202.

Comment
The sensitivity of ^{67}Ga for detection of Hodgkin's disease and non-Hodgkin's lymphoma is very high, 95% and 95%, respectively, particularly when SPECT is used. In many posttherapy cases, CT scanning shows a residual chest or abdominal mass. The differential diagnosis includes a partial incomplete response to chemotherapy with residual viable tumor, which requires further treatment, versus a nonviable mass of fibrosis and necrosis. ^{67}Ga scanning can make this distinction very accurately. This patient's tumor was treated effectively. Differentiating normal colonic clearance from tumor is a common diagnostic dilemma. Although bowel cleansing with laxatives and hydration can be helpful, delayed imaging at 4 to 7 days often is required to fully evaluate the abdomen and pelvis. The colon has the highest radiation absorbed dose (target organ). The higher dose of ^{67}Ga administered for patients with tumors compared with those evaluated for infection and inflammation allows for better quality planar images and SPECT. SPECT is performed routinely at most institutions because it allows detection of disease that might not be seen on planar imaging, particularly in the chest and abdomen. SPECT increases the image contrast by eliminating overlying and underlying activity. It improves detection of small lesion and deep lesion. Imaging is performed 48 to 72 hours after injection.

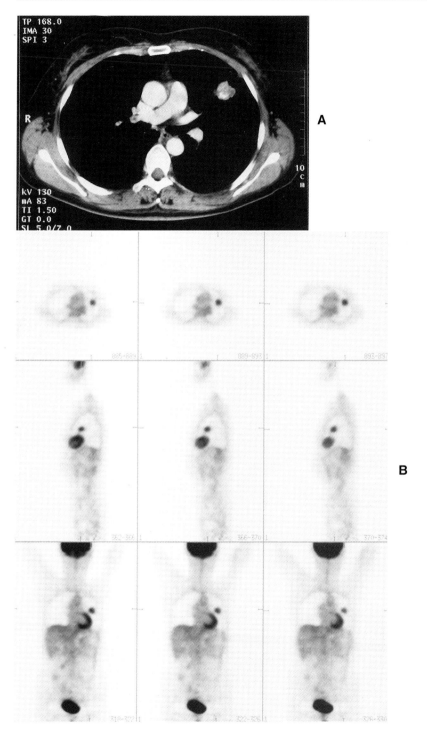

A 67-year-old man has a 2.5-cm left upper lobe lung lesion detected on chest radiographs and confirmed with CT *(A)*. [18]F fluorodeoxyglucose positron emission tomography (FDG-PET) scan is shown *(B)*.

1. What percentage of all newly discovered pulmonary nodules are malignant?

2. What percentage of single pulmonary nodules are indeterminate in etiology after chest radiography and CT examination? What percentage ultimately are benign?

3. What is the likelihood of lung cancer in this case?

4. What are causes for false-negative/false-positive ^{18}F FDG-PET studies?

Oncology: FDG-PET—Single Pulmonary Nodule

1. Only 20% to 30% are malignant overall. However, the incidence is as high as 50% in smokers.

2. By radiographic/CT criteria, 30% to 40% are indeterminate; 50% percent of these are benign.

3. High.

4. False-negative findings are uncommon and usually are the result of small lesion size (<1.0 cm), bronchoalveolar carcinoma, and carcinoid tumors. False-positive findings can be caused by benign tumor, and inflammatory or infectious disease, e.g., histoplasmosis, tuberculosis. Typically inflammatory lesions have less uptake than malignant tumors, but overlap exists.

Reference

Gould MK, Maclean CC, Kuschner WG, et al: Accuracy PET for diagnosis of pulmonary nodules and mass lesions: a meta-analysis, *JAMA* 285;936-937, 2001.

Cross-Reference

Nuclear Medicine: THE REQUISITES, ed 2, pp 209-210.

Comment

Of approximately 130,000 pulmonary lung nodules diagnosed annually, one third are malignant. CT scans can further characterize the lesion. However, after CT, 30% to 40% are indeterminate; 50% of these ultimately are malignant. If characteristic benign changes are not seen in a low-risk patient, multiple follow-up CT scans are performed over 2 years to confirm that the lesion is benign. Various invasive procedures are used to make the diagnosis, including bronchoscopy, percutaneous biopsy, and video-assisted thoracoscopy and thoracotomy. Resection of pulmonary nodules has associated risk. A noninvasive method to preoperatively determine which patients require a more invasive diagnostic procedure would avoid unnecessary surgery, morbidity, and even death for many patients. [18]F FDG-PET can help differentiate benign from malignant lesions. Data from 17 investigations and 588 patients show 96% sensitivity for the diagnosis of malignancy in single pulmonary nodules, specificity of 88%, and overall accuracy of 94%. A negative FDG-PET study result obviates the need for diagnostic surgery in patients at high risk for surgery who have chronic obstructive pulmonary disease (COPD) or other serious medical problems and young patients at low risk for malignancy.

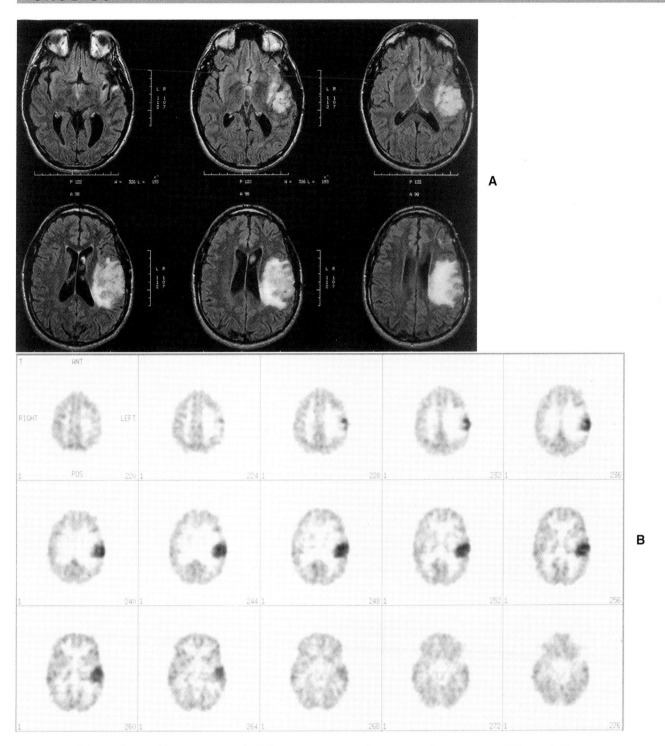

A 38-year-old man had a diagnosis of grade I-II astrocytoma and was treated 11 years ago. He has had a recent onset of seizures. MRI showed no definite change from the many prior studies *(B)*.

1. What FDG-PET scan findings are expected with a low-grade glioma?

2. What is the finding on this FDG-PET scan *(A)?*

3. Interpret this study.

4. Would ⁹⁹ᵐTc HM-PAO show a similar appearance?

Primary Brain Tumor

1. Low-grade gliomas typically have poor or no uptake.

2. Intense uptake in the large temporoparietal mass.

3. Transformation of a low-grade to a high-grade glioma.

4. No. Malignant tumors usually do not have receptors for binding of the radiopharmaceutical, which is necessary before intracellular incorporation.

References

Delbeke D, Myerowitz C, Lapidus RL, et al: Optimal cutoff levels of F-18 FDG uptake in the differentiation of low-grade from high-grade brain tumors with PET, *Radiology* 195:47-52, 1995.

Langleben DB, Segall GM: PET in differentiation of recurrent brain tumor from radiation injury, *J Nucl Med* 41:1861-1867, 2000.

Cross-Reference

Nuclear Medicine: THE REQUISITES, ed 2, pp 314-316.

Comment

Primary brain tumors were first imaged with FDG-PET by Dr. Di Chiro in 1982. These tumors have increased glucose metabolism demonstrated by ^{18}F FDG-PET. The degree of FDG uptake correlates with the tumor grade and the patient's prognosis. Low-grade tumors (grade I-II astrocytomas) have poor or no uptake. High-grade tumors (grade III anaplastic astrocytomas and grade IV glioblastoma multiforme) have uptake greater than gray matter. Because gray matter metabolism is three to four times that of white matter, white matter typically is seen as having no uptake on the scans. Biopsy is invasive and often provides limited information. Because gliomas are not homogeneous and contain areas of necrosis, biopsy is subject to sampling error.

FDG-PET has been used to direct stereotactic biopsy in heterogeneous tumors. FDG-PET also is helpful in the differential diagnosis of intracranial masses in patients with acquired immunodeficiency syndrome (AIDS). Tumors, such as lymphoma, take up the FDG, whereas infection, e.g., toxoplasmosis, usually does not have significant uptake. FDG-PET also may be important in the evaluation of the effectiveness of therapy. The uptake or absence of uptake of FDG after therapy can determine whether the tumor has responded to radiation therapy. Areas of radiation necrosis have very low glucose metabolism, whereas ineffective therapy is indicated by uptake. Finally, FDG-PET can be used to detect transformation of a low-grade tumor to a high-grade tumor before changes are seen on MRI, as in this case.

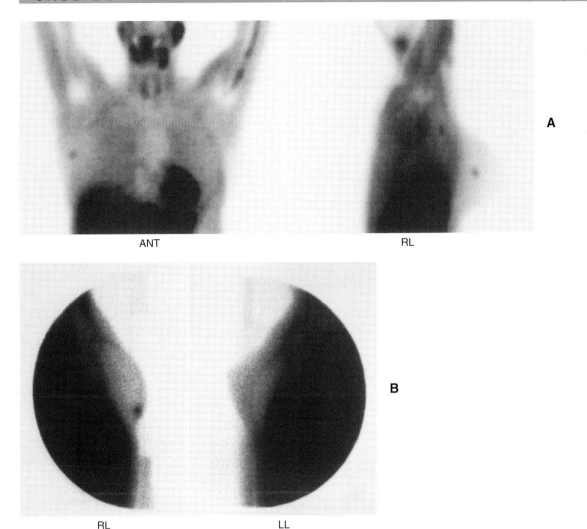

ANT   RL   **A**

RL   LL   **B**

Scintimammography in two different patients; *A,* a mammographically detected right breast mass; *B,* a palpable mass adjacent to a right breast prosthesis.

1. What is the radiopharmaceutical? What is its mechanism of uptake?
2. Describe the imaging findings and give an interpretation.
3. What is the accuracy of conventional mammography and scintimammography for breast cancer?
4. What are causes of false-negative and false-positive findings on scintimammography?

Oncology: Scintimammography

1. ^{99m}Tc sestamibi lipophilicity allows it to enter the cell where it is concentrated in the mitochondrial region related to charge.

2. Patient A has prominent focal uptake in a right breast mass. Patient B has definite focal uptake at the periphery of the breast prosthesis.

3. Accuracy of conventional mammography: sensitivity, 70% to 95%; positive predictive value for cancer, 20% to 30%. Scintimammography multicenter trial: sensitivity/specificity, 75%/83%. Palpable lesion sensitivity, 87%; nonpalpable lesion sensitivity, 71%.

4. Most false-negative findings are in lesions less than 1 cm. False-positive findings occur in fibroadenomas and benign and malignant tumors other than breast cancer.

References

Khalkali I, Villaneuva-Meyer J, Edell SL, et al: Diagnostic accuracy of ^{99m}Tc-sestamibi breast imaging: multicenter trial results, *J Nucl Med* 41:1973-1979, 2000.

Taillefer R: The role of ^{99m}Tc-sestamibi and other conventional radiopharmaceuticals in breast cancer diagnosis, *Semin Nucl Med* 29:16-40, 1999.

Cross-Reference

Nuclear Medicine: THE REQUISITES, ed 2, pp 204-206.

Comment

Mammography has good sensitivity for detection of malignancy; its sensitivity is lower in patients with dense breasts, implants, or after breast surgery or radiotherapy. Of greater concern is its poor positive predictive value. Many women require biopsy because of the limitations of mammographic diagnosis. Only one third to one fourth of breast biopsies demonstrate cancer. Ultrasonography can differentiate a cyst from a solid tumor but has limitations for solid masses. MRI is quite sensitive, but its specificity is low. The role of scintimammography (SM) is evolving. Because its negative predictive value (10% to 15%) is not adequate to exclude malignancy with confidence, biopsy is still needed. Better imaging devices, including dedicated breast scanners, are being developed with the goal of improved sensitivity for small lesions. SM is clinically useful for patients with nondiagnostic mammograms, those with dense breasts, patients with breast implants, previous surgery, nodular breasts, and fibrocystic disease. ^{99m}Tc tetrofosmin, a cardiac imaging agent similar to ^{99m}Tc sestamibi, has been used for SM and has similar accuracy.

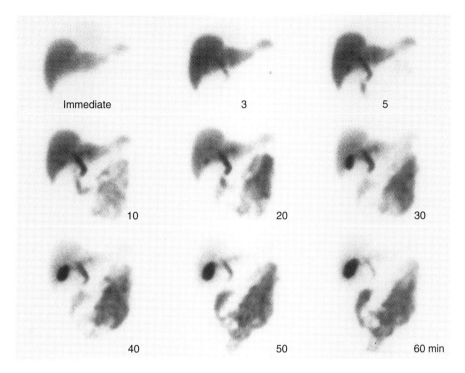

Immediate   3   5

10   20   30

40   50   60 min

A 39-year-old woman had acute upper abdominal pain. Cholescintigraphy was requested.

1. What patient preparation is required before cholescintigraphy?

2. Which hepatobiliary radiopharmaceuticals are available in the United States?

3. What are the radiopharmaceuticals mechanisms of uptake and their differences?

4. Has acute cholecystitis been ruled out? With what degree of certainty?

Hepatobiliary System: Cholescintigraphy— Normal Study

1. No oral intake for 3 to 4 hours before radiopharmaceutical injection.

2. ^{99m}Tc disofenin (DISIDA), Hepatolite. ^{99m}Tc mebrofenin (BrIDA), Choletec.

3. Both are iminodiacetic acid (IDA) analogues, extracted and excreted by hepatocytes into the biliary system. Mebrofenin has higher hepatocyte extraction (98% vs. 88%).

4. Yes. Acute cholecystitis (cystic duct obstruction) is ruled out with a high degree of certainty. The false-negative rate is 1% to 5%.

References

Ziessman HA, Zeman RK, Akin EA: Cholescintigraphy: correlation with other hepatobiliary imaging modalities. In Sandler MP, editor: *Diagnostic nuclear medicine,* ed 4, Philadelphia, 2002, Lippincott Williams & Wilkins.

Freitas JE: Cholescintigraphy. In Murray IPC, Ell PH, editors: *Nuclear medicine in clinical diagnosis and treatment,* ed 2, London, 1998, Churchill Livingstone, pp 83-92.

Cross-Reference

Nuclear Medicine: THE REQUISITES, ed 2, pp 229-231.

Comment

Fasting for 3 to 4 hours is required before initiating cholescintigraphy. If the patient has eaten recently, the gallbladder may be contracted as a result of endogenously stimulated cholecystokinin (CCK). The time required before gallbladder relaxation depends on the size and type of meal and the rate of gastric emptying. Conversely, if the patient has not eaten for 24 hours and thus has had no stimulus to contraction, the gallbladder is likely to be full of viscous concentrated bile that can prevent entry of the radiotracer and result in a false-positive study (nonfilling of the gallbladder in a patient without cholecystitis). A CCK analogue, sincalide (Kinevac), should be infused to empty the gallbladder. ^{99m}Tc IDA is injected 30 minutes after completion of the sincalide infusion to allow time for gallbladder contraction and relaxation.

This case is a normal study. Hepatic function is good, as determined by the prompt background (heart blood pool) clearance by 5 minutes. The common duct is visualized by 5 minutes. The gallbladder begins filling at 5 to 10 minutes and is filled by 60 minutes, at which time the liver has mostly washed out. Normal biliary-to-bowel clearance is seen by 10 minutes, and the common duct is clearing by 50 to 60 minutes. Gallbladder filling and common duct visualization by 60 minutes is defined as normal.

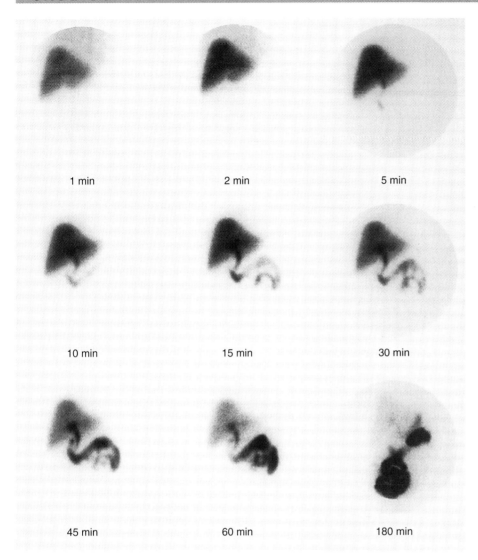

1 min   2 min   5 min

10 min   15 min   30 min

45 min   60 min   180 min

A 45-year-old woman with clinically suspected acute cholecystitis.

1. *A,* Is the study normal or abnormal at 60 minute? *B,* Is it diagnostic of acute cholecystitis at 60 minutes? *C,* Is it diagnostic of acute cholecystitis at 180 minutes?

2. *A,* What is the diagnostic accuracy of cholescintigraphy for acute calculous cholecystitis? *B,* What is the diagnostic accuracy of cholescintigraphy for acute acalculous cholecystitis?

3. What is the relative accuracy of cholescintigraphy versus ultrasonography?

4. What are the most common causes for false-positive cholescintigraphy results in the evaluation of acute cholecystitis?

Hepatobiliary System: Acute Cholecystitis

1. *A,* Abnormal. *B,* No. *C,* Yes.

2. *A,* Sensitivity 98%, specificity 95%. *B,* Greater than 90%.

3. The few direct comparisons published have shown cholescintigraphy superior to ultrasonography.

4. Prolonged fasting, hyperalimentation, serious concurrent illness, chronic cholecystitis, and hepatic insufficiency.

References

Samuels BI, Freitas JE, et al: Comparison of radionuclide hepatobiliary imaging and real-time ultrasound for the detection of acute cholecystitis, *Radiology* 147:207-210, 1983.

Swayne LC: Acute acalculous cholecystitis: sensitivity in detection using technetium-99m iminodiacetic acid cholescintigraphy, *Radiology* 160:33-38, 1986.

Cross-Reference

Nuclear Medicine: THE REQUISITES, ed 2, pp 237-240.

Comment

Nonvisualization of the gallbladder at 60 minutes is abnormal, but it is not diagnostic of acute cholecystitis. Traditionally, delayed images for up to 3 to 4 hours have been acquired to make or exclude the diagnosis. The majority of patients with delayed gallbladder visualization (nonvisualization at 4 hours, but visualization at 3 to 4 hours) have chronic cholecystitis. The advantage of cholescintigraphy is that the pathophysiological abnormality is detected, i.e., cystic duct obstruction. Ultrasonography shows secondary and less specific findings, e.g., gallbladder wall thickening, pericholecystic fluid. If an imaging study is ordered to confirm acute cholecystitis, cholescintigraphy is indicated. If the cause of upper abdominal pain is less certain, ultrasonography may be more appropriate as the initial study. Acute acalculous cholecystitis occurs in sick hospitalized patients, e.g., those with severe trauma, sepsis, or shock. It has a high morbidity and mortality. In many patients the cystic duct is obstructed by inspissated bile and inflammatory debris; however, sometimes the gallbladder is inflamed hematogenously from infection or toxins, but without obstruction. Because the cystic duct is patent the sensitivity for detection with cholescintigraphy might be expected to be somewhat less than with acute calculous cholecystitis. If the gallbladder fills in a patient with a high clinical suspicion for cholecystitis and a false-negative outcome is suspected, cholecystokinin can be administered. Acutely or chronically diseased gallbladders do not contract. A radiolabeled leukocyte study may be helpful to confirm or exclude the diagnosis.

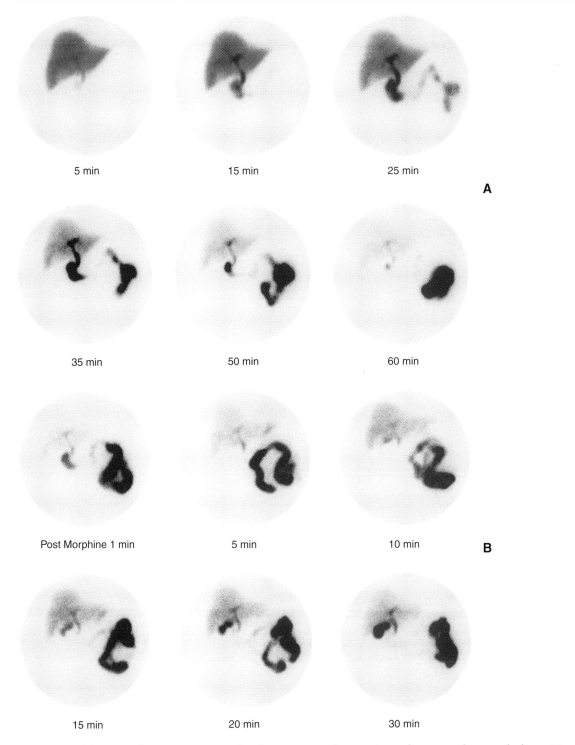

5 min

15 min

25 min

A

35 min

50 min

60 min

Post Morphine 1 min

5 min

10 min

B

15 min

20 min

30 min

A 53 year-old woman has recent onset of right upper quadrant pain and suspected acute cholecystitis. *A,* 60-minute cholescintigraphy. *B,* 30-minute postmorphine acquisition.

1. Why is morphine used as an alternative to 3- to 4-hour delayed imaging?

2. In a patient with nonvisualization of the gallbladder at 60 minutes, what must be determined before morphine is administered?

3. What is the accuracy of morphine cholescintigraphy?

4. What is the dose of morphine, and how long after injection is the image obtained?

Hepatobiliary System: Morphine-Augmented Cholescintigraphy

1. Morphine produces contraction of the sphincter of Oddi, which increases intraluminal common bile duct pressure. Bile and excreted radiotracer then preferentially flow through the cystic duct into the gallbladder if the cystic duct is patent.

2. Exclude drug allergy. Do not give if evidence of common duct obstruction, e.g., delayed filling or clearance of the common duct or delayed biliary-to-bowel transit, exists.

3. The accuracy is at least as good, if not better, than the delayed imaging method.

4. Intravenous administration of 0.04 mg/kg morphine, e.g., 2.4 mg for a 60-kg patient. Images are acquired for an additional 30 minutes.

References

Kim CK, Kevin KM, et al: Cholescintigraphy in the diagnosis of acute cholecystitis: morphine augmentation is superior to delayed imaging, *J Nucl Med* 34:1866-1870, 1993.

Kistler AM, Ziessman HA, Gooch D: Morphine-augmented cholescintigraphy in acute cholecystitis: alternative to delayed imaging, *Clin Nucl Med* 16:404-406, 1991.

Cross-Reference

Nuclear Medicine: THE REQUISITES, ed 2, pp 238-239.

Comment

The 60-minute study *(A)* shows nonfilling of the gallbladder, near-complete washout of the liver, and normal biliary-to-bowel transit. A repeat half-dose of ^{99m}Tc IDA was administered at the same time as morphine infusion *(B)*. Note the increasing hepatic uptake at 5 to 10 minutes. The gallbladder promptly visualizes, ruling out acute cholecystitis. With the rapid washout often seen with IDA radiopharmaceuticals, delayed imaging can be problematic. In addition, a 3- to 4-hour test is not optimal in a seriously ill patient. Morphine-augmented cholescintigraphy is routinely used in many nuclear medicine laboratories to confirm the diagnosis of acute cholecystitis. However, the handling of narcotics requires accountability and can be a logistical problem on weekends and nights at some hospitals. The reinjection of the radiotracer at the time of morphine infusion sometimes is necessary because the liver often has washed out by 60 minutes. Because morphine causes a functional partial common duct obstruction, the diagnosis of common duct obstruction cannot be made once it is given. Thus common duct obstruction must be excluded before morphine administration. After intravenous infusion of morphine the gallbladder fills promptly, if the cystic duct is patent. Thus the entire study takes only 90 minutes. Nonfilling of the gallbladder 30 minutes after morphine administration is consistent with cystic duct obstruction and acute cholecystitis.

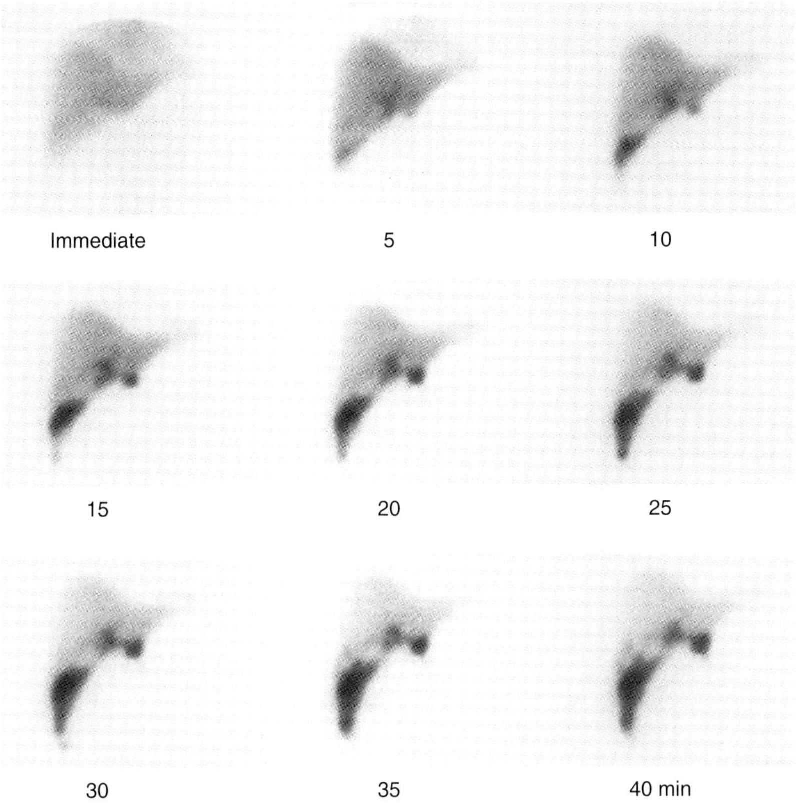

Immediate   5   10

15   20   25

A

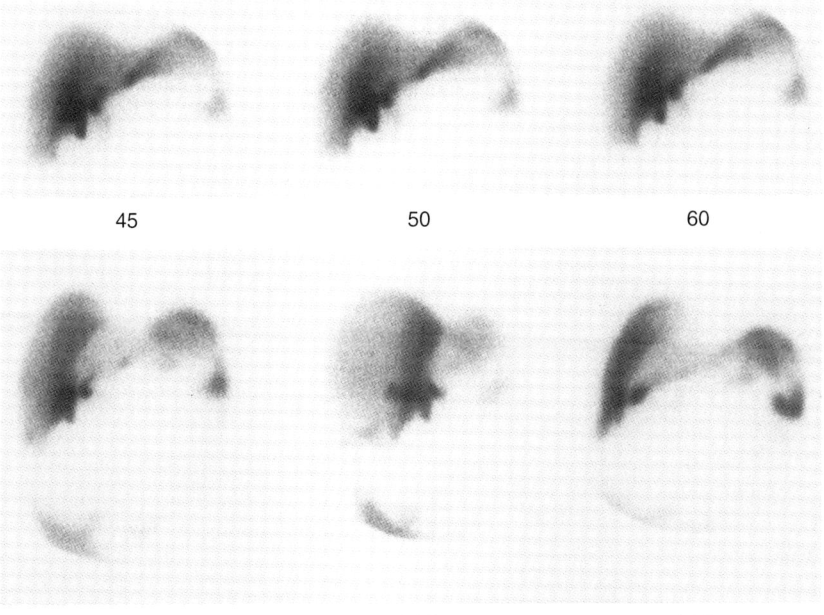

30   35   40 min

45   50   60

B

120 min   RAO   LAO

A 43-year-old woman has a low-grade fever and abdominal discomfort 2 days after cholecystectomy.

1. Describe the cholescintigraphic findings.

2. Interpret the study.

3. What are possible causes for this problem?

4. What unique information does cholescintigraphy provide that is not obtainable from other diagnostic imaging procedures?

Hepatobiliary System: Biliary Leak

1. Rapid bile leakage probably originating from the region of the ligated cystic duct and extending toward the right colonic gutter and with time, over the dome of the liver.

2. Rapid biliary leak.

3. The most common cause is disruption of the cystic duct ligature after cholecystectomy. Other causes for leak include disruption of a surgical anastomosis, blunt or penetrating trauma, interventional radiographic procedures, tumor, or inflammatory processes.

4. Confirm that fluid collections seen by anatomical imaging modalities are biliary in nature. The rate of leakage also can be estimated.

Reference

Rosenberg DJ, Brugge WR, Alavi A: Bile leak following an elective laparoscopic cholecystectomy: the role of hepatobiliary imaging in the diagnosis and management of bile leaks, *J Nucl Med* 32:1777-1781, 1991.

Cross-Reference

Nuclear Medicine: THE REQUISITES, ed 2, pp 244-245.

Comment

Biliary tract injury resulting in bile leakage occurs in less than 1% of patients undergoing cholecystectomy. However, the complication can have dire consequences. A reduction in morbidity and mortality can be achieved by early detection. Sterile slow biliary leaks often seal spontaneously, whereas larger and more rapid leaks often require surgical intervention. Cholescintigraphy is a very sensitive and specific noninvasive method for detection of a bile leak and estimation of the leakage rate. Bile leakage can result in peritonitis, subhepatic fluid collection, abscess, and fistula formation.

Ultrasonography and CT can reliably detect fluid collections but often cannot determine whether they contain bile or freely communicate with the biliary tree. Because a frequent cause of postoperative bile leakage is incomplete cystic duct ligation, the most common site of bile collection is in the gallbladder fossa, although subcapsular and intraperitoneal locations may be seen. Bilomas often appear photopenic initially; however with time they fill in and become more obvious. Multiple views are often helpful to accurately locate and confirm the leak. Delayed views beyond the routine 60-minute imaging period may be required to detect a slow leak or one that is obscured by enteric activity. If immediate surgery is not clinically indicated, cholescintigraphy may be repeated on a later day to confirm improvement or resolution of the biliary leak.

Immediate

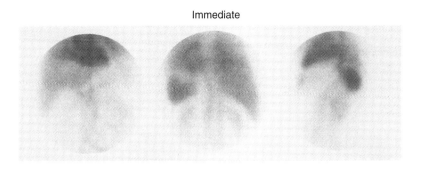

Delayed

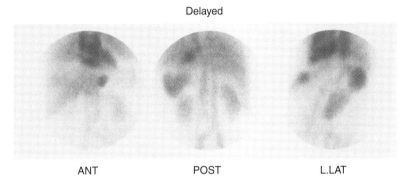

ANT   POST   L.LAT

A 59-year-old man is referred with abdominal pain. CT reportedly showed a lesion of uncertain origin in the left lobe of the liver.

1. What is the radiopharmaceutical? What is the study?

2. What are the findings and the likely diagnosis?

3. How large must this lesion be to be seen on planar scintigraphy?

4. What are the advantages/disadvantages and accuracy of the radionuclide study?

Hepatobiliary System: Cavernous Hemangioma of the Liver

1. [99mTc]-labeled red blood cells (RBCs). RBC liver scintigraphy.

2. Immediate images show no definite abnormality. Delayed images show increased focal uptake in the left lobe consistent with a cavernous hemangioma.

3. At least 2 cm.

4. Very specific (>99%) for hemangioma. Poor sensitivity for small lesions.

Reference

Birnbaum BA, Weignreb JC, Meigibow AJ, et al: Definitive diagnosis of hepatic hamartomas: MR versus [99mTc] labeled RBC SPECT, *Radiology* 176:95-101, 1990.

Ziessman HA, Silverman PM, Patterson J, et al: Improved detection of small cavernous hemangiomas of the liver with high-resolution three-headed SPECT, *J Nucl Med* 32:2086-2091, 1991.

Cross-Reference

Nuclear Medicine: THE REQUISITES, ed 2, pp 250-253.

Comment

Cavernous hemangiomas are the most common benign liver tumor, second in occurrence only to hepatic metastases. They are composed of abnormally dilated endothelial lined vascular channels of varying size separated by fibrous septae. Hemangiomas are not hypervascular but have increased vascular space (blood pool) compared with normal tissue. The explanation for the characteristic change in appearance from immediately after injection until 1- to 2-hour delayed images is the time required for the labeled RBCs to exchange and equilibrate with the large, relatively stagnant, nonlabeled blood pool of the hemangioma. Blood flow usually is normal.

Ultrasonography has poor specificity for the diagnosis of hemangiomas. When strict CT criteria are used, sensitivity is only 55% to 70%. With less strict criteria, sensitivity is higher but specificity is considerably poorer. MRI accuracy is high, probably greater than 90%; however, false-positive results occur because of a variety of benign and malignant tumors. Direct comparison studies of MRI and SPECT have shown similar accuracy, although MRI is superior for small hemangiomas and those adjacent to major vessels. The positive predictive value of the RBC study is higher.

Planar images can detect hemangiomas to a size of approximately 2 cm, and smaller if they are superficial. SPECT is superior to planar imaging. Multiheaded SPECT cameras allow detection of most hemangiomas 1.4 cm or larger in size. A major advantage of the RBC technique is its very high specificity for hemangioma. False-positive results are rare.

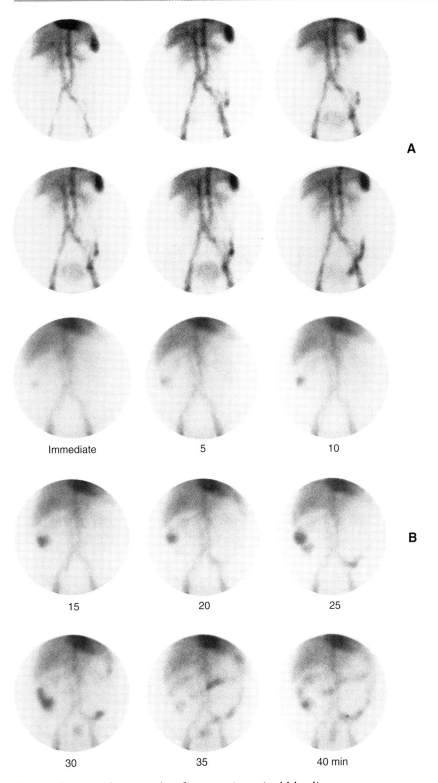

A

Immediate   5   10

B

15   20   25

30   35   40 min

Two patients undergo studies for gastrointestinal bleeding.

1. What radiopharmaceutical is used?

2. Determine the site of bleeding in study A.

3. Determine the site of bleeding in study B.

4. What is the slowest rate of bleeding that can be detected with scintigraphy and with contrast angiography?

Gastrointestinal System: 99mTc RBC Colonic Bleeding

1. 99mTc-labeled RBCs.

2. *A,* Left colon, rectosigmoid region.

3. *B,* Right colon, hepatic flexure. It moves rapidly to the left colon.

4. RBC scintigraphy, 0.1 ml/min; contrast angiography (1.0 ml/min).

References

Maurer AH: Gastrointestinal bleeding and cine-scintigraphy, *Semin Nucl Med* 26:43-50, 1996.

Gutierrez C, Mariano M, Laan TV, et al: The use of Tc-labeled erythrocyte scintigraphy in the evaluation and treatment of lower gastrointestinal hemorrhage, *Am Surg* 64:989-992, 1998.

Cross-Reference

Nuclear Medicine: THE REQUISITES, ed 2, pp 280-287.

Comment

The purpose of the radionuclide gastrointestinal bleeding study is to diagnose the approximate site of bleeding so that the angiographer can minimize time and contrast in pinpointing the exact site. The apparent site of active bleeding usually is described as at the cecum, hepatic flexure, transverse colon, splenic flexure, or rectosigmoid region. The angiographer and surgeon need to know whether the bleeding site is in the distribution of the celiac, superior, or inferior mesenteric artery. The radionuclide bleeding study allows for a more rapid and safer angiographic procedure by the time saved in locating the site and thus minimizing the amount of contrast media required.

99mTc sulfur colloid also has been used to diagnose gastrointestinal bleeding. After intravenous injection, it is cleared from the vascular system within 15 to 20 minutes because of rapid extraction by the reticuloendothelial system (RES), particularly the liver and spleen. With active bleeding, radiotracer extravasates at the bleeding site into the bowel lumen. The target/background ratio is high. However, because of the intermittent nature of gastrointestinal bleeding, colloid scintigraphy has limitations. Bleeding must occur during the 20- to 30-minute study and be detected. Delayed imaging is not possible, unless the 99mTc sulfur colloid injection is repeated. Comparative studies of 99mTc–sulfur colloid and 99mTc-labeled erythrocytes have consistently shown the superiority of the labeled cells.

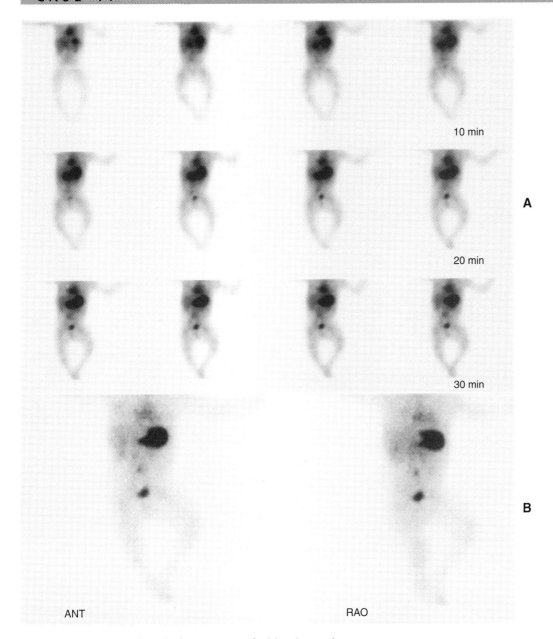

10 min

20 min

A

30 min

B

ANT   RAO

A 5-year-old girl is referred after passage of a bloody stool.

1. What is the radiopharmaceutical, its mechanism of uptake, and study type?
2. Which pharmacological drugs can be used to enhance detectability? What is their mechanism?
3. Provide an interpretation.
4. Why is bleeding a common complication of this disease entity?

Gastrointestinal System: Meckel's Diverticulum

1. ^{99m}Tc pertechnetate Meckel's scan. The radiopharmaceutical is taken up and secreted by gastric mucosa.

2. Pentagastrin increases rapidity, intensity, and duration of uptake. It is used with glucagon, which has an antiperistaltic effect that inhibits the rapid dispersion effect of pentagastrin. Cimetidine, a histamine antagonist, increases and prolongs uptake because of inhibition of ^{99m}Tc pertechnetate secretion from gastric mucosal cells. It is commonly used because of its lack of side effects.

3. Increasing focal uptake in the mid-abdomen suspicious for Meckel's diverticulum; however, atypical timing of uptake lessens the certainty. The uptake should be coincident with gastric uptake in cases of Meckel's diverticulum. This may be a false-positive scan.

4. Acid and pepsin secretion by the gastric mucosa produces inflammation and ulceration of adjacent bowel mucosa.

Reference

Treves ST, Grand RJ: Gastrointestinal bleeding. In Traves ST, editor: *Pediatric nuclear medicine,* ed 2, New York, 1994, Springer-Verlag, pp 179-189.

Cross-Reference

Nuclear Medicine: THE REQUISITES, ed 2, pp 288-290.

Comment

Meckel's diverticulum occurs in 1% to 3% of the population. This most common gastrointestinal congenital anomaly is caused by failed closure of the omphalomesenteric duct in the embryo. It is a true diverticulum and arises on the antimesenteric side of the small bowel, usually 80 to 90 cm proximal to the ileocecal valve. Gastric mucosa occurs in 10% to 30% of cases, in 60% of symptomatic patients, and in 98% of patients with bleeding.

The pattern of uptake in this case is atypical for a Meckel's diverticulum, which typically demonstrates uptake simultaneously with the stomach. In this case the uptake is delayed relative to gastric uptake and is not as intense as usual. False-positive studies can occur, most commonly related to accumulation of tracer in the urinary tract, e.g., extrarenal pelvis, hydronephrosis, reflux, bladder diverticulum. Other causes include local intestinal hyperemia and inflammation, e.g., inflammatory bowel disease, abscess, appendicitis, and tumors. Gastric mucosa also may be found in Barrett's esophagus, retained gastric antrum, and gastrointestinal duplications. These can be distinguished from Meckel's diverticulum by clinical history and epigastric location. False-negative results occasionally occur because of the rapid ^{99m}Tc washout or lack of sufficient gastric mucosa, e.g., less than 2 cm. The overall accuracy is 85% sensitivity and 95% specificity.

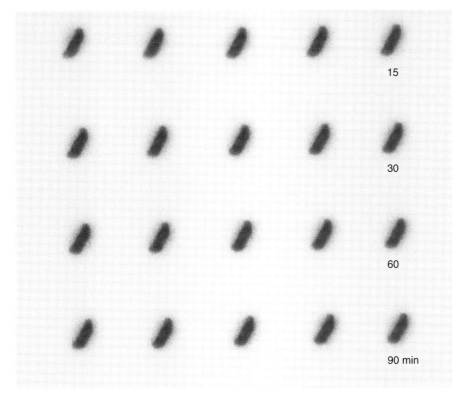

15

30

60

90 min

A patient with insulin-dependent diabetes has chronic symptoms of early satiety, postprandial bloating, and abdominal discomfort. A gastric emptying study is conduct 90 minutes after a solid meal.

1. What is the diagnosis?
2. What are normal values for solid meal gastric emptying?
3. What is the advantage of a solid radiolabeled meal over a liquid meal?
4. Why is attenuation correction recommended for accurate quantification of gastric emptying?

Gastrointestinal System: Diabetic Gastroparesis

1. Consistent with severe diabetic gastroparesis. Obstruction cannot be ruled out.

2. Normal values are meal specific and depend on its volume/composition, the method of acquisition, attenuation correction, processing, and quantification. Normal values must be determined in each clinic or results of a published method should be followed closely.

3. Solid (meat) or semisolid (egg) gastric emptying meals are more sensitive for detection of mild to moderate delay in emptying than studies conducted after a liquid meal.

4. Activity is detected with greatest efficiency close to the camera. The anterior view alone underestimates emptying, and the posterior view overestimates it because of variable attenuation as the meal moves through the stomach from the posterior gastric fundus to the more anterior gastric antrum.

Reference

Ziessman HA: Keep it simple—it's only gastric emptying! In Freeman LM, editor: *Nuclear Medicine Annual 2000,* Philadelphia, 2000, Lippincott Williams & Wilkins, pp 233-260.

Cross-Reference

Nuclear Medicine: THE REQUISITES, ed 2, pp 273-279.

Comment

Diabetic gastroparesis is a complication of diabetes caused by vagal nerve damage in a generalized autonomic neuropathy. Symptoms are nonspecific and often indistinguishable from other diabetic problems, e.g., poor glucose control and infection. Solid emptying can be underestimated unless attenuation correction is performed. This is a particular problem in obese patients, but occurs in nonobese patients as well. Correction cannot be done after the test. The geometric mean method is the most accurate, requiring both anterior and posterior acquisition and then mathematical correction at each time point. If a single-headed camera is used, sequential anterior and posterior views can be obtained. Alternatively, the study can be acquired in the left anterior oblique (LAO) projection. In this view the stomach contents move roughly parallel to the detector, thus compensating for attenuation without the need for mathematical correction. Accuracy using the LAO projection compares favorably with the geometric mean. Time-activity curves are used to quantify emptying. The pattern of solid emptying is characterized by an initial lag phase followed by linear emptying. The lag phase is the time required for the antrum to grind up solid food into small enough particles (1 to 2 mm) to pass through the pylorus. The fundus is primarily responsible for liquid emptying, which occurs rapidly (half-life [$t_{1/2}$] of 10 to 20 minutes) in an exponential pattern.

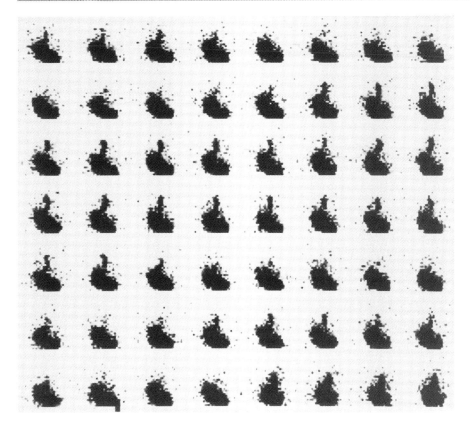

A 3-month-old infant was referred with symptoms of gastroesophageal reflux. A radionuclide gastroesophageal reflux study (milk study) was performed (posterior view).

1. What are common symptoms and problems in children associated with reflux?

2. What other method is used by pediatricians for detection of reflux?

3. What radiolabel and what meal is used for this study?

4. How frequently should images be acquired to maximize sensitivity of this test?

Gastrointestinal System: "Milk" Study—Gastroesophageal Reflux

1. Vomiting, pulmonary symptoms, asthma, pneumonia, sudden death, failure to thrive, anemia.

2. 24-hour pH monitoring.

3. ^{99m}Tc sulfur colloid (1 mCi) in the child's usual feeding, formula, or milk.

4. 5 to 10 seconds/frame.

Reference

Piepsz A: Recent advances in pediatric nuclear medicine, *Semin Nucl Med* 25:165-182, 1995.

Cross-Reference

Nuclear Medicine: THE REQUISITES, ed 2, pp 270-273.

Comment

Gastroesophageal reflux is a common clinical pediatric problem. Although this occurs in healthy infants, it usually resolves by approximately 8 months and rarely causes serious medical problems. However, some children have symptomatic reflux that can persist into adulthood. Symptoms associated with reflux can be serious, including failure to thrive, esophagitis with stricture, anemia, aspiration, recurrent respiratory infections, asthma, and sudden death syndrome.

The 24-hour pH probe monitoring technique often is considered the gold standard. However, comparative studies of the two techniques have shown similar sensitivity for detection of gastroesophageal reflux by scintigraphy (milk study) and pH probe. The disadvantages of the pH probe are that children younger than 5 years must be hospitalized and possible underestimation of reflux because a small volume of acid reflux may adhere to the probe, preventing subsequent events from being recorded. Conversely, the milk study is most sensitive when the stomach is full. As it empties, the detected reflux events decline. The milk study is a simple study to perform. After ingesting the milk or formula feeding, the study is acquired for 1 to 2 hours with the child supine on the gamma camera. Reflux events can be detected easily on computer review of the study. Various quantitative methods have been used; the most simple and straightforward is counting the number of reflux events and categorizing them as high (greater than half the distance to the mouth) or low and short (less than 10 seconds) or long events. This case study has frequent short and long reflux events. The patient has many high and long recurrent reflux events.

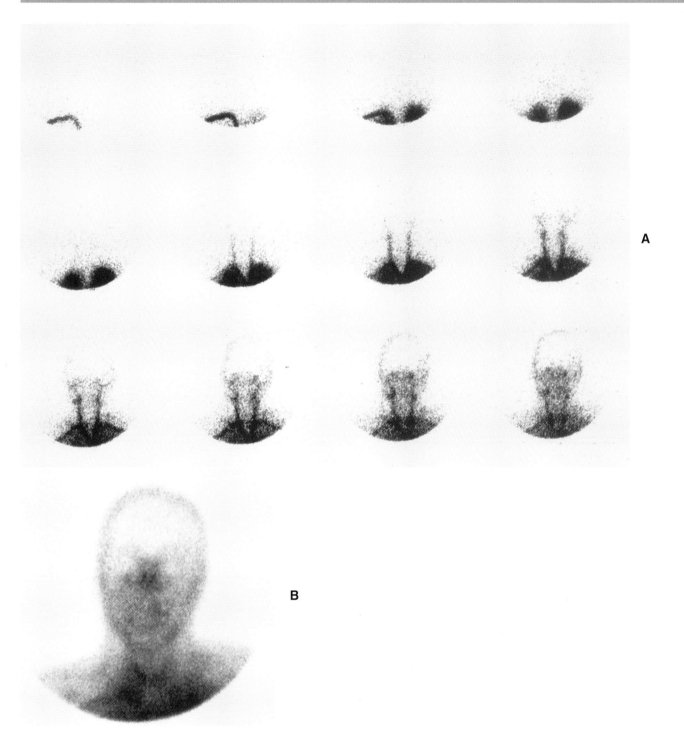

A

B

A 35-year-old man has been comatose for 2 weeks since a recent severe head injury. The electroencephalogram (EEG) is flat and he is being considered as an organ donor.

1. If the EEG is a flat line, why is another study indicated?

2. What are the clinical findings of brain death?

3. List two different types of radiopharmaceuticals with different mechanisms that could be used for this study.

4. What are the scintigraphic findings and the diagnosis?

Central Nervous System: Brain Death

1. An isoelectric flat EEG can be caused by barbiturates, depressive drugs, or hypothermia.

2. Deep coma, no brain stem reflexes or spontaneous respiration, exclusion of reversible causes, and the cause of the brain dysfunction must be diagnosed.

3. ^{99m}Tc diethylenetriaminepentaacetic acid (DTPA) or ^{99m}Tc pertechnetate can be used as a brain flow study (radionuclide angiogram). However, ^{99m}Tc HM-PAO and ^{99m}Tc ethyl-cysteinate dimer (ECD) have the advantage of irreversible cellular binding on the first pass, allowing for delayed images.

4. No blood flow to the cerebral cortex. Brain blood flow study consistent with brain death. This is a ^{99m}Tc DTPA study. ^{99m}Tc HM-PAO would show salivary uptake. With normal brain perfusion, cerebral cortical activity would be seen.

Reference

Rikofsky RS, Masanori I, Seibyl JP, et al: Functional brain SPECT imaging: 1999 and beyond. In Freeman LM, editor: *Nuclear medicine annual 1999,* Philadelphia, 1999, Lippincott Williams & Wilkins.

Cross-Reference

Nuclear Medicine: THE REQUISITES, ed 2, pp 305-306, 312-313.

Comment

Specific criteria required to make the diagnosis of brain death have been published and are listed above. The diagnosis is primarily clinical. The findings of brain death must be present for at least 24 hours. Ancillary tests are used to increase the diagnostic certainty. A single EEG does not adequately confirm the diagnosis. At least one additional confirmatory study is required. Increased intracranial pressure sufficient to overcome arterial blood pressure prevents cerebral blood flow, which is diagnostic of brain death. The radionuclide study is ordered when the diagnosis is uncertain.

Although ^{99m}Tc pertechnetate and ^{99m}Tc DTPA have been used successfully for years to evaluate for brain death, they have limitations. Technical problems, e.g., a bad bolus, or camera or computer failure during acquisition, can complicate interpretation. However, the new cerebral perfusion agents, ^{99m}Tc HM-PAO and ECD fix intracellularly in brain cells. A flow study is not mandatory. Static images after the flow show whether the radiopharmaceutical is taken up by the cerebral cortex. If cortical uptake does not occur, the diagnosis of brain death is confirmed. This is the only use of the ^{99m}Tc-labeled brain perfusion agents where SPECT is not required.

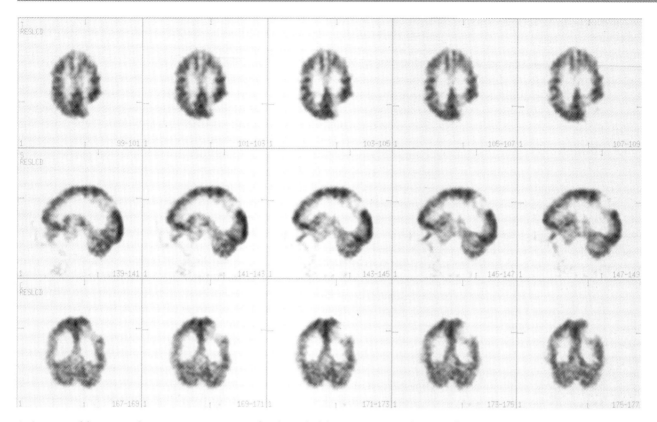

A 65-year-old man with recent acute onset of right-sided hemiparesis undergoes ^{18}F FDG-PET scanning.

1. What is the radiopharmaceutical used for metabolic cerebral imaging with PET, and what is the mechanism of uptake?

2. What are the radiopharmaceuticals used for PET cerebral perfusion imaging?

3. Describe this patient's PET imaging findings (above, transverse; middle, sagittal; bottom, transverse)?

4. What is the differential diagnosis?

Central Nervous System: Cerebral Infarct

1. ^{18}F PET-FDG is dependent on glucose metabolism.

2. SPECT ^{99m}Tc HM-PAO and ECD are cerebral perfusion agents that are lipid soluble, distribute according to cerebral blood flow (gray to white matter, 3:1 to 4:1), and fix intracellularly.

3. Wedge-shaped severe decreased metabolism in the left posterior parietal region in a vascular posterial parietal distribution.

4. Cerebral hemorrhage, infarct, and neoplasm.

References

Saha GB, MacIntyre WJ, Go RT: Radiopharmaceuticals for brain imaging, *Semin Nucl Med* 24:324-349, 1994.

Van Heertum RL, Drocea C, Ichise M, et al: Single photon emission of CT and positron emission tomography in the evaluation of neurologic disease, *Radiol Clin North Am* 39:1007-1034, 2001.

Cross-Reference

Nuclear Medicine: THE REQUISITES, ed 2, pp 309-311.

Comment

Seventy-five percent of cerebral strokes are ischemic in nature. Ischemic infarctions may be embolic or, more commonly, thrombotic. Emboli may originate from the heart or, most commonly, from the carotid arteries from thrombi caused by atheromatous plaques. Hypertension is an important known risk factor.

Cerebral perfusion SPECT agents, ^{99m}Tc HM-PAO and ECD, usually result in images similar to those obtained with FDG-PET because blood flow follows metabolism in most disease states. In acute cerebral infarction, SPECT and PET demonstrate hypoperfusion and hypometabolism, respectively, within 24 hours, a period when CT and MRI often still show normal findings. The early phase (3 to 7 days) after an acute stroke is an exception in which blood flow does not match metabolism. Blood flow is preserved is the setting of no metabolism because of failed cerebrovascular autoregulation. Perfusion may appear normal in this period ("luxury perfusion"). Crossed-cerebellar diaschisis is a possible finding after stroke for both PET and SPECT. The cerebellum contralateral to the side of the stroke has decreased uptake because of the loss of afferent stimuli. This may have accompanying clinical cerebellar symptoms that may be reversible.

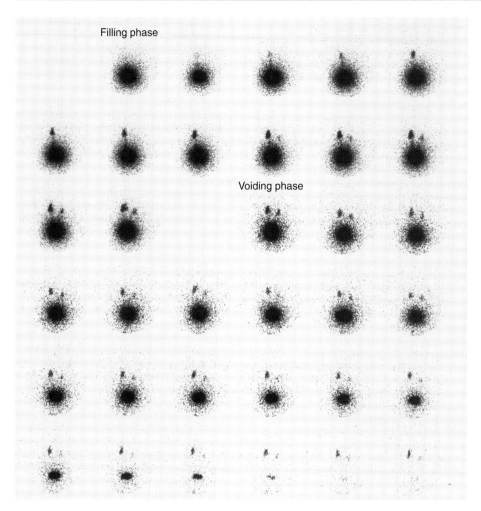

Filling phase

Voiding phase

A 5-year-old girl has had two urinary tract infections in the past 6 months.

1. Which radiopharmaceuticals commonly are used for cystography?

2. What is the advantage of radionuclide cystography over the contrast study?

3. What is the difference between indirect and direct radionuclide cystography?

4. How is reflux graded with radionuclide cystography?

Radionuclide Cystography

1. ^{99m}Tc DTPA and ^{99m}Tc sulfur colloid are the two most commonly used.

2. Radionuclide cystography is more sensitive in detection of vesicoureteral reflux (VUR) and results in 50 to 200 times less radiation exposure to the gonads compared with the contrast study.

3. The direct method is commonly used and requires urinary catheterization and instillation of radiotracer into the bladder through a catheter. The indirect method is performed after routine renography with ^{99m}Tc DTPA/mercaptylacetyltriglycine (MAG3). When the bladder is full, a previoiding image is obtained, followed by dynamic images during and after voiding.

4. Grading criteria are similar to those used with contrast cystography; however, the radionuclide study's limited resolution does not permit assessment of calyceal morphology. Mild reflux: confined to the ureter. Moderate: reaches the pelvicocalyceal system. Severe: distorted collecting system and dilated tortuous ureter.

References

Eggli DF, Tulchinsky M: Scintigraphic evaluation of pediatric urinary tract infection, *Semin Nucl Med* 23:199-218, 1993.

Cooper JA: Kidney infection in children: role of nuclear medicine. In Freeman LM, editor: *Nuclear medicine annual 1998,* Philadelphia, 1998, Lippincott-Raven.

Cross-Reference

Nuclear Medicine: THE REQUISITES, ed 2, pp 355-357.

Comment

VUR is caused by failure of physiological valve function. The ureter normally passes obliquely through the bladder wall and submucosa to its opening at the trigone. As urine fills the bladder, the valves passively close, preventing reflux. If the intramural ureteral length is too short compared with its diameter, the valve does not close and reflux results. In more than 80% of cases the abnormality resolves as the child grows. Untreated reflux and pyelonephritis may result in renal scarring, hypertension, and renal failure. The combination of VUR and infected urine are required to produce injury to the kidneys. The goal of therapy is to prevent renal damage until the reflux resolves spontaneously or is surgically corrected. In many centers, contrast cystography is reserved for the initial evaluation because of better anatomical detail, particularly for male patients, to exclude posterior urethral valves. This case shows early VUR on the left (posterior view) reaching the renal pelvis during the later bladder filling phase and lesser reflux into the right pelvis. VUR decreases slowly over the voiding phase with residual activity in the pelves, particularly the left, at the end of the study. Radionuclide cystography is acquired dynamically on computer. The 10-second/frame acquisition rate allows for very high sensitivity for detection of VUR.

A

B

Furosemide

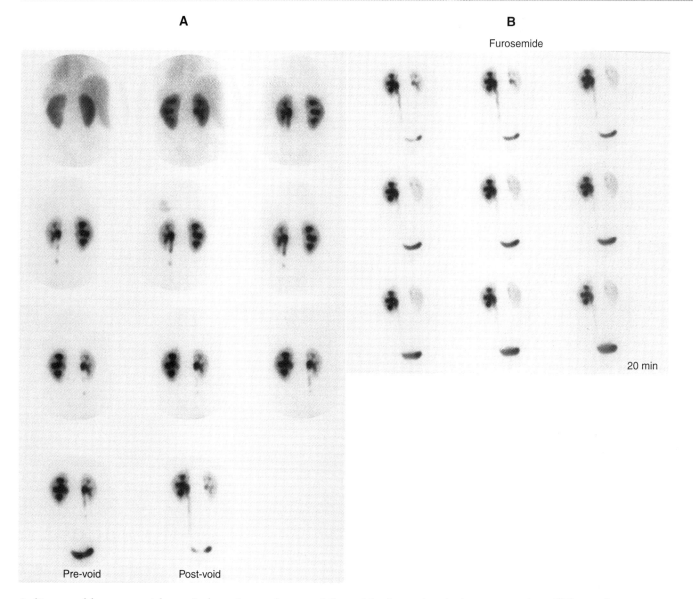

20 min

Pre-void   Post-void

A 45-year-old woman with cervical carcinoma has new bilateral hydronephrosis demonstrated on CT scanning.

1. Describe the scintigraphic findings before and after furosemide administration.

2. Interpret the study before laser administration.

3. Interpret the study after laser administration.

4. List some limitations of diuretic renography.

Diuretic Renography: Unilateral Obstruction

1. Good symmetrical cortical uptake and prompt excretion into collecting systems bilaterally. Retention of activity in left renal collecting system, apparent cutoff in the upper ureter, and very poor response to furosemide. The right side shows a prominent collecting system but washes out spontaneously before furosemide administration.

2. Hydronephrosis of the left kidney. Rule out obstruction.

3. Consistent with significant obstruction of the left kidney.

4. Dehydration, renal insufficiency, inadequate diuretic dose, full bladder, large collecting system.

References

Connolly LP, Zurakowski D, Peters CA, et al: Variability of diuresis renography interpretation due to method of post-diuretic renal pelvic clearance half-time determination, *J Urol* 164:467-471, 2000.

Roarke MC, Sandler CM: Provocative imaging: diuretic renography, *Urol Clin North Am* 25:227-249, 1998.

Cross-Reference

Nuclear Medicine: THE REQUISITES, ed 2, pp 340-348.

Comment

The limitations of diuretic renography must always be considered. The patient must receive a sufficient furosemide dose. The diuretic dose needed is greater with renal insufficiency, but the exact dose is only an estimate. Renal insufficiency poses a major problem in interpretation and is a common reason for an indeterminate study.

An obstructed kidney shows very poor or no washout ($t_{1/2} > 20$ minutes). A nonobstructed kidney shows prompt washout. However, some patient studies show partial washout, defined as indeterminate for obstruction. An indeterminate response often is seen in patients who have had previous intervention for obstruction but still have a very dilated system. These patients can be monitored over time to ensure that no deterioration in renal function or diuretic response occurs. Calculation of a washout half-time can be valuable for serial studies. Poor renal function or dehydration often contributes to an intermediate response. A functional bladder outlet obstruction may be a factor if the bladder cannot be emptied before furosemide administration; in such cases a urinary catheter may be necessary. Catheterization is routine in many clinics in children who will not or cannot void on instruction.

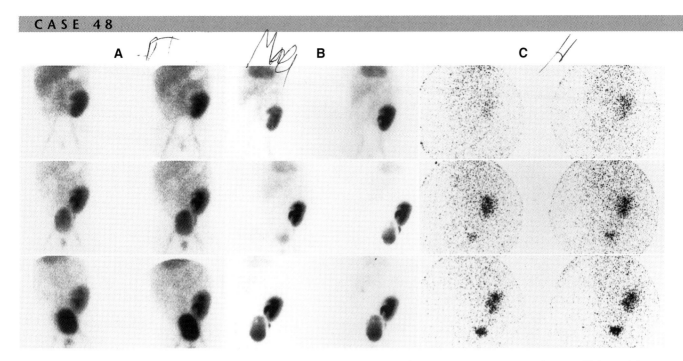

A 35-year-old renal transplant patient has three renal studies (sequential images over 30 minutes) using ^{99m}Tc DTPA on one day and ^{99m}Tc MAG3 and ^{131}I hippuran 1 week later.

1. Which renal radiopharmaceutical is used for each study: *A, B,* and *C?*

2. What is the mechanism of uptake of the three radiopharmaceuticals?

3. What are the advantages and disadvantages of each radiopharmaceutical?

4. Can a blood flow (radionuclide angiogram) study be done with all three agents? Why?

CASE 48

Renal Radiopharmaceuticals

1. *A*, ^{99m}Tc DTPA; *B*, ^{99m}Tc MAG3; *C*, ^{131}I hippuran.

2. DTPA: glomerular filtration; MAG3: tubular secretion; hippuran: 20% glomerular, 80% tubular.

3. DTPA is inexpensive, provides a good image quality, but has low extraction efficiency (10% to 20%) and poor quality images with renal insufficiency. MAG3 has a high extraction rate (60%), good target to background, and good-quality images with renal insufficiency. Hippuran has good extraction efficiency, high target-to-background, poor image quality, poor cortical/collecting system differentiation, and delivers a high radiation dose in renal insufficiency.

4. No. The administered dose of ^{131}I hippuran is too low (200 to 300 µCi), limited by the high radiation absorbed dose. A dose of 5 mCi is needed for good blood flow images.

References

Taylor A: Radionuclide renography: a personal approach, *Semin Nucl Med* 29:102-127, 1999.

O'Malley JP, Ziessman HA, Chantarapitak N, et al: ^{99m}Tc MAG3 as an alternative to ^{99m}Tc DTPA and I-131 hippuran for renal transplant evaluation, *Clin Nucl Med* 18:22-29, 1993.

Cross-Reference

Nuclear Medicine: THE REQUISITES, ed 2, pp 324-328.

Comment

The ^{131}I hippuran study is easy to recognize because of its poor-resolution images. However, it does provide valuable functional information and time-activity curves (not shown) similar to ^{99m}Tc MAG3. ^{99m}Tc DTPA and ^{99m}Tc MAG3 studies look fairly similar because of the high-resolution ^{99m}Tc agents. Both are superior to ^{131}I hippuran for discriminating cortex from collecting system. Uptake is greater and background less with the ^{99m}Tc MAG3 than DTPA because DTPA has a first-pass extraction fraction of only 10% to 20% compared with 60% for MAG3. Thus MAG3 has an important advantage for patients with renal insufficiency. This transplant patient has moderate renal dysfunction demonstrated by the slow clearance. Both ^{99m}Tc agents result in a low radiation absorbed dose to the patient compared with ^{131}I hippuran and allow for a blood flow study. ^{99m}Tc MAG3 is the agent most commonly used for renal scintigraphy in the United States. ^{99m}Tc DTPA results in high-quality images and provides useful functional information for patients with normal or mildly decreased renal function and has a relatively low cost.

A   B

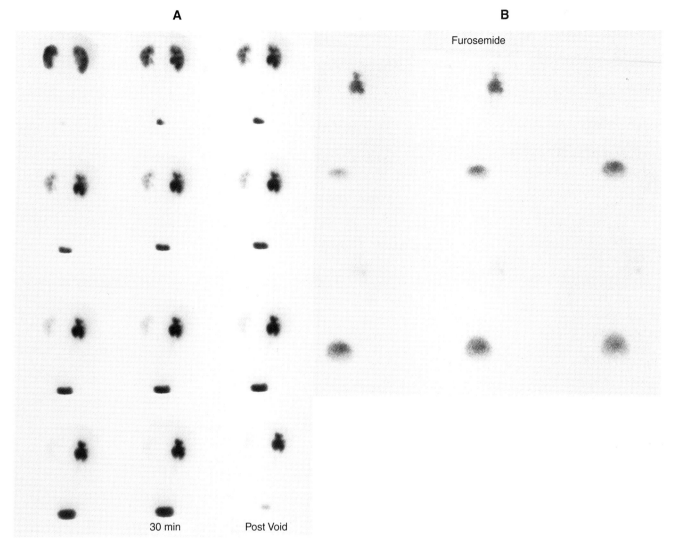

Furosemide

30 min   Post Void

A 31-year-old man with a history of congenital ureteropelvic junction obstruction had surgical correction several years ago. The most recent diuretic renogram was interpreted as right renal obstruction. This scan was obtained after the second surgical correction.

1. Describe the scintigraphic imaging findings before and after administration of furosemide.

2. What is your interpretation of the study?

3. Can ureteropelvic vs. ureterovesical obstruction be distinguished from this study?

4. What is the Whittaker test?

Genitourinary System: Diuretic Renography/Nonobstructed Hydronephrosis

1. Bilateral prompt cortical uptake and excretion into collecting systems. Retention in the right collecting system at 30 minutes with good post-furosemide washout.

2. Good response to surgical correction. Negative for obstruction.

3. Not with certainty. Ureteral nonvisualization is not diagnostic of ureteropelvic junction obstruction because a standing column of ureteral urine can prevent radiotracer entry.

4. It measures pressure-flow relationships and requires fluoroscopically guided trocar or spinal needle insertion into the renal pelvis. Basal and pressure measurements during infusion of a contrast solution at a set rate are recorded. Obstruction pressure is defined as greater than 15 cm water, no obstruction as less than 10 to 12 cm water.

References

Mandell GA, Cooper JA, Leonard JC, et al: Procedure guideline for diuretic renography in children, *J Nucl Med* 38:1647-1650, 1997.

Piepsz A, Arnello F, Tondeur M, et al: Diuretic renography in children, *J Nucl Med* 39:2015-2016, 1998.

Cross-Reference

Nuclear Medicine: THE REQUISITES, ed 2, pp 340-348.

Comment

Contrast intravenous urography, ultrasonography, and conventional radionuclide renography are not reliable in differentiating obstructive from nonobstructive hydronephrosis. Dilation, delayed opacification, and delayed washout are seen with obstruction on contrast urography but also may be seen with nonobstructive hydronephrosis. Similarly, ultrasonography can depict hydronephrosis but cannot distinguish between obstruction and nonobstruction. The Whittaker test is rarely used today because it is invasive and unnecessary; diuretic renography has similar accuracy and is now the standard diagnostic test. The increased urine flow as a result of furosemide diuresis produces prompt washout in a nonobstructed system. With a fixed obstruction the capacity to augment outflow is limited, resulting in prolonged washout.

An intermediate furosemide renography result may indicate some component of obstruction but is most informatively reported, since obstruction cannot be excluded. The majority of diuretic renographic studies are for patients with incomplete obstructions (high-grade defined as renal uptake but no excretion into the collecting system). The rapid washout with furosemide proves that surgery was successful in relieving the obstruction in this patient.

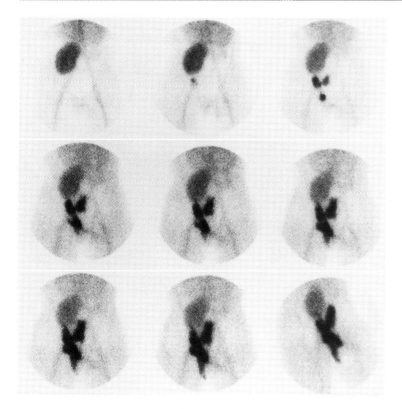

A 30-year-old kidney transplant recipient has decreasing postoperative urine output, fullness and tenderness around the graft, and scrotal swelling 24 hours after surgery.

1. Describe the findings on the 25-minute dynamic renal scintigraphy.

2. What is the diagnosis?

3. What are other causes of postoperative fluid collections adjacent to the graft?

4. What are other common complications during the first weeks after transplantation?

Genitourinary System: Transplant Kidney
Urinary Leak

1. Rapid leakage of urine just inferior to the transplanted kidney and extravasating into the scrotum.

2. Urinary leak caused by disruption of the surgical anastomosis.

3. Hematomas and abscesses occur in the early postoperative course, whereas lymphoceles generally are noted 4 to 8 weeks after surgery.

4. Acute tubular necrosis, acute rejection, obstruction. Cyclosporin toxicity usually occurs months after transplantation.

Reference

Choyke PL, Becker JA, Ziessman HA: Imaging the transplanted kidney. In Pollack HM, McLennan BL: *Clinical urology,* ed 2, Philadelphia, 2000, WB Saunders, pp 3091-3118.

Cross-Reference

Nuclear Medicine: THE REQUISITES, ed 2, pp 351-353.

Comment

Urinomas usually are diagnosed within the first or second postoperative week. They usually are located between the transplanted kidney and the bladder, although they may occur in the scrotum or thigh. Ureteral breakdown is usually caused by vascular insufficiency leading to ureteral necrosis but also can be caused by increased urinary pressure from distal obstruction. Large urinomas can rupture intraperitoneally to produce urinary ascites. They can become infected and form abscesses.

Urinary fistulas generally develop in the posttransplantation period. They are managed by reimplantation of the ureter or another reconstructive procedure. Urinomas result from the continued, slow extravasation of urine from the renal pelvis, ureter, or ureteroneocystostomy site. Large urinomas and urinary leaks can be a serious complication of renal transplantation. Smaller leaks often result in walled-off collections that may or may not produce symptoms and can resolve spontaneously. Larger and more rapid leaks require prompt intervention. An abrupt halt in urine output from a transplant that was functioning initially after surgery suggests a urinary leak. On ultrasound imaging, urinomas are well-defined, anechoic fluid collections. The radionuclide study can confirm their urinary origin. With a slower leak, delayed images may be required to detect the urinary collection.

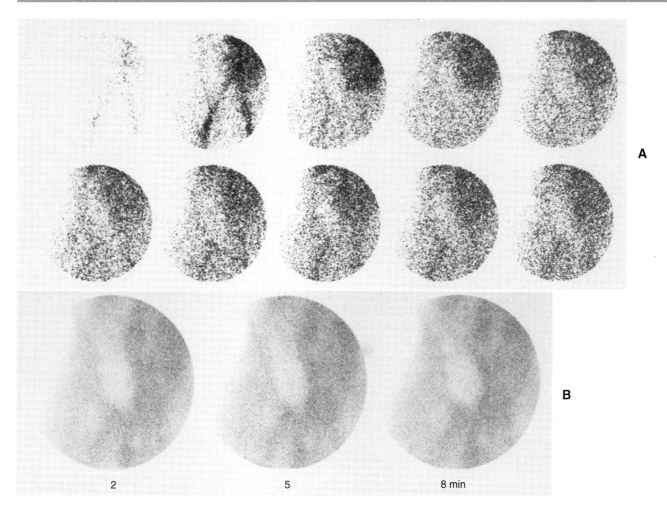

A

B

2   5   8 min

Radionuclide blood flow and early dynamic images at 24 hours after transplantation.

1. What are the scintigraphic findings?
2. What is your physiologic interpretation?
3. What is the differential diagnosis?
4. What therapy would be appropriate?

Genitourinary System: Nonviable Kidney After Transplantation

1. No blood flow to the transplanted kidney. No renal uptake. A photopenic region in the shape of the transplanted kidney.

2. Nonviable kidney.

3. Arterial or venous thrombosis, severe irreversible rejection, acute cortical necrosis.

4. Removal of the nonviable transplanted kidney.

References

Choyke PL, Becker JA, Ziessman HA: Imaging the transplanted kidney, In Pollack HM, McLennan BL: *Clinical urology,* ed 2, Philadelphia, 2000, WB Saunders, pp 3091-3118.

Russell CD, Yang H, Gastron RS, et al: Prediction of renal transplant survival from early postoperative radioisotope studies, *J Nucl Med* 41:1332-1336, 2000.

Cross-Reference

Nuclear Medicine: THE REQUISITES, ed 2, pp 349-350.

Comment

A major benefit of scintigraphy is that radionuclide angiography can be performed and blood flow at the capillary level demonstrated. Acute arterial thrombosis is an uncommon complication that presents as anuria posttransplantation. It is an emergency when it does occur. Acute kinking of the transplanted artery may present similarly. Acute venous thrombosis may look identical to arterial thrombosis because of the lack of normal lymphatic drainage after transplantation.

Hyperacute rejection is a rapidly progressive irreversible process first detected immediately after implantation of the transplanted kidney. The kidney turns blue in the operating room. The precipitating factor is the presence of preformed antibodies. Immediately after anastomosis an antibody-antigen reaction takes place in the graft, leading to rapid thrombosis of the vascular bed and complete functional destruction within minutes to hours. However, this is uncommon because of the current careful prescreening to determine immunological compatibility. Renal artery stenosis can occur at any time but usually occurs 3 months or later after transplantation.

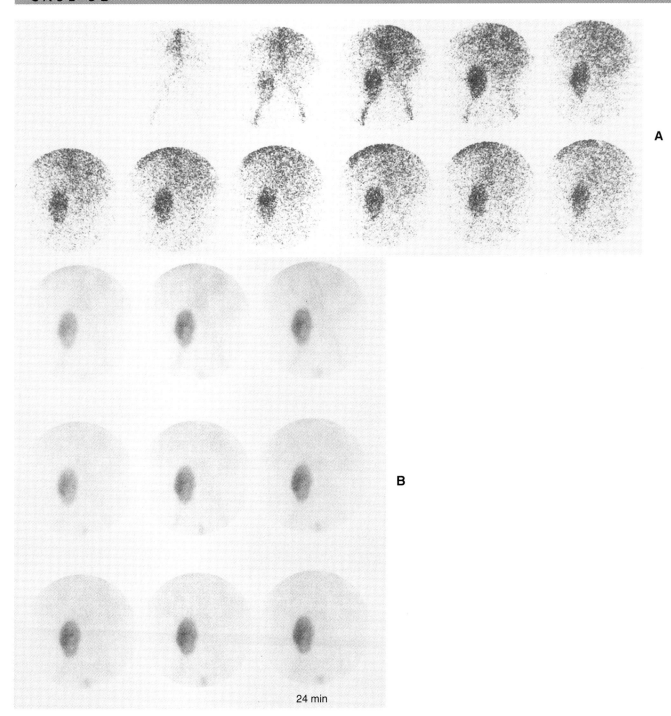

A

B

24 min

A 25-year-old man undergoes imaging 3 days after a renal cadaver transplant.

1. Which postoperative complications occur in the first week of renal transplantation?

2. During which postoperative period does acute rejection typically occur?

3. What are the scintigraphic findings in this case?

4. What is the diagnosis?

Genitourinary System: Renal Transplant with Acute Tubular Necrosis

1. Acute tubular necrosis, accelerated acute rejection, urinary leak, urinary obstruction.

2. The second postoperative week. Accelerated rejection may occur during the first week in patients who have had previous transplants or received multiple transfusions.

3. Normal blood flow, very poor function, no excretion. Base of penis seen inferiorly.

4. The pattern of normal blood flow but poor function during the first week after transplantation is typical of acute tubular necrosis (ATN).

References

Dubovsky EV, Russell CD, Bischof-Delaloye A, et al: Report of the radionuclides in nephrourology committee for evaluation of transplanted kidney, *Semin Nucl Med* 29:175-188, 1999.

Brown ED, Chen MY, Wolfman NT, et al: Complications of renal transplantation: evaluation with ultrasound and radionuclide imaging, *Radiographics* 20:607-622, 2000.

Cross-Reference

Nuclear Medicine: THE REQUISITES, ed 2, pp 305-308.

Comment

ATN occurs invariably after transplantation with cadaver allografts and frequently with living related donor grafts. An extended time between salvaging the donor kidney and transplantation increases the likelihood and severity of ATN. The scintigraphic findings of ATN are visible within 24 hours of transplantation. ATN usually resolves over 1 to 3 weeks. Sometimes ATN becomes superimposed on other postoperative complications, e.g., acute rejection, which begin the second week after transplantation. Acute rejection usually begins 5 to 7 days after transplantation and usually is associated scintigraphically with decreased blood flow. Obstruction cannot be excluded totally in this case. However, the absence of initial photopenia representing a full renal pelvis does not support obstruction.

^{99m}Tc MAG3 is the radiopharmaceutical of choice for renal transplant evaluation. ^{131}I hippuran also provides reliable information about function, but blood flow studies cannot be performed because of the low administered dose (300 μCi). ^{99m}Tc DTPA can provide blood flow information but cannot detect improvement or deterioration in function when the serum creatinine concentration is elevated, e.g., greater than 2.5 mg/dl. ^{99m}Tc MAG3 allows evaluation of both blood flow and function even in the setting of very poor renal function. The radionuclide study can be particularly valuable when renal function is difficult to determine clinically, e.g., in patients undergoing dialysis. Improvement in renal function often can be detected 24 to 48 hours before changes in the serum creatinine level.

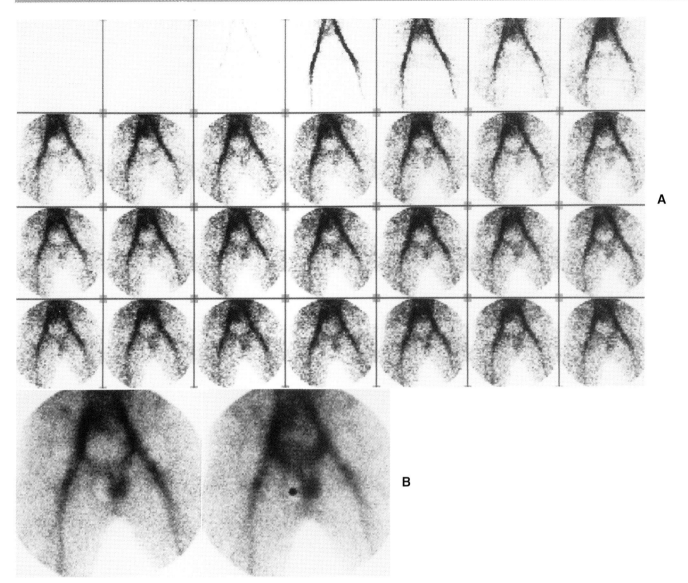

A

B

An 8-year-old boy has acute onset of right testicular pain.

1. What is the radiopharmaceutical and mechanism of distribution?
2. What are the most common causes of acute testicular pain?
3. What is the mechanism of testicular torsion?
4. What are the imaging findings, and what is the diagnosis in the case?

Genitourinary System: Testicular Torsion

1. ^{99m}Tc pertechnetate, initial blood flow, and then the radiotracer distributes in the extracellular fluid space (intravascular and interstitial).

2. Acute epididymitis, testicular torsion, torsion of the testicular appendage.

3. Developmental abnormality of testicular descent and attachment predisposes to spermatic cord torsion. The most common anatomical abnormality is "bell-clapper" testis.

4. Decreased blood flow to the right testicle and a photopenic right testicle consistent with acute testicular torsion.

Reference

Paltiel HJ, Connolly LP, Atala A, et al: Acute scrotal symptoms in boys with an indeterminate clinical presentation: comparison of color Doppler, sonography, and scintigraphy, *Radiology* 207:223-231, 1998.

Cross-Reference

Nuclear Medicine: THE REQUISITES, ed 2, pp 357-362.

Comment

Patients with a high likelihood of testicular torsion usually undergo immediate surgery without diagnostic imaging. Testicular torsion is a surgical emergency because testicular atrophy may occur as early as 4 hours after the acute event and is inevitable by 10 hours. However, some patients have an indeterminate likelihood of torsion based on symptoms and clinical signs. Approximately 70% of patients have conditions other than testicular torsion that do not require surgery. Imaging typically is performed in patients with equivocal clinical findings to help the urologist decide whether surgery is indicated.

The bell clapper testis is a congenital abnormality, usually bilaterally, in which the tunica vaginalis completely invests the testes. The normal posterior mesorchial anchor is absent, allowing the testis to twist on its vascular pedicle.

The reported accuracy of scintigraphy is approximately 95%. Recently, color Doppler ultrasonography has become a commonly used imaging modality for evaluation of acute scrotal symptoms. Direct comparison of the two diagnostic studies does not show a significant difference in interpretative accuracy. Doppler often is more rapid and easily obtained in the acute emergency department setting. Scintigraphy may be particularly helpful when Doppler studies show equivocal flow. Potassium perchlorate may be administered to children before the scintigraphic study to prevent thyroid uptake and radiation exposure. Scintigraphy is not indicated for chronic or painless disorders of the scrotum.

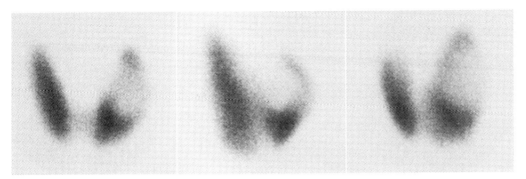

A 55-year-old woman is referred for a thyroid scan to evaluate a palpable thyroid nodule. Left to right views are anterior, right anterior oblique, and left anterior oblique.

1. What are the two radiopharmaceuticals used for thyroid scintigraphy, their photopeaks, and physical half-lives?
2. What is the likelihood of thyroid cancer in this patient?
3. What would you recommend as the next diagnostic or therapeutic procedure?
4. What imaging method is used here? What is its image resolution?

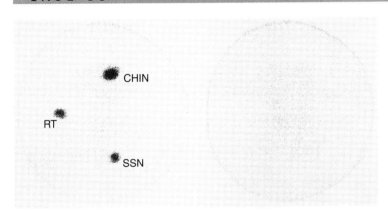

A 48-year-old woman has recent onset of neck tenderness and hyperthyroidism (thyroid-stimulating hormones [TSH] <0.05 μU/ml); ^{123}I scan uptake (radioactive iodine uptake [RAIU]) $\leq$1%). Right side *(R)*; suprasternal notch *(SSN)*.

1. What is the clinical differential diagnosis of hyperthyroidism?
2. What is the clinical purpose of the thyroid scan and RAIU tests in hyperthyroidism?
3. How is the RAIU calculated?
4. What is the likely diagnosis in this patient?

CASE 54

Endocrine System: Cold Thyroid Nodule

1. Intravenous ^{99m}Tc pertechnetate, 140 keV, 6 hours; oral sodium ^{123}I, 159 keV, 8 hours.

2. A single cold nodule has a 15% to 20% chance of malignancy.

3. Aspiration needle biopsy.

4. Pinhole collimator. 4 to 6 mm.

References

Freitas JE, Freitas AE: Thyroid and parathyroid imaging, *Semin Nucl Med* 24:234-245, 1994.

Cases JA, Surks MI: The changing role of scintigraphy in the evaluation of thyroid nodules. *Semin Nucl Med* 30:81-87, 2000.

Cross-Reference

Nuclear Medicine: THE REQUISITES, ed 2, pp 364-375.

Comment

^{123}I is trapped and organified by thyroid follicular cells. ^{99m}Tc has a similar uptake mechanism, but it is not organified. ^{99m}Tc is advantageous for children because of its short imaging time related to the high-count rate and low radiation absorbed dose to the thyroid. The adult administered dose is 3 to 5 mCi intravenously versus 200 to 300 µCi orally for ^{123}I. ^{123}I is used most commonly in adults. Images are obtained at 2 to 6 hours and uptakes at 24 hours after oral administration of the capsule.

Photopenic regions on thyroid scintigraphy scan are caused by various conditions, e.g., cysts, colloid nodules, new or old thyroiditis, Hashimoto's disease, and hematoma. The incidence of thyroid cancer is less than 5% in a multinodular goiter (multiple cold nodules) and less than 1% for a hot nodule.

A pinhole collimator is used with thyroid imaging for magnification. However, it results in distortion and magnification. In the oblique images the lobe farther from the pinhole (left lobe in the right anterior oblique, right lobe in the left anterior oblique) is distorted. The resolution depends on the size of the pinhole insert, usually 4 to 6 mm (4 to 6 mm resolution). Size is difficult to judge with a pinhole collimator because of the magnification factor. Size markers are sometimes used but are unreliable because of the changing magnification with depth. Physical examination is the commonly used method to estimate size, although it is subjective and open to interobserver differences.

Notes

CASE 55

Endocrine System: Hyperthyroidism/ Thyroiditis

1. Graves' disease, toxic nodule(s), thyroiditis (subacute, silent, postpartum), iatrogenic thyroid hormone ingestion, iodine-induced (Jod Basedow), trophoblastic tumors (hydatidiform mole and choriocarcinoma), Hashitoxicosis, ectopic hyperfunctioning thyroid tissue (struma ovarii).

2. Aid in the differential diagnosis of hyperthyroidism.

3. A nonimaging gamma probe obtains counts/time from the neck and a phantom-containing activity equal to the orally administered dose (µCi) to convert the gamma probe counts to µCi. %RAIU = neck (µCi) divided by the total administered dose (µCi) after background correction.

4. Subacute thyroiditis based on the history of neck tenderness, laboratory finding, and RAIU.

Reference

Sarkar SD: Thyroid pathophysiology. In Sandler MP, Coleman RE, Wachers FJTh, et al: *Diagnostic nuclear medicine,* ed 3, Baltimore, 1996, Williams & Wilkins, pp 899-908.

Cross-Reference

Nuclear Medicine: THE REQUISITES, ed 2, pp 368-378.

Comment

Thyroiditis and Graves' disease are the most common causes of hyperthyroidism and often are difficult to distinguish clinically. Hyperthyroidism is diagnosed by a suppressed TSH level. Thyroxine (T_4) and triiodothyronine (T_3) may or may not be elevated. The scan and RAIU aid in the differential diagnosis. The scan can distinguish nodular disease from Graves' disease or thyroiditis. The RAIU differentiates diseases with increased uptake, e.g., Graves', hashitoxicosis, from those with low uptakes (most other diseases listed in answer 1, e.g., thyroiditis). These latter diseases do not have autonomous function. The RAIU can be misleadingly low because of ingestion of thyroid hormone, stable iodine in foods, medications, vitamins, and iodinated contrast agents.

Subacute thyroiditis is a granulomatous disease that initially manifests as hyperthyroidism and neck tenderness. Silent thyroiditis has no pain but a similar clinical course. The patient history can suggest postpartum thyroiditis. During the acute phase of thyroiditis, hormone is released from the inflamed cells, producing symptoms of hyperthyroidism. Antithyroid antibodies are elevated. Although Hashimoto's disease usually presents with goiter and hypothyroidism in middle-aged women, a subgroup of patients have an acute hyperthyroid phase (Hashitoxicosis). In these cases the thyroid scan and uptake are indistinguishable from Graves' disease.

Notes

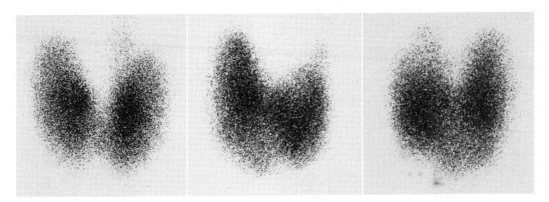

A 35-year-old woman with hyperthyroidism. Radioactive iodine uptake was 94% at 4 hours and 81% at 24 hours.

1. Describe the difference between Graves' disease and euthyroid scan appearance.

2. What is the appropriate therapy for Graves' disease?

3. What are the usual administered doses of radiotracer for ^{131}I uptakes, ^{123}I scans, and Graves' disease therapy?

4. What are the short-term and long-term side effects of ^{131}I therapy for hyperthyroidism?

C A S E   5 7

A

ANT   POST

B

CHIN

RIGHT

Suprasternal Notch

A 39-year-old woman 6 weeks previously underwent total thyroidectomy for thyroid cancer. Scanning was done 7 days after therapy for thyroid ablation with 75 mCi of ^{131}I.

1. Describe and interpret the scintigraphic images.

2. What is the reason for the star artifact pattern in the neck in scan *A*?

3. What collimator was used for image *B*?

4. Why is the liver seen in image *A*?

CASE 56

Endocrine System: Graves' Disease

1. Scan appearance may be similar. With a large goiter the scan often has a plumper appearance with convex borders. The pyramidal lobe may be seen, as in this case.

2. Surgery is seldom performed because of the high risk. Propylthiouracil (PTU) and methimazole (Tapazole) sometimes are used initially, particularly in patients with severe disease who require "cooling down," young children, and pregnant patients. Most of these are treated with radioactive iodine after 6 to 12 months of antithyroid medication. Many patients are treated initially with ^{131}I.

3. ^{131}I uptake (10 μCi), ^{123}I scan and uptake (300 μCi), Graves' disease therapy: ^{131}I (5 to 15 mCi)

4. Short-term: occasional exacerbation of hyperthyroidism, cardiac symptoms in elderly, very rare thyroid storm. Long-term: hypothyroidism. There is no increased incidence of secondary cancers, reduction in fertility, or congenital defects in offspring.

References

Kaplan MM, Meier DA, Dworkin HJ: Treatment of hyperthyroidism with radioactive iodine, *Endocrinol Metab Clin North Am* 27:205-223, 1998.

Wartofsky L: Radioiodine therapy of Graves' disease: case selection and restrictions recommended to patients in North America, *Thyroid* 7:213-216, 1997.

Cross-Reference

Nuclear Medicine: THE REQUISITES, ed 2, pp 369-374.

Comment

Uptake measurements with a gamma (nonimaging) probe are made at 4 (2 to 6) or 24 hours, or both. Most commonly there is a continual increase in uptake from 4 to 24 hours. Sometimes the uptake plateaus between 4 and 24 hours; in other cases, the 24-hour uptake is lower than at 4-hours because of rapid iodine turnover. For therapy for Graves' disease, an arbitrary dose, e.g., 10 to 15 mCi, is used by some clinicians. Others adjust for the two variables that determine the radiation dose to the gland: gland size and the RAIU. Some use an equation to calculate the therapy dose: gram size of gland × 50 to 200 μCi/gm divided by the RAIU. With lower μCi/gm doses the radiation dose is minimized, but the recurrence rate is higher. With higher μCi/gm doses the need for retreatment is low, but onset of hypothyroidism is earlier and more likely. Many endocrinologists prefer the higher doses because of the lack of serious side effects and the inevitability of hypothyroidism. Doses of 33 mCi or greater can be used routinely on an outpatient basis per revised Nuclear Regulatory Commission (NRC) regulations.

Notes

CASE 57

Endocrine System: ^{131}I Star Artifact

1. *A,* Posttherapy ^{131}I whole-body scan shows intensive uptake in the neck with a "star" artifact, diffuse liver activity, and bladder clearance. The mediastinum is difficult to visualize because of the artifact. *B,* Pinhole image of the neck with three foci of uptake.

2. Septal penetration of high-energy ^{131}I gamma rays through the collimator septa.

3. Pinhole collimator centered on the thyroid.

4. Radiolabeled thyroid hormone is metabolized in the liver. This usually is seen only on the posttherapy scans.

Reference

Tsui BMW, Gunter DL, Beck RN, et al: Physics of collimator design. In Sandler MP, Coleman RE, Wackers FJTh, et al, editors: *Diagnostic nuclear medicine,* ed 3, Baltimore, 1996, Williams & Wilkins, pp 67-69.

Cross-Reference

Nuclear Medicine: THE REQUISITES, ed 2, pp 364-368.

Comment

The star artifact, most commonly seen with ^{131}I scans, is seen only with high-dose administration and intense focal uptake, e.g., thyroid remnants in patients with thyroid cancer after thyroidectomy. The purpose for near-total thyroidectomies for thyroid cancer is to remove tumor and as much thyroid tissue as possible, but to leave the parathyroids, which requires leaving some adjacent tissue. Thus the patient is made hypothyroid (patient has elevated TSH levels) to ensure good therapeutic iodine uptake. To enable patient follow-up with measurements of serum thyroglobulins and ^{131}I scans postoperatively is then feasible.

The therapeutic ^{131}I dose is administered to ablate the remaining normal thyroid, to treat any remaining thyroid cancer, or both. In patients with thyroid cancer the dose for ablation of residual normal tissue ranges from 30 to 100 mCi. The thyroid cancer therapy dose in patients with metastases ranges from 100 to 200 mCi. Higher doses sometimes are administered but usually only after dosimetric studies that ensure no excess radiation to the bone marrow, the critical organ.

The star artifact makes interpretation of the neck and upper chest difficult. The pinhole collimator magnifies because of its geometry. Resolution is better with the pinhole collimator than the high-energy collimator used for whole body imaging. Thus the pinhole collimator makes interpretation of the neck possible, but the upper chest region can still be problematic.

Notes

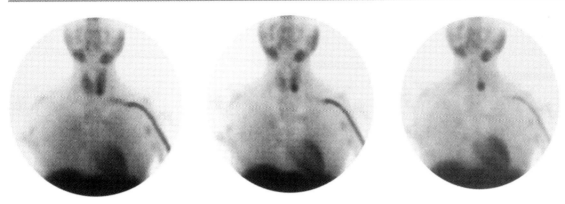

A 55-year-old man with hypercalcemia has an elevated serum PTH level. Images are taken at 5 minutes and at 1 and 2 hours.

1. Which radiopharmaceutical is being used, and what is the rationale for this technique?

2. What is the diagnosis?

3. What is the accuracy of this study?

4. What is the most common cause for a false-positive study result?

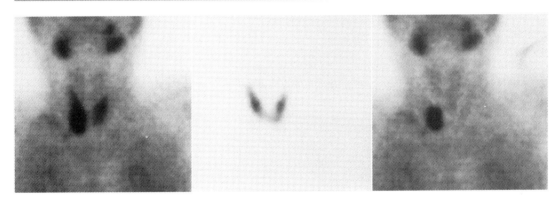

A patient has elevated serum calcium and parathyroid hormone levels and normal findings on neck examination.

1. What other protocol in addition to dual-phase (early and delayed) ^{99m}Tc sestamibi imaging can be used to evaluate for parathyroid disease?

2. Describe how that procedure is performed.

3. Describe the findings. Left: ^{99m}Tc sestamibi; middle: ^{123}I; right: subtraction.

4. List the differential diagnosis and the most likely diagnosis.

CASE 58

Endocrine System: Hyperparathyroidism

1. ^{99m}Tc sestamibi (MIBI) is taken up by the thyroid and parathyroid tissue, but washes out more rapidly from the thyroid.

2. Parathyroid adenoma in the region of the left lower lobe of the thyroid.

3. Greater than 90% predictive value for preoperative localization of parathyroid adenoma; lower test accuracy for hyperplasia and small tumors.

4. Thyroid follicular adenoma.

References

Taillefer R, Boucher Y, Potvin C, et al: Detection and localization of parathyroid adenomas in patients with hyperparathyroidism using a single radionuclide imaging procedure with ^{99m}Tc sestamibi (double-phase study), *J Nucl Med* 33:1801-1805, 1992.

Rauth JD, Sessions RB, Ziessman HA: Comparison of ^{99m}Tc MIBI and ^{201}Tl/^{99m}Tc for diagnosis of primary hyperparathyroidism, *Clin Nucl Med* 21:602-608, 1996.

Cross-Reference

Nuclear Medicine: THE REQUISITES, ed 2, pp 384-387.

Comment

Before the availability of ^{99m}Tc MIBI, ^{201}Tl and ^{99m}Tc pertechnetate were used for parathyroid scintigraphy. ^{201}Tl is taken up by both normal thyroid and hyperfunctioning parathyroid tissue, but ^{99m}Tc by the thyroid only. Computer subtraction was performed. The method has limitations, e.g., poor imaging characteristics of ^{201}Tl, patient movement, and computer subtraction artifacts.

^{99m}Tc MIBI is a nonspecific tumor-imaging agent taken up by a variety of benign and malignant tumors. Follicular adenoma of the thyroid is the most common false-positive finding, but other tumors, e.g., lymphoma, may have similar uptake. ^{99m}Tc MIBI has a higher accuracy for detection of parathyroid tumors than other imaging modalities, e.g., ^{201}Tl/^{99m}Tc, ultrasonography, or MRI. In addition to the superior imaging characteristics of ^{99m}Tc compared with those of ^{201}Tl, MIBI has useful pharmacokinetic characteristics, i.e., it washes out from parathyroid tumors at a slower rate than thyroid tissue, as seen in this case. It also often has higher initial uptake compared with the thyroid. A variety of techniques have been used, including computer subtraction with ^{123}I and SPECT. The simple early-late method sequence used in this case often is adequate for localization. Thyroid imaging may be helpful occasionally in patients with anatomical abnormalities or thyroid adenomas. Preoperative parathyroid scintigraphy can save operative time. Intraoperative gamma probes currently are used by many surgeons.

Notes

CASE 59

Endocrine System: Parathyroid Adenoma

1. Dual-isotope imaging with subtraction, in the past using ^{201}Tl and ^{99m}Tc pertechnetate, and more recently using ^{123}I and ^{99m}Tc sestamibi (MIBI).

2. ^{123}I by mouth. After a delay of 2 to 3 hours, an anterior ^{123}I thyroid scan is obtained. Without moving the patient, an image is obtained after intravenous injection of ^{99m}Tc MIBI. The ^{123}I image is computer subtracted from the ^{99m}Tc MIBI image.

3. The ^{123}I thyroid scan appears normal, although the left lobe extends more inferiorly *(middle)*. The MIBI image *(left)* shows an asymmetrical bulbous configuration in the region of the right lower pole of the thyroid. Subtraction demonstrates focal radiotracer compatible with parathyroid adenoma at the lower pole of the right thyroid *(right)*.

4. Parathyroid, thyroid adenoma, parathyroid, thyroid carcinoma, metastatic carcinoma.

Reference

Haney TP, editor. Rehm PKR: Nuclear medicine: oncology—conventional tumor imaging, Reston, Va, 1997, *Nuclear medicine self-study program IV,* unit 2, Society of Nuclear Medicine, pp 32-34.

Cross-Reference

Nuclear Medicine: THE REQUISITES, ed 2, pp 363, 384-387.

Comment

Parathyroid scintigraphy may be performed successfully using a variety of different protocols. Based on pooled data, MIBI/thyroid scanning subtraction techniques have greater sensitivity than ^{201}Tl/thyroid subtraction imaging (87% vs. 71%) because of the better image resolution of ^{99m}Tc MIBI compared with ^{201}Tl. The latter has suboptimal imaging characteristics because of its low energy (69 to 83 keV) and low administered dose (3 mCi). Either ^{99m}Tc or ^{123}I can be used for the thyroid imaging portion of the subtraction technique. ^{123}I has the advantage of a different photopeak (159 keV) compared with ^{99m}Tc-labeled MIBI. Some variability in washout occurs with the two-phase MIBI technique. The addition of the thyroid scan and subtraction images offers some advantages. It can confirm the thyroid rather than parathyroid origin of the uptake, e.g., follicular adenomas, and can be helpful in patients with anatomical variants, prior thyroid surgery, or those receiving thyroid hormone causing thyroid suppression. However, subtraction techniques sometimes produce artifacts because of patient motion or misregistration of images. Computer subtraction images should always be interpreted as an adjunct to image analysis, not in isolation.

Notes

Fair Game Cases

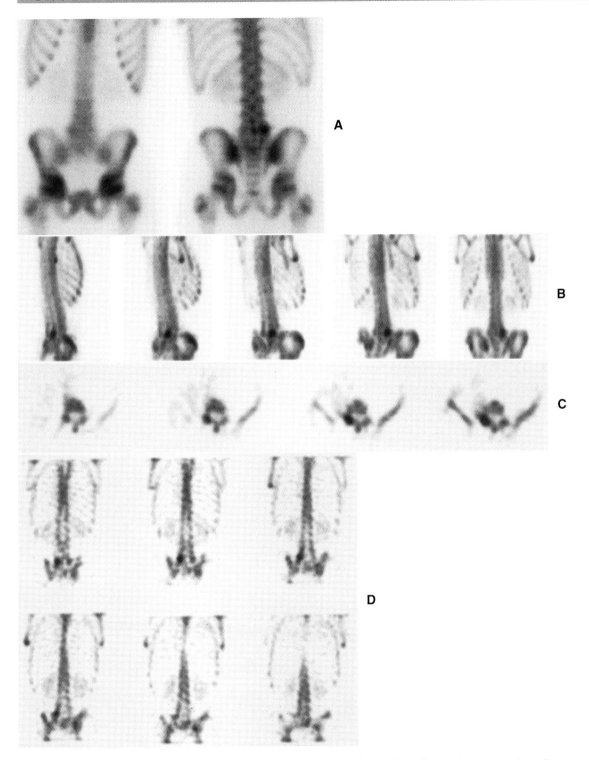

A 12-year-old boy has recent onset of back pain. The report of outside radiographs was equivocal.

1. Describe the bone scan findings on the planar images *(A)* and reprojection SPECT *(B)* images.
2. Describe the findings on the transverse and coronal SPECT slices (*C* and *D*).
3. Provide a differential diagnosis and the most likely diagnosis.
4. This entity may be associated with an abnormality of alignment. Describe it.

Skeletal System: L5 Pars Interarticularis Defect

1. The bone scan demonstrates focal increased uptake in the lateral aspect of L5 vertebra.

2. The finding is better demonstrated and better localized on the SPECT images, where the abnormal uptake is clearly seen in the region of the left pars interarticularis/facet joint.

3. L5 unilateral pars interarticularis defect, degenerative or posttraumatic facet disease. Pars defect is the most likely diagnosis in this age group.

4. Spondylolisthesis or slippage of the vertebrae out of normal alignment can occur if the defect is bilateral.

Reference

Collier BD, Krasnaw AZ, Hellman RS: Bone scanning. In Collier BD, Fogelman I, Rosenthall L, editors: *Skeletal nuclear medicine,* St Louis, 1996, Mosby, pp 51-56.

Cross-Reference

Nuclear Medicine: THE REQUISITES, ed 2, pp 128-132.

Comment

Spondylolysis is a fracture of the neural arch of the vertebra involving the pars interarticularis. Currently it is believed to represent a stress fracture caused by repetitive injury between infancy and early adult life, rather than a single trauma, although the latter may occur. Spondylolysis is most frequent in the lumbar spine; the majority of cases involve the fifth vertebra, as in this case. It may be unilateral or bilateral and may be associated with slippage, or spondylolisthesis of the vertebra with respect to adjacent vertebrae.

Spondylolysis may cause symptoms, prompting an imaging diagnosis, but it may be asymptomatic and discovered incidentally on radiographic studies. Localization of increased uptake on planar images is often difficult. SPECT allows for determining whether abnormal uptake is in the body, pedicle, or posterior elements. SPECT has significantly higher sensitivity than planar imaging (85% vs. 62%) for detection of a pars defect. Thus SPECT should be performed even after negative planar study findings when the diagnosis is suspected, particularly in young patients with low back pain. An abnormality seen on bone scintigraphy has significant patient management implications. Inappropriate early manipulation or too early a return to sports could convert the stress-related parts defect into a frank fracture, possibly leading to unstable spondylolisthesis.

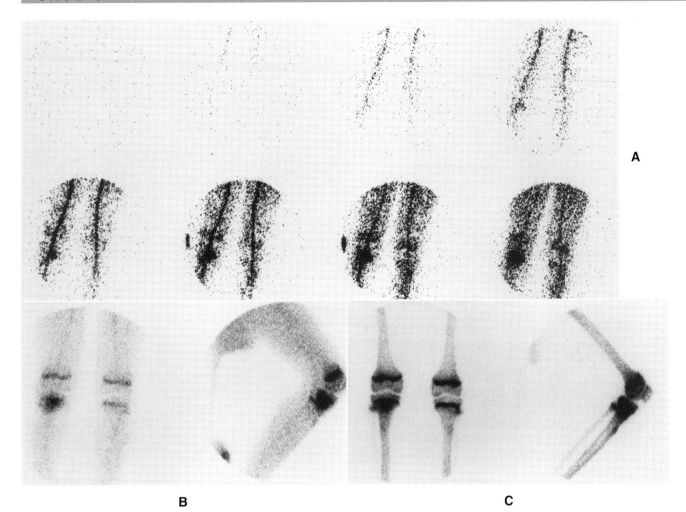

A 5-year-old boy with low-grade fever and pain in the right knee was referred for a three-phase bone scan.

1. Describe the three-phase scintigraphic findings.

2. Provide a differential diagnosis.

3. Do these findings suggest a septic arthritis?

4. What other radionuclide study could confirm or exclude infection?

Bone: Tibial Osteomyelitis—Three-Phase Positive Bone Scan

1. Increased blood flow *(A)*, blood pool *(B)*, and uptake on delayed images *(C)* in the proximal metaphyseal region of the right tibia.

2. Osteomyelitis, bone tumor, fracture/osteotomy.

3. No. A bone scan with septic arthritis shows increased uptake at the end of long bones symmetrically on both sides of the joint. An asymmetrical appearance may be seen if osteomyelitis and septic arthritis coexist; however, this study reveals normal findings on the femoral side.

4. ^{99m}Tc HM-PAO–labeled leukocyte study in a child.

Reference

Palestro CJ, Torres MA: Radionuclide imaging in orthopedic infections, *Semin Nucl Med* 27:334-343, 1997.

Cross-Reference

Nuclear Medicine: THE REQUISITES, ed 2, pp 134-138, 186-189.

Comment

Bone infection is usually bacterial in origin (most commonly staphylococcal) and reaches the bone by hematogenous spread, direct extension from a contiguous skin site of infection, or direct introduction by surgery or trauma. In acute hematogenous osteomyelitis, infection involves the red marrow of long bones as a result of the relatively slow blood flow in metaphyseal sinusoidal veins and the relative lack of phagocytes. In adults the long bones rarely are affected because adipose tissue has replaced red marrow. Infection most often occurs in the spine with septicemia as the initiating event. Direct extension from contiguous sites of infection is a very common cause of osteomyelitis, usually as a result of soft tissue infection after trauma, radiation therapy, burns, or pressure sores. Direct introduction of bacteria may occur during open fractures, open surgical reduction, or penetrating trauma by foreign bodies.

The bone scan is very sensitive for making the diagnosis. However, a positive three-phase bone scan is not specific for osteomyelitis. Fracture, tumor, and Charcot joints may be three-phase positive. The specificity of the bone scan is even poorer in patients with underlying conditions such as previous bone infection, fractures, orthopedic implants or devices, and neuropathic joints. The patient's history, radiographs, radiolabeled leukocytes, and biopsy frequently are necessary to make a definitive diagnosis in nonvirgin bone. The bone scan has a high negative predictive value and thus a negative study result can rule out bone disease.

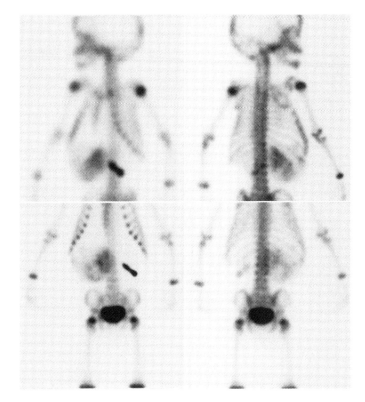

An 11-month-old infant has a hepatic mass on ultrasound. Bone scan ordered to exclude bone metastases.

1. Describe the scintigraphic findings.

2. Besides a neoplastic process, what other conditions could be associated with the findings?

3. Name another likely origin of the tumor other than the liver.

4. What is the most likely diagnosis?

Notes

Skeletal System: Hepatoblastoma

1. Nonuniform abnormal soft tissue right upper quadrant uptake that cannot be clearly separated from the right kidney.

2. Trauma to soft tissue or organs, in this case, the liver, resulting in contusion or hematoma, ischemic injury (although the pattern appears round rather than suggestive of a vascular distribution), chronic abscess.

3. Adrenal: neuroblastoma.

4. Given that it is a hepatic mass, hepatoblastoma is most likely based on the patient's age and uptake of bone radiotracer.

References
Buomono C, Taylor GA, Share JC, et al: Gastrointestinal tract. In Kirks DR, editor: *Practical pediatric imaging,* ed 3, Philadelphia, 1998, Lippincott-Raven, pp 960-969.

Blickman H: *Pediatric radiology: the requisites,* ed 2, St Louis, 1998, Mosby, pp 137-138.

Cross-Reference
Nuclear Medicine: THE REQUISITES, ed 2, pp 112-115, 124-125.

Comment
Because this is a hepatic mass, hepatoblastoma is most likely based on the patient's age and uptake of bone radiotracer. After the kidney and the adrenals, the liver is the third most common site of abdominal malignancies in infants and children, of which one third are benign. In many cases, imaging cannot reliably determine the tumor type and pathological study is required. In children younger than 5 years of age the most likely tumors are hepatoblastoma, mesenchymal hamartoma, and hemangioma. Hepatoblastoma is the most common primary hepatic tumor of childhood; two thirds of cases occur in children younger than 2 years of age. Similar to patients with neuroblastoma, abdominal radiographs of patients with hepatoblastoma show calcification in up to 50% of cases, which accounts for the deposition of bone radiopharmaceutical. The bone scan is used to diagnose metastases.

In adults, bone radiopharmaceutical uptake in tumors most commonly is seen in metastases from colon, breast, and lung. Hepatic necrosis, metastatic calcification, and amyloidosis are other reported causes.

A   B

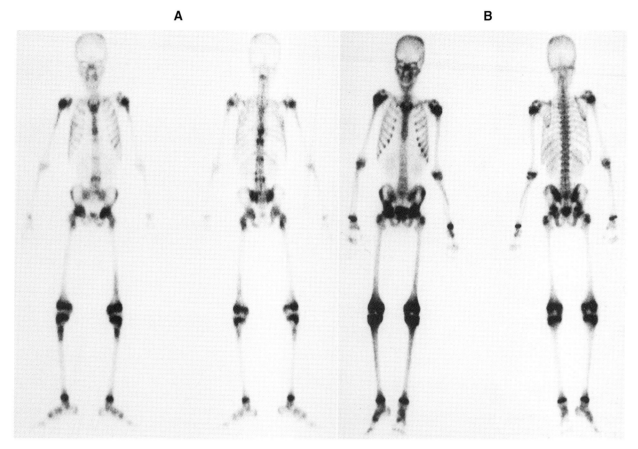

A 13-year-old girl adolescent with sickle cell disease, low-grade fever, arm, leg, and back pain was referred for a bone scan *(A)*. The scan was repeated 1 year later; the patient now has arm and back pain *(B)*.

1. Describe the scintigraphic bone and soft tissue findings.

2. What is the likely diagnosis?

3. What other nuclear medicine study can detect sickle infarcts?

4. How can osteomyelitis be differentiated from bone infarct?

CASE 63

Skeletal System: Sickle Cell Disease

1. *A,* Abnormal increased uptake in the proximal right humerus, left distal femur, multiple sites in the thoracic and lumbar spine. *B,* Uptake in the right ulna and left posterior ninth rib. Subtle soft tissue uptake is present in the region of the spleen.

2. Sickle cell crises with infarcts.

3. ^{99m}Tc sulfur colloid bone marrow scan.

4. Combined ^{99m}Tc bone scan and marrow scan early in the acute crisis.

Reference

Alavi A, Heyman S, Tse KM, Munz D: Bone marrow imaging. In Sandler MP, Coleman RE, Wackers FJTh, et al, editors: *Diagnostic nuclear medicine,* ed 3, Baltimore, 1996, Williams & Wilkins, pp 845-864.

Cross-Reference

Nuclear Medicine: THE REQUISITES, ed 2, pp 134-138, 186-189.

Comment

Bone and joint complaints are quite common in patients with sickle cell hemoglobinopathies. Symptoms may be transient, but they are related to marrow infarctions that occur as part of a sickle crisis. Often these resolve without radiographic changes. Radionuclide scans are the most sensitive imaging technique for early detection and evaluation of the extent of damage. A ^{99m}Tc sulfur colloid bone marrow scan can detect bone marrow infarctions early; the lesion appears as a cold defect. Conversely, marrow scanning often cannot detect infarcts in the mid-spine, lower ribs or sternum. Thus bone scanning is the technique most commonly used. During the first few days after a vasoocclusive crisis with infarction, decreased uptake may be seen on the bone scan. Soon increased uptake is evident, starting as a rim of increased activity around the infarct. Often only increased uptake will be seen because the bone scan usually is not obtained during the acute phase. Avascular necrosis of the head of the femur is the most disabling bone lesion, and early diagnosis is important. Combined bone scans and marrow studies, if obtained early in the course, may be used to differentiate aseptic osteonecrosis and osteomyelitis. With infarction the marrow defect is larger than the bone scan abnormality; however, with infection the marrow study results are positive only after 5 to 6 days, whereas the bone scan is positive early.

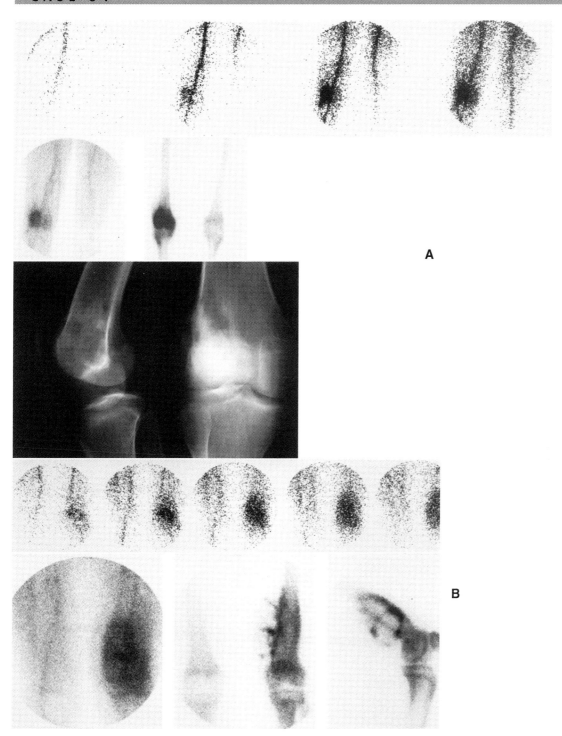

Two patients have knee pain, with no fever or calor. Patient *A:* bone scan and radiograph. Patient *B:* bone scan.

1. Describe the abnormal three-phase bone scan findings for patients *A* and *B.*

2. What other general information about the patients is evident from the bone scans?

3. Provide a differential diagnosis and the most likely diagnoses for each patient.

4. What term is commonly used to describe the pattern seen on delayed images in *B?*

Skeletal System: Osteosarcoma

1. *A,* Increased blood flow *(above)* and blood pool *(below, left)* to the right distal femur and increased uptake on delayed images in the distal femoral metaphysis extending to the joint surface *(below, right).* Mild increased uptake in the proximal tibia probably the result of hyperemia. *B,* Radiograph: mixed lytic-sclerotic lesion of the distal femur with cortical destruction and indistinct margins. No periosteal reaction. *C,* Abnormal increased flow and blood pool to the left distal femur with delayed increased uptake in spiculated pattern extending beyond the femoral contour.

2. The patients are skeletally immature but near the mature stage. Physes are seen faintly on delayed images, indicating that fusion is imminent. These are teenagers.

3. *A,* Monostotic primary neoplasm, e.g., osteosarcoma, secondary neoplasm, or osteomyelitis. *B,* Characteristic sunburst pattern of osteosarcoma.

4. Sunburst pattern.

Reference
Rehm PK: Nuclear medicine self-study program IV, unit 2. In Haney TP, Rehm PK, editors: *Nuclear medicine: oncology-conventional tumor imaging,* Reston, Va, 1997, Society of Nuclear Medicine, pp 7-9, 20-22.

Cross-Reference
Nuclear Medicine: THE REQUISITES, ed 2, pp 125-127, 136.

Comment
Osteosarcoma (osteogenic sarcoma) is the most common malignant primary tumor in children and adolescents. The intraosseous tumor usually arises in the metaphyses of long bones, the distal femur (44%), proximal tibia (22%), and proximal humerus (9%). It can extend into the diaphysis, epiphysis, or both. Two thirds of patients initially are seen with a large metaphyseal tumor as the primary focus. Radiographically the lesion may be predominantly osteosclerotic (25%), osteolytic (25%), or mixed (50%). A coexistent soft tissue mass characterized by the production of osteoid or bone usually is present. A periosteal reaction of interrupted or spiculated type frequently occurs.

Bone scintigraphy is indicated before initiation of therapy to detect skip lesions, multicentric osteosarcoma, or a primary lesion with multiple metastases. In the presence of multiple lesions, limb amputation is no longer appropriate. On bone scan, osteosarcoma avidly accumulates the radiotracer with or without extension into adjacent soft tissue. Occasionally an extended or augmented pattern may imply extensive marrow extension or transarticular involvement. Bone scintigraphy is poor in defining intraosseous tumor length. The extended pattern is attributed to circulatory changes in bone that simulate regional osteoblastic activity. Preoperative assessment is now based on MRI.

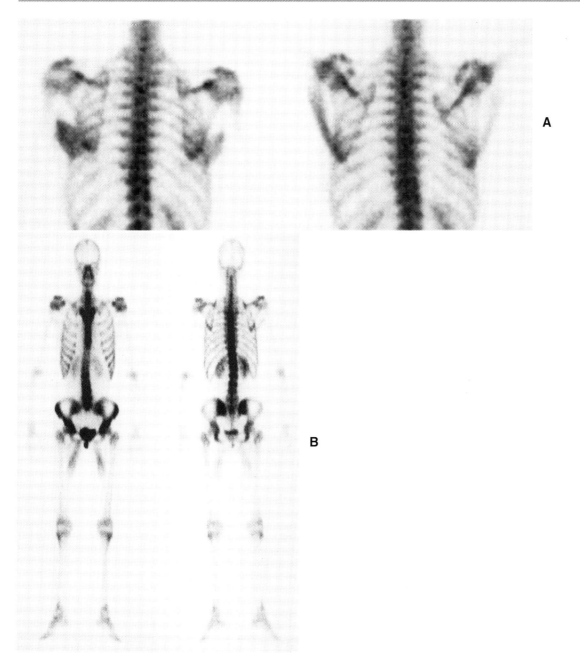

A

B

Two young adults were referred for a bone scan. Patient *A* has thoracic pain, and patient *B* has hip pain.

1. Describe the scintigraphic findings in both patients.
2. What is the diagnosis and cause for this pattern of uptake in these patients?
3. What is the mechanism of radiopharmaceutical uptake?
4. What are other causes of uptake in muscle?

Skeletal System: Muscle Injury

1. *A,* Uptake in teres major muscles bilaterally. *B,* Bilateral uptake in the adductor magnus muscles of the thighs.

2. Soft tissue muscle injury caused by repetitive stress; weight lifting in *A,* and stair climber exertion in *B.*

3. Soft tissue deposition of ^{99m}Tc-labeled diphosphonates is caused by binding to microcalcifications at sites of injury and possibly binding to injured immature collagen.

4. Rhabdomyolysis, iron dextran injection, polymyositis, myositis ossificans, ischemia, electrical injuries, direct trauma.

Reference

Brill DR: Radionuclide imaging of nonneoplastic soft tissue disorders, *Semin Nucl Med* 11:277-288, 1981.

Cross-Reference

Nuclear Medicine: THE REQUISITES, ed 2, pp 130-133.

Comment

A good general rule when reviewing bone scans is to first scrutinize the scan for renal and soft tissue abnormalities before focusing on the bones. Although kidney abnormalities are more commonly noted, soft tissue abnormalities are not uncommon. Patients usually are referred to confirm or exclude bone abnormalities, e.g., stress fractures and shin splints; however, the bone scan occasionally provides specific soft tissue diagnosis, as in these cases. Overexertion injuries to the musculoskeletal system are common. Many are associated with overexertion repetitive stress injuries.

The proposed mechanism of uptake is absorption to denatured proteins or binding to mitochondrial calcium, which is increased in ischemic tissues. The cause of muscle localization is believed to be rhabdomyolysis. Muscle localization of bone tracers has been reported after a variety of exercises. In downhill runners, uptake occurs in the buttocks, hamstrings, and quadriceps, whereas uphill runners have increased uptake in the thigh adductors. Uptake in the thighs can be seen in bicycle riders and in the abdominal muscles after push-up contests. Bilateral activity posteriorly in the teres major muscle has been reported in weight lifters.

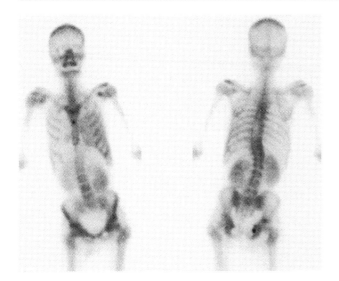

1. Describe the bone scan findings.
2. Name structures where the tracer could be deposited.
3. Provide the differential diagnosis.
4. What other information would be helpful?

Skeletal System: Pleural Uptake

1. Abnormal soft tissue uptake in the anterior left hemithorax; scoliosis and mild arthritic changes in both hips.

2. Starting on the inside working outward: in the lung parenchyma, in a primary or secondary tumor in the lung, in the pleural or pleural effusion, in the soft tissue of the chest wall.

3. Extensive pleural calcification, fibrothorax, prior radiation.

4. History, chest radiograph, or SPECT.

Reference

Gray HW, Krasnow AZ: Soft tissue uptake of bone agents. In Collier DB Jr, Fogelman I, Rosenthall L, editors: *Skeletal nuclear medicine,* St Louis, 1996, Mosby, p 383.

Cross-Reference

Nuclear Medicine: THE REQUISITES, ed 2, pp 112-115, 142-143.

Comment

The curvilinear inferior margin follows the contour of the diaphragm, suggesting that the uptake relates to pleura. The finding is evident on the anterior view only, indicating it is located anteriorly; therefore pleural effusion is unlikely unless it is loculated anteriorly. Prior radiation is unlikely to involve the anterior and spare posterior structures, or have a rounded superior margin, as in this case. Similarly, uptake in a soft tissue mass within the thorax or arising from the chest wall is unlikely to have an inferior margin that parallels the diaphragm. This patient had a history of prior left empyema and subsequently developed a fibrothorax.

In general the most common reason for unilateral uptake in soft tissues within the thorax is malignant pleural effusion. If the effusion is free-flowing, the scintigraphic pattern can change with changes in patient position, as it does when radiographs are taken with the patient erect and supine or in the decubitus position.

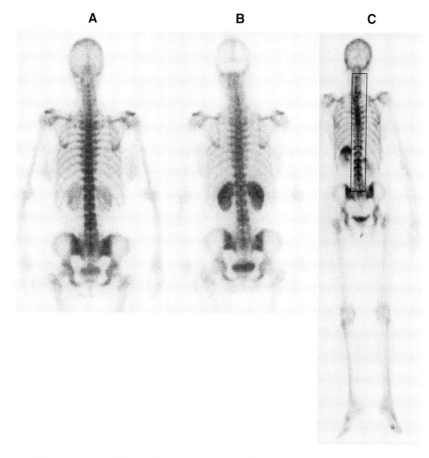

A   **B**   **C**

1. What are possible explanations for the change in the patient's bone scan from *A* to *B?*
2. List three questions that would be helpful to limit the differential diagnosis in *A/B.*
3. Describe the bone scan findings in patient *C.* Ignore the rectangular region of interest.
4. Provide the most likely diagnosis for the scans *A/B* and *C.*

Skeletal System: Hot Kidneys, Radiation Nephritis, and Spinal Photopenia

1. Increased radiotracer is present in both renal cortices in a bilateral symmetrical pattern on the follow-up study that was not seen on the initial study.

2. Has the patient been treated with a new medication in the interval since the prior bone scan? Has the patient had recent intravenous contrast media? Has the patient had restricted fluid intake?

3. Increased activity in the upper portions of both kidneys and cold lower thoracic spine.

4. *A/B,* Chemotherapy-induced interstitial nephritis. *C,* Prior radiation therapy to the spine with radiation nephritis.

Reference

Siddiqui AR: Increased uptake of technetium-99m-labeled bone imaging agents in the kidney, *Semin Nucl Med* 12:101-102, 1982.

Cross-Reference

Nuclear Medicine: THE REQUISITES, ed 2, p 115.

Comment

Dehydration can cause "hot" kidneys on bone scan that resolves on repeat study with good hydration. It may be seen transiently in patients with acute tubular necrosis. Most commonly, it is caused by renal toxicity as a result of medications such as chemotherapy, nephrotoxic antibiotics, or radiographic contrast. The kidneys return to a normal appearance on subsequent scans. The pattern may be persistent in chronic conditions, such as iron overload and multiple myeloma.

Radiation can lead to parenchymal ischemia as a result of small-vessel arteritis, which can be followed by renal atrophy. Radiation nephritis is seen less commonly with modern radiation therapy techniques but may occur. Effects in bone are related to dose, patient age, site, and specifics of the radiation technique. Radiation osteitis refers to a variety of appearances, including growth arrest, periostitis, and abnormalities of mineralization. When immature bone is inadvertently in the radiation treatment field, long-term outcome may include scoliosis and undergrowth of irradiated bone. Although some debate exists, vascular injury is the likely underlying mechanism for bone injury. Increased radiotracer uptake in bone associated with hyperemia is present during the first weeks after radiation greater than 30 Gy (3000 rads). This phase usually is missed because the diagnosis is known and treatment under way, and no clinical need exists for a scan. With time the scan pattern evolves to photopenia that usually resolves completely or remains at most slightly decreased compared with normal adjacent bones.

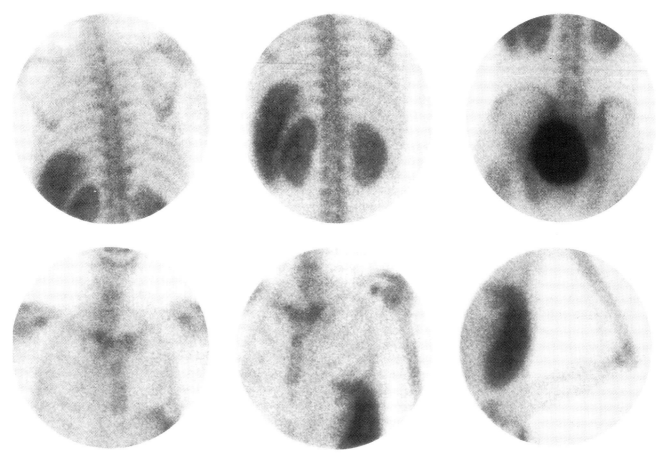

1. Describe the advantage of whole body imaging for the technologist compared with spot imaging, which was used in this case.

2. Describe the advantage of whole body imaging for the physician.

3. Describe the abnormality

4. Provide the differential diagnosis.

Skeletal System: Splenic Uptake

1. Less camera repositioning and time for the technologist.

2. Easier for the physician to check for quality assurance and for interpretive review.

3. Intense abnormal uptake in a structure that appears to be an enlarged spleen by its location and configuration.

4. Blood dyscrasias, including sickle cell disease, sickle thalassemia, thalassemia major; hemosiderosis; extensive subcapsular splenic hematoma.

Reference

Silberstein EB, McAfee JG, Spasoff AP: *Diagnostic patterns in nuclear medicine,* Reston, Va, 1998, Society of Nuclear Medicine, p 228.

Cross-Reference

Nuclear Medicine: THE REQUISITES, ed 2, pp 133-134.

Comment

Whole body images are easier for the physician to review. When the study is performed as multiple spots, the physician must be careful to ensure that no gaps between the scanned regions exist where a lesion may be missed. The whole body format ensures that the whole area has been imaged, and the whole body study is easier for the technologist to perform. The technologist positions the patient and sets up the whole body scanner, which then does a "sweep" without further technologist intervention. In contrast, the technologist must reposition the patient for each of the multiple spots using the other technique.

The most common cause of splenic uptake of bone tracer is sickle cell disease. However, the spleen would be expected to be shrunken, as a result of autoinfarction, in a patient who is skeletally mature, as in this case. In a child with sickle cell disease the spleen may not be small. Bone findings suggesting bone infarcts would support the diagnosis of sickle cell disease, although depending on the age of the bone infarct, they may be difficult or impossible to identify. If multiple fractures or uptake in soft tissue contusions were demonstrated, splenic trauma would be a likely possibility. Because of the perfect configuration of the tracer in a spleenlike appearance and the lack of other findings, subcapsular hematoma would seem unlikely. Therefore sickle thalassemia, thalassemia major, or hemosiderosis are the best diagnoses. This patient had sickle thalassemia.

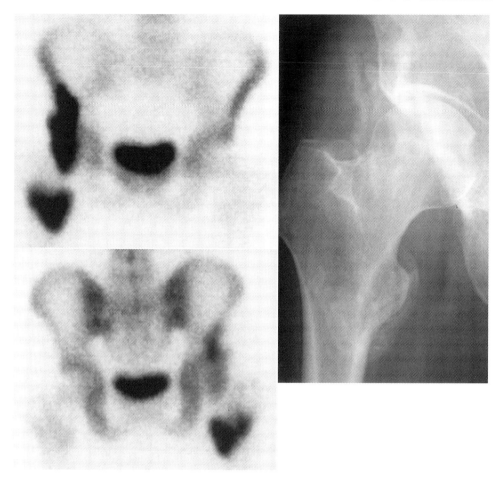

The bone scan image and radiograph of a paraplegic patient are provided.

1. Describe the bone scan findings.
2. Provide a differential diagnosis.
3. What interventions could be performed if artifact is suspected?
4. Radiograph of the right hip was obtained after the bone scan. What is the most likely diagnosis?

Skeletal System: Heterotopic Ossification

1. Radiotracer in a full urinary bladder obscures the central portion of the bony pelvis. Intense activity is seen overlying the right acetabulum with a separate area of uptake overlying the proximal right femur.

2. Urinary contamination; fracture with exuberant callus; heterotopic ossification or myositis ossificans; soft tissue injury (contusion).

3. If urinary contamination is suspected: remove clothing and overlying bed sheets; wash the patient's skin in the area of suspected contamination.

4. Heterotopic ossification.

Reference
Greenspan A: *Orthopedic radiology: a practical approach,* Philadelphia, 2000, Lippincott Williams & Wilkins, p 648.

Cross-Reference
Nuclear Medicine: THE REQUISITES, ed 2, pp 124-125.

Comment
The terms *heterotopic ossification of myositis ossificans* and *heterotopic bone formation* frequently are used interchangeably. Some restrict the term *myositis ossificans* to cases in which new bone arises as a result of inflammation of muscle and reserve *heterotopic ossification* or *heterotopic new bone formation in soft tissue* in the absence of well-defined cause. The proposed mechanism is that primitive mesenchymal cells differentiate into osteoblasts that deposit matrix that ossifies. The radiographic appearance in this patient is typical. The lesion frequently is seen adjacent to the cortex of a long bone or flat bone. It shows dense, well-organized bone at the periphery with less organized bone at the center. A well-defined separation of the lesion from the cortex of the adjacent bone is present. Alternatively, the condition appear as a veil-like lesion that is less well delineated. Biopsy of myositis ossificans/heterotopic ossification early after onset can lead to histological confusion with sarcoma. Appropriate correlation with the radiographic appearance is critical to avoid unnecessary biopsy or further intervention if biopsy is inadvertently performed.

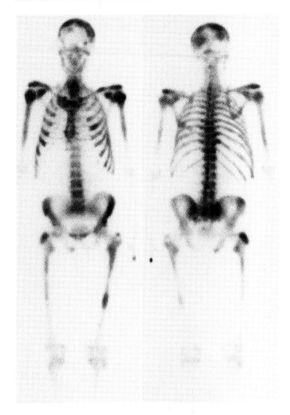

Elevated alkaline phosphatase level.

1. Describe the bone scan findings.

2. Name two other nonosseous systems that should be evaluated on the bone scan.

3. Describe any other findings.

4. What term can be applied to this case?

Skeletal System: Superscan Secondary to Metastatic Prostate Cancer

1. Increased radiotracer in the large majority of the visualized bones, with nonuniform involvement particularly evident in both femurs, both humeri, and skull.

2. Soft tissues and genitourinary tract.

3. The kidneys are not visualized, but faint activity is seen in the urinary bladder. Little soft tissue activity is seen.

4. Superscan.

References

Siegel BA, Chang A: Osteoporotic insufficiency fractures. In Thrall JH, section editor: *Nuclear radiology* (fourth series) *test and syllabus,* Reston, Va, 1990, American College of Radiology, p 230.

McAfee JG, Reba RC, Majd M: The musculoskeletal system. In Wagner HN, Szabo Z, Buchanan JW: *Principles of nuclear medicine,* ed 2, Philadelphia, 1995, WB Saunders, pp 991-994.

Cross-Reference
Nuclear Medicine: THE REQUISITES, ed 2, p 121.

Comment

The term *superscan* refers to a bone scan pattern with increased radiopharmaceutical uptake relative to soft tissue background and renal activity. Soft tissue, kidneys, and bladder appear to have decreased uptake. The superscan can occur in any diffuse skeletal disorder in which tracer uptake is markedly increased in the skeleton. Because less of the tracer is available for renal excretion, faint or no visualization of the kidneys results. Optimization of the imaging parameters for the skeletal activity level contributes to the apparent nonvisualization of renal activity.

Widespread metastatic disease is the most frequent cause of a superscan. The primary tumors responsible include carcinomas of the breast, lung, and prostate, although it may occur with lymphoma and bladder cancer. Superscan occurs in late-stage metastatic disease of bone with diffuse involvement. This patient had prostate cancer. Usually some inhomogeneity or hot spots in the pattern suggest tumor as the cause. A single radiograph of an involved bone such as the pelvis or femur usually provides easy confirmation of metastatic involvement. The other major causes of a superscan are metabolic bone diseases, e.g., renal osteodystrophy, osteomalacia, and hyperparathyroidism. Myelofibrosis and systemic mastocytosis can result in a similar pattern. In this case, additional clinical information such as the absence of chronic renal failure and primary hyperparathyroidism increase the likelihood of metastatic disease as the likely diagnosis.

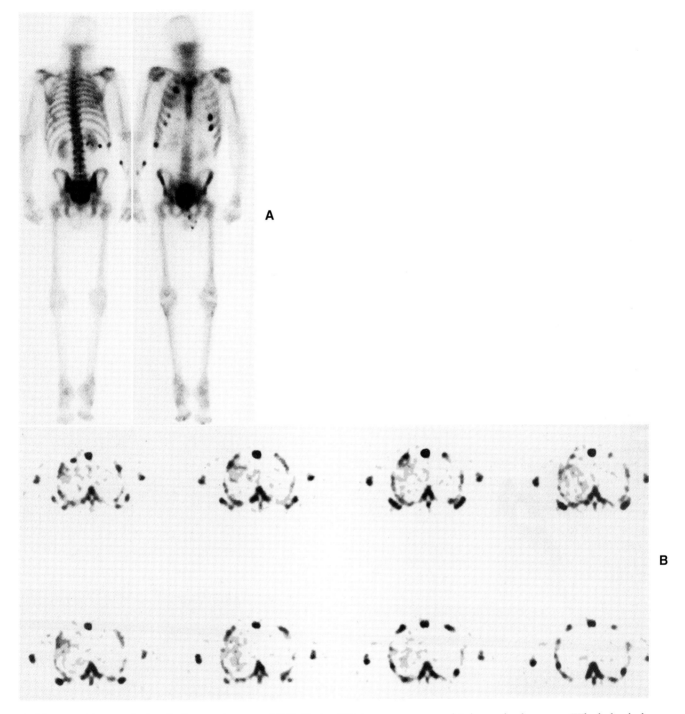

A 56-year-old was admitted after a seizure and fall. Brain CT demonstrates multiple cerebral masses. Whole body bone scan *(A)* and multiple transverse SPECT images of the chest *(B)* are shown.

1. Describe the skeletal abnormalities.

2. Describe any other abnormalities.

3. What is the most likely diagnosis?

4. Name 3 liver primary or metastatic tumors that have increased bone tracer uptake.

Skeletal System: Soft Tissue Uptake in Lung Mass

1. Focal abnormal uptake in the right and left anterior ribs, right upper posterior rib, and sternum.

2. Abnormal diffuse radiotracer uptake in the right upper chest on the anterior and posterior views, which does not conform to normal bone configuration. Selected SPECT images demonstrate the uptake to be in a large ovoid mass within the right lung.

3. Lung cancer with brain metastases. The bone scan abnormalities are likely traumatic because of the distribution and history of a fall.

4. A high percentage of neuroblastomas involving the liver have bone tracer uptake, and a much smaller percent of metastases from lung, breast, and colon cancer, especially mucinous cancers.

Reference

Peller PJ, Ho VB, Kransdorf MJ: Extraosseous Tc-99m MDP uptake: a pathophysiologic approach, *Radiographics* 13:715-734, 1993.

Cross-Reference

Nuclear Medicine: THE REQUISITES, ed 2, pp 124-125.

Comment

Bone scintigraphy may demonstrate abnormal soft tissue uptake in a wide variety of nonosseous disorders, including neoplastic, hormonal, inflammatory, ischemic, traumatic, excretory, and artifactual entities. Thoracic uptake on bone scans often is seen in patients with cancer of the lung. However, in contrast to this study, it is more commonly the result of pleural involvement and malignant pleural effusion. The distribution characteristically extends to the diaphragmatic costal margin, particularly if the patient is standing or sitting up. On the other hand, benign effusions typically cause attenuation and thus decreased uptake is seen on that side. Ascites can result in similar findings in the abdomen, with increased or decreased uptake depending on whether the peritoneal process is malignant or benign.

Metastatic tumors to the spleen occasionally show uptake on bone scanning. Patients with sickle cell disease often have splenic bone tracer uptake until the spleen atrophies. Primary breast cancers may have uptake, particularly if they are large or inflammatory. Preliminary studies suggest that the sensitivity for detection of primary breast cancer with bone radiotracers is similar to ^{99m}Tc sestamibi. Bilateral uptake is more likely the result of fibrocystic disease and other benign causes.

Notes

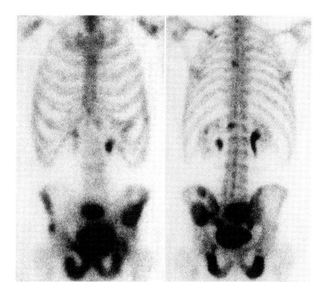

A 55-year-old man has low back pain and no prior history. Bone scan images, anterior and posterior views.

1. Provide a general distribution for the bone abnormalities.
2. Describe the findings.
3. List three factors that help limit the differential diagnosis.
4. What is the most likely diagnosis?

Skeletal System: Prostate Cancer Bone Metastases, Axial Distribution

1. Spine and pelvis.

2. Abnormal focal and regional activity is seen in multiple sites in the sacrum, both ilium, both inferior pubic rami, right superior pubic ramus, mid-thoracic and lower thoracic spine. Note the incidental calcification of costochondral cartilage.

3. Multiple lesions, axial predominance, older adult man.

4. Multiple skeletal metastases from prostate cancer.

Reference

Jacobson AF: Bone scanning in metastatic disease. In Collier BD Jr, Fogelman I, Rosenthall L, editors: *Skeletal nuclear medicine,* New York, 1996, Mosby, pp 90, 108-109.

Cross-Reference

Nuclear Medicine: THE REQUISITES, ed 2, pp 121-122.

Comment

In this case the findings of multiple lesions that are distributed in the axial skeleton, and not at sites that suggest degenerative change, suggest skeletal metastatic disease. With patient information (older man) and a knowledge of the most prevalent cancers, the most likely diagnosis can be determined. The pattern of bone metastases of most tumors (except primary lung cancers) shows a predominance in the axial skeleton and pelvis, although not exclusively. The distribution is not in proportion to arterial blood flow, suggesting that this is not the likely mode of dissemination of tumor emboli. General agreement exists that the vertebral venous plexus is an important factor in the predilection of bone metastases to the axial skeleton. Tumor cells originating below the diaphragm can move through the vertebral venous plexus to the pelvis, abdomen, and chest while bypassing the inferior vena cava. Interconnections between Batson's plexus and the intercostal veins provide a route of spread to ribs. Retrograde flow through the valveless plexus can occur from increased pressure resulting from coughing or straining. In this case, radiographs of the pelvis revealed multiple sclerotic lesions, and prostate biopsy confirmed the diagnosis.

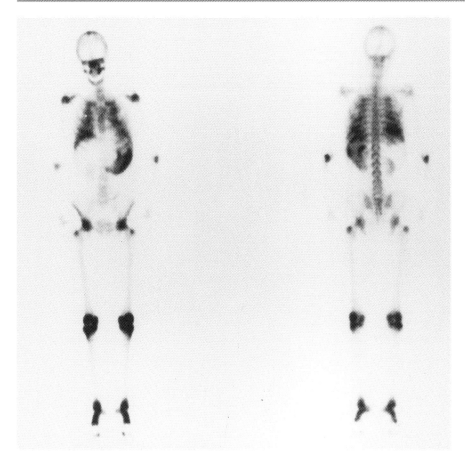

A 53-year-old woman with hypercalcemia was referred to rule out metastatic bone disease.

1. Describe the bone scan findings.
2. Give a differential diagnosis.
3. Provide the most likely diagnosis.
4. Could this pattern be caused by free ^{99m}Tc pertechnetate? Why?

Skeletal System: Hyperparathyroidism

1. Abnormal diffuse uptake in the lungs and stomach. Poor visualization of small kidneys and bladder, increased uptake in the shoulders, hips, knees, and ankles.

2. Hyperparathyroidism, metastatic calcification caused by hypercalcemia, renal failure or both, metabolic bone disease.

3. This particular pattern of metastatic calcification is characteristic of long-standing hyperparathyroidism. Although other causes of metabolic bone disease, e.g., osteomalacia and renal osteodystrophy, result in abnormal bone scans, they do not have this characteristic pattern. This scan pattern is seen in hyperparathyroidism.

4. Free ^{99m}Tc pertechnetate has gastric, thyroid, and salivary gland uptake. The latter two are not seen in this patient, who also shows large uptake.

Reference

Siegel BA, editor: *Nuclear radiology* (syllabus, second series), Reston, Va, 1978, American College of Radiology, pp 410-424.

Cross-Reference

Nuclear Medicine: THE REQUISITES, ed 2, pp 112, 121, 138.

Comment

The mechanism of altered bone radiotracer uptake in hyperparathyroidism is related to the increase in bone resorption and secondary increased bone turnover, causing increased osteoblastic activity in the skeleton with less radiotracer available for renal excretion. The bone scan in primary hyperparathyroidism often appears normal or may have subtle abnormalities of diffuse increased bone uptake detectable only by quantitative techniques. When present, bone scan abnormalities usually correspond to areas with radiographic demineralization or erosion, e.g., in the calvaria, mandible, acromioclavicular areas, sternum, lateral humeral epicondyles, and hands. If brown tumors are present, they typically show uptake. As the disease advances, extraskeletal mineralization of soft tissues can occur in the cornea, cartilage, joint capsules, tendons, and periarticular regions. Bone scans in patients with severe, long-standing hyperparathyroidism may have soft tissue uptake, characteristically in the lungs, stomach, and often kidneys as a result of metastatic calcification. Interestingly, all these organs with uptake are involved with acid-base metabolism. In addition, scintigraphy may show diffusely increased uptake in bone, low soft tissue, and renal activity, and prominent uptake in the skull, acromioclavicular joints, mandible, sternum, and the periarticular areas of large joints.

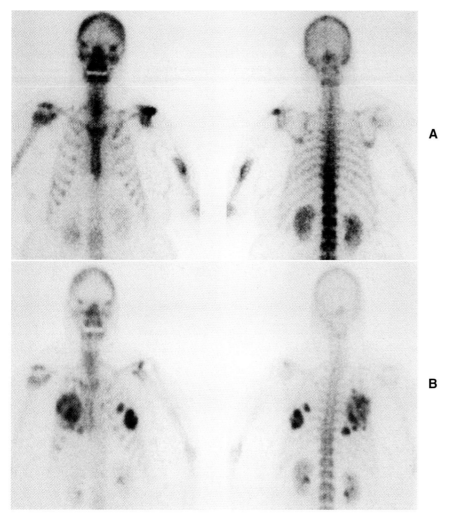

An initial bone scan *(A)* and repeat study 2 years later *(B)*.

1. Describe the bone scan abnormalities on the initial study *(A)*.

2. Describe the skeletal abnormalities on the follow-up study *(B)*.

3. List the differential diagnoses.

4. Provide the most likely diagnosis.

Bone: Osteosarcoma Metastatic to Lung

1. *A,* Abnormal decreased and increased uptake in the left humerus (proximal and mid, respectively).

2. *B,* Irregular uptake in the chest anterior and posterior views indicates location midway between in the lung parenchyma. Uptake is nodular and masslike. Rib abnormalities cannot be excluded, but the pathological condition extends across the rib spaces. Left shoulder arthroplasty is shown by photopenia.

3. The differential diagnosis for abnormal lung activity in a focal pattern includes primary lung tumors and metastases, especially for tumors with calcific or ossific components. For abnormal lung activity in a regional pattern, not evident in this case, the differential diagnosis includes malignant pleural effusion, fibrothorax, or radiation therapy-induced pneumonitis.

4. Osteosarcoma of the left proximal humerus, status/post-arthroplasty, with lung metastases.

References

Link MP, Eilber F: Osteosarcoma. In Pizzo PA, Poplack DG, editors: *Pediatric oncology,* Philadelphia, 1989, Lippincott, pp 706-707.

Sartoris DJ: *Musculoskeletal imaging: the requisites,* St Louis, 1996, Mosby, pp 244-254.

Cross-Reference

Nuclear Medicine: THE REQUISITES, ed 2, pp 126, 207.

Comment

Distant metastases are found at initial staging of osteosarcoma in only 2% of patients. Osseous metastases occur at a rate of 1% per month between 5 and 29 months after diagnosis, with a decrease in the rate thereafter. Before the advent of adjuvant chemotherapy, bone metastases usually were detected before pulmonary metastases. However, the natural course of the disease has been altered; bone metastases now appear before pulmonary metastases in only 15% of cases. Metastases to other sites, including liver, kidney, and lymph nodes, occasionally are demonstrated by skeletal scintigraphy.

The primary tumor and metastases avidly produce osteoid that results in bone tracer uptake. Although bone scintigraphy often can demonstrate lung metastases, both planar and SPECT imaging are less sensitive than CT for detection of lung metastases from osteosarcoma. The increasing use of surgical resections of lung metastases, especially in children, has contributed to improved survival. The most widely used excisional procedures for lung metastases are for osteosarcoma. The surgery is rather unique: the individual metastasis is excised with a minimal margin of surrounding lung tissue with the goal of preserving the maximum amount of lung tissue.

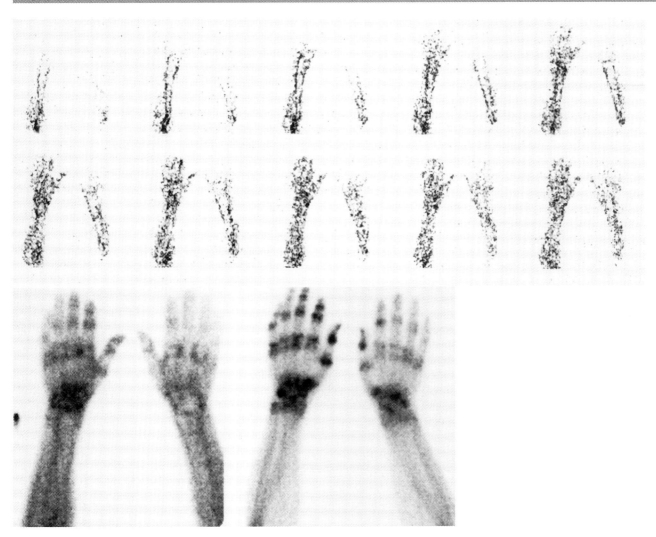

Diffuse upper extremity pain was noted 3 months after thoracotomy. Hand radiographs show normal findings. The remainder of the bone scan is normal.

1. Describe the scintigraphic bone scan findings in this case (palms down on the camera).

2. Provide the differential diagnosis.

3. What is the likely diagnosis in this case?

4. Discuss the pathogenesis.

Skeletal System: Reflex Sympathetic Dystrophy

1. Three-phase study demonstrates abnormal increased blood flow and blood pool of the distal right upper extremity. The delayed bone phase shows increased activity in the bones in the same distribution, with a striking increase in periarticular activity causing the joints to stand out.

2. Reflex sympathetic dystrophy syndrome (RSDS), disuse of a limb of new onset, e.g., recent stroke or immobilization by orthopedic cast or splint.

3. Shoulder-hand syndrome, a frequently encountered form of RSDS.

4. Neurogenic origin with loss of sympathetic autonomic tone is the generally accepted explanation, although not firmly established.

References

Sartoris DJ: *Musculoskeletal imaging: the requisites,* St Louis, 1996, Mosby, pp 290-292.

Fournier RS, Holder LE: Reflex sympathetic dystrophy: diagnostic controversies, *Semin Nucl Med* 28:116-123, 1998.

Cross-Reference

Nuclear Medicine: THE REQUISITES, ed 2, pp 136-137.

Comment

Other causes of increased periarticular uptake include inflammatory osteoarthritis, e.g., rheumatoid, early postarthroplasty changes, or prosthesis complicated by infection or loosening. However, these entities generally do not involve the entire limb, so they would be inappropriate considerations in this case. Also referred to as Sudeck's atrophy, or causalgia, reflex sympathetic dystrophy syndrome is an entity that includes pain, swelling, osteoporosis, and late atrophy of the limb. The cause is thought to be neurogenic, and often it is associated with trauma, surgery, or illness.

Radiographs may demonstrate soft tissue swelling and osteoporosis. Bone scintigraphy often demonstrates abnormalities before clinical or radiographic findings. Classically the entire distal extremity demonstrates scintigraphic abnormalities. The typical pattern of reflex sympathetic dystrophy is increased perfusion, blood pool, and uptake on delayed images in the affected extremity. Typically prominent and characteristic diffuse periarticular uptake is present. However, the perfusion and blood pool phases are not as reliable as the delayed images. Increased flow and blood pool is seen in approximately 50% of patients with RSDS, whereas more than 95% are abnormal on delayed images.

A   B

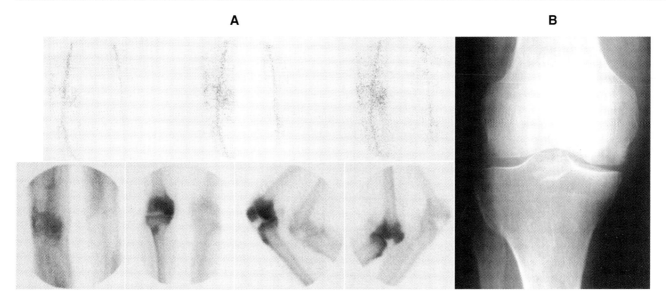

An elderly patient has had right knee pain for 3 months. Radiographs at onset were reported as normal.

1. Describe the bone scan findings. *A, above:* flow; *A, below:* blood pool and delayed images.

2. Based on the scan findings, provide a differential diagnosis.

3. A radiograph then was obtained *(B).* Given all available information, what is the most likely diagnosis?

4. What are common causes for this condition in the femoral head?

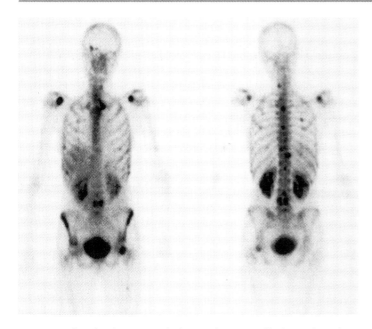

A patient has back pain and elevated serum alkaline phosphatase concentration.

1. What is the mechanism of uptake of bone scan agents?

2. Describe the bone findings. Describe any other soft tissue findings.

3. What is the most likely diagnosis?

4. List three possible primary neoplasms.

Skeletal System: Spontaneous Osteonecrosis of Distal Femur

1. Increased activity in the medial femoral condyle on all three phases of the bone scan.

2. Osteonecrosis, fracture, osteoarthritis, primary bone neoplasm (unlikely with prior normal radiograph).

3. Spontaneous osteonecrosis of the medial femoral condyle.

4. Trauma, steroid therapy, vasculitis, infarction (sickle cell, Gaucher's disease), alcoholic, caisson disease.

References

Sartois DJ: *Musculoskeletal imaging: the requisites,* St Louis, 1996, Mosby, p 25.

O'Mara RE: Benign bone disease. In Sandler MP, Coleman RE, Wackers FJTh, editors: *Diagnostic nuclear medicine,* ed 3, Baltimore, 1996, Williams & Wilkins, pp 669-705.

Cross-Reference
Nuclear Medicine: THE REQUISITES, ed 2, pp 32-34.

Comment

Juxtaarticular lesions that are three-phase positive on scintigraphy and result in subchondral sclerosis and deformity of the articular contour on radiographs include osteonecrosis and osteochondritis desiccans. Most bones have a dual blood supply that includes a network of periosteal vessels and one or more nutrient arteries that supply the marrow, the trabecular bone, and an endosteal portion of the cortex. Bones that lack the periosteal supply because they are covered with articular cartilage or enclosed within the joint capsule are more vulnerable to ischemic insults and osteonecrosis (also called avascular necrosis). Osteonecrosis can be idiopathic or result from an underlying cause. This patient demonstrates idiopathic osteonecrosis, a spontaneous disorder of the knee that occurs with sudden onset in older patients. It usually involves the medial femoral condyle. Bone scan abnormalities may precede the development of radiographic abnormalities, although they were present in this patient, probably because of the duration of symptoms. Osteonecrosis resulting from an underlying cause such as steroid use can create a similar pattern, but it usually involves multiple sites, including the medial and lateral femoral condyles, humeral and femoral heads, and talus. Osteochondritis dessicans is a condition that occurs in children and adults; it usually involves the lateral surface of medial femoral condyle, although it may involve other bones, including the talus and capitellum.

Notes

Skeletal System: Metastases to Bone and Liver

1. Uptake is dependent on blood flow and adsorption to the hydroxyapatite crystal.

2. Abnormal focal uptake in the skull, scapulae, ribs, spine, pelvis, and left femur. Diffuse uptake in the majority or entire liver.

3. Malignant metastases to bone and liver.

4. Breast, colon, lung.

Reference

Silberstein EB, McAfee JG, Spasoff AP: *Diagnostic patterns in nuclear medicine,* Reston, Va, 1998, Society of Nuclear Medicine, p 227.

Cross-Reference
Nuclear Medicine: THE REQUISITES, ed 2, pp 117-125.

Comment

Uptake on bone scans is very dependent on blood flow. The radiopharmaceutical must be delivered to the bone surface before uptake can occur. The amount of uptake depends somewhat on the amount of blood flow. The greater the flow, the higher the uptake. ^{99m}Tc phosphonates become adsorbed on the hydroxyapatite matrix of the bone. The radiopharmaceutical localizes in the mineral phase of bone at active sites of bone formation (remodeling), particularly at the osteoid mineral interfaces, and is incorporated into the crystalline structure. The binding sites for diphosphonates can be saturated by administration of diphosphonates.

The polyostotic distribution of multiple focal abnormalities strongly suggests skeletal metastases. To ascribe all the findings to one disease entity, the liver abnormality should be considered as an additional site of involvement. In addition, the long list of tumors that metastasize to bone and liver can be shortened by considering only those whose soft tissue metastases are likely to show uptake of bone radiotracer. Many of these are adenocarcinomas. Therefore the shortened differential diagnosis list includes common malignancies such as breast, colon, lung, and less common malignancies such as ovarian, and adenocarcinomas arising from other gastrointestinal organs, e.g., pancreas, gastric.

Notes

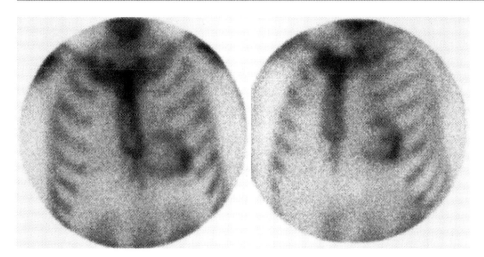

A bone scan was ordered because an elderly man "hurts all over." The remaining bone scan (not shown) was otherwise normal.

1. Describe the ^{99m}Tc disphosphonate bone scan findings.

2. In terms of anatomical location, where is the abnormal radiotracer uptake?

3. What other radiopharmaceutical would give a similar appearance?

4. What is the differential diagnosis?

Skeletal System: Myocardial Uptake

1. Curvilinear "horseshoe" pattern of uptake in the anterior chest that does not correspond to normal bony anatomy and therefore is most likely abnormal soft tissue uptake.

2. Cardiac uptake, either the myocardium or pericardium.

3. ^{99m}Tc pyrophosphate.

4. Idiopathic or secondary cardiomyopathy, e.g., due to cardiotoxic drugs, myocarditis, cardioversion injury, myocardial contusion, ventricular aneurysm, infarction, severe unstable angina, pericarditis with or without calcification, amyloidosis.

Reference

Gray HW: Soft tissue uptake of bone agents. In Collier BD, Fogelman I, Rosenthall L, editors: *Skeletal nuclear medicine,* St Louis, 1996, Mosby, p 383.

Cross-Reference

Nuclear Medicine: THE REQUISITES, ed 2, pp 105-107, 124-125.

Comment

Bone scanning agents have evolved over the past 40 years. Different ^{99m}Tc-labeled phosphorous-based radiopharmaceuticals have been developed. They can be classified on the basis of their phosphate linkage, e.g., polyphosphate (P-O-P), imidophosphates (P-N-P), pyrophosphates (P-P), and phosphonates (P-C-P). The image quality of polyphosphates was limited because of in vivo hydrolysis. This led to the use of the more stable P-N-P or P-C-P linkage compounds. The diphosphonates, which incorporate P-C-P grouping, are now the most commonly used skeletal agents. Pyrophosphate (P-P) is used when the question specifically relates to myocardial necrosis because the radiopharmaceutical has more soft tissue uptake, although the findings can be similar with both radiotracers. P-P is used when the electrocardiogram and enzyme study results are inconclusive. Large cerebral or intestinal infarcts also may show bone tracer uptake.

Normal uptake in nonosseous structures often is seen on bone imaging, including uptake in thyroid cartilage, calcifications in blood vessels, and calcified costal cartilages. Abnormal uptake occurs in patients with heterotopic calcification, rhabdomyolysis, and soft tissue calcification seen in scleroderma and dermatomyositis, in addition to more diffuse lung uptake caused by metastatic calcification, e.g., hyperparathyroidism, milk-alkali syndrome. Some primary and metastatic tumors characteristically take up bone radiotracers, e.g., metastatic osteosarcoma to the lung and neuroblastoma.

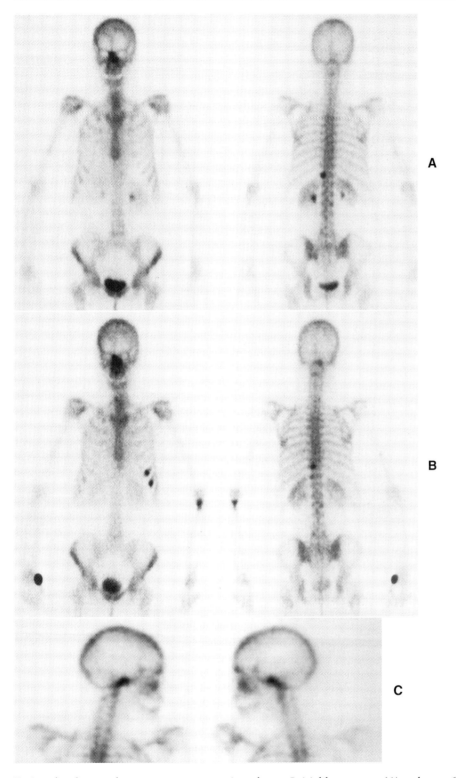

A

B

C

Patient has known breast cancer metastatic to bone. Initial bone scan *(A)* and scan 6 months later *(B* and *C)* are submitted.

1. Describe any interval change.
2. Describe the findings in *C.*
3. Where is the skull abnormality most likely located?
4. What is the most likely explanation?

Skeletal Metastases: Metastasis to Clivus

1. Increased intensity of activity is seen in the nasal region on the anterior view and midline occiput on the posterior view and left sixth and seventh costochondral junctions and left radial head uptake (not injection site).

2. The skull abnormally increased activity projects over the temporomandibular joint region on the right and left lateral skull images.

3. Skull base in the midline.

4. Metastasis to clivus; other skeletal metastases appear stable.

Reference

McAfee JG, Reba RC, Majd M: The musculoskeletal system. In Wagner HN, Szabo Z, Buchanan JW, editors: *Principles of nuclear medicine,* ed 2, Philadelphia, 1995, WB Saunders, pp 991-994.

Cross-Reference

Nuclear Medicine: THE REQUISITES, ed 2, p 121.

Comment

Recognition of the typical appearance and distribution of benign findings (e.g., degenerative and arthritic changes) is important for the correct identification of metastatic lesions. The findings in the clivus on the first scan were not initially interpreted as suspicious for metastasis. However, the lesion became more obvious on the subsequent examination and was associated with symptoms. Failure of response to therapy commonly is associated with an interval increase in the extent or intensity of a metastatic lesion, as in this case. However, "flare" caused by healing of metastases secondary to therapy can result in an increase in the intensity or extent of previously demonstrated lesions, or reveal "new" lesions that were scintigraphically occult on prior scans. Many benign lesions, e.g., fractures, show a decrease on serial examinations. Degenerative lesions frequently remain stable, although they can increase in intensity if they progress. However, the distribution and appearance of degenerative lesions is usually helpful but not always definitive.

This case is a good example of how triangulation of findings from orthogonal views is necessary for accurate location using planar images. This important principle also applies in interpretation of radiographs; the prevalence of cross-sectional techniques, e.g., CT, SPECT, should not dull our thinking.

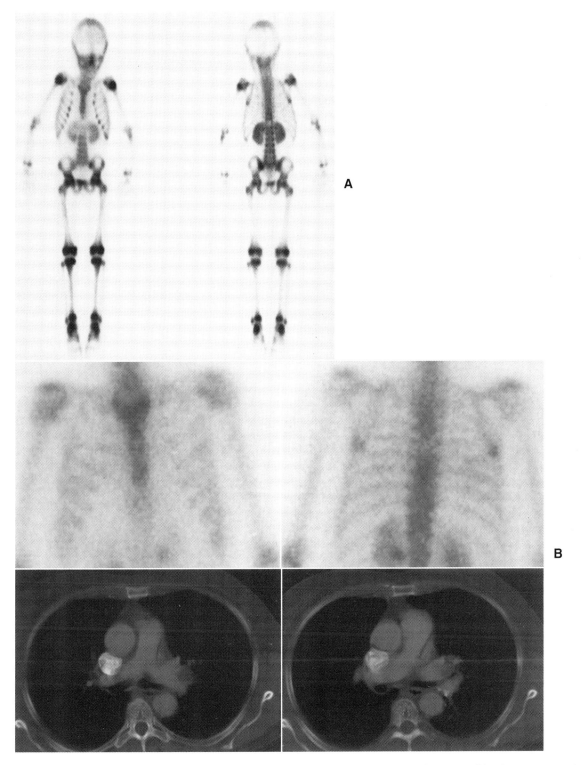

A

B

Two patients are shown. *A,* A 10-year-old boy was referred for a bone scan because of back pain. *B,* A 60-year-old man with new lung cancer. Bone scan and CT scan are provided.

1. Describe the bone scan findings in both patients.

2. Give a differential diagnosis for these abnormalities.

3. Describe the extraosseous soft tissue abnormality in *B.*

4. What are the two most likely causes for the soft tissue abnormality?

Skeletal System: Cold Spine Defects

1. *A,* Cold defect in T11. *B,* Decreased activity at approximately T6.

2. Benign or malignant tumor, osteomyelitis, avascular necrosis, congenital or surgical defect, artifact, radiation therapy.

3. Intense renal cortical uptake (cortical staining).

4. Nephrotoxic antibiotics or chemotherapeutic agents associated with interstitial nephritis.

References

Sopov V, Liberson A, Gorenberg M, et al: Cold vertebrae on bone scintigraphy, *Semin Nucl Med* 31:82-83, 2001.
Blickman H: *Pediatric radiology: the requisites,* ed 2, St Louis, 1998, Mosby, p 234.

Cross-Reference

Nuclear Medicine: THE REQUISITES, ed 2, pp 115-135.

Comment

Patient *A* had leukemia, the cause of the cold defect in this case. Patient *B* had a hemangioma. Common causes for a cold defect on bone scan are avascular necrosis, e.g., posttraumatic, sickle cell disease, but also radiation therapy, malignant tumors, particularly osteoclastic or lytic lesions, e.g., multiple myeloma, renal cell and thyroid cancer. Osteomyelitis may appear as a cold defect, particularly in children. Chordoma, plasmocytoma, and prior orthopedic surgery are other causes of cold defects. Attenuation may be caused by jewelry, belt buckles, clothing snaps, coins, or barium in the gastrointestinal tract.

Renal cortical uptake as a result of chemotherapy or nephrotoxic antibiotics is a common finding on bone scans, particularly in patients receiving nephrotoxic chemotherapy or antibiotics. High-grade bilateral renal obstruction may show this renal pattern. In that case, no activity would be seen in the bladder and background would be high. Patients with sickle cell anemia may have increased cortical uptake as a result of microcalcifications.

The CT shows an intact vertebral body with prominent trabeculae, widely spaced and sclerotic without soft tissue component. Hemangiomas often cause no symptoms and usually represent an incidental finding. On bone scans, they display the full spectrum of uptake, most commonly are isointense, and are unrecognized; however, they may be photopenic (as in *B*) or even have increased uptake. Intraosseous hemangiomas are most commonly found in the spine (75%) but also occur in skull and facial bones.

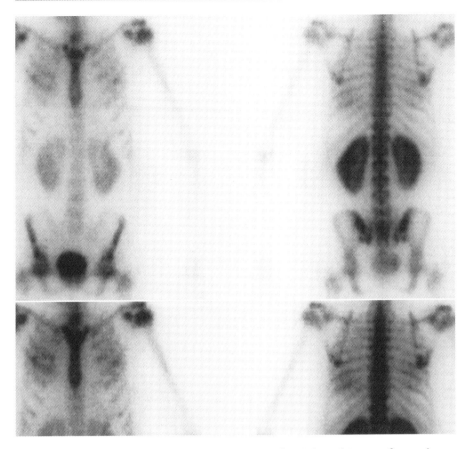

A patient has abnormal blood chemistry test results. Selected images from a bone scan are submitted printed in normal and dark modes.

1. Describe the findings.
2. Name two features that help to narrow the diagnosis.
3. List other findings outside the chest that can help to narrow the differential diagnosis.
4. Provide the most likely diagnosis.

Skeletal System: Metastatic Calcification in Lungs and Kidneys

1. Abnormal bilateral lung activity; increased activity in the renal parenchyma; kidneys appear enlarged.

2. The findings are bilateral and uniform. Two different organs are involved.

3. Tracer uptake in the stomach would suggest hyperparathyroidism.

4. Metastatic calcification caused by hypercalcemia associated with renal insufficiency.

Reference

Alderson PO, editor: *Nuclear radiology* (set 20, third series syllabus), Chicago, Ill, 1993, American College of Radiology, pp 564-579.

Cross-Reference

Nuclear Medicine: THE REQUISITES, ed 2, pp 112-115, 142-143.

Comment

Renal cortical uptake greater than the spine uptake is abnormal. It can be seen after radiation therapy and is thought to reflect ischemic tissue damage caused by radiation-induced vascular occlusion. Renal uptake also may be seen after therapy with cyclophosphamide (Cytoxan), vincristine (Oncovin), or doxorubicin (Adriamycin) and is seen most commonly within 7 days of therapy. It may be caused by a transient nephrotoxic response to the drugs. Abnormal retention may be seen in sickle cell anemia, other hemoglobinopathies, and iron overload syndromes.

In patients with diffuse lung uptake of ^{99m}Tc bone tracers due to hypercalcemia, calcium precipitates in the alveolar septa. Metastatic calcification occurs in the presence of renal failure when the solubility product for calcium and phosphate is exceeded. This process is reversible with the correction of the cause for hypercalcemia. The differential diagnosis for abnormal lung activity includes metastatic calcification, fibrothorax, metastases, pleural effusion, primary lung tumors, radiation therapy, and alveolar microlithiasis. Because the abnormality is diffuse, bilateral, and symmetrical, causes that typically are focal or unilateral can be discounted, narrowing the differential diagnosis to: metastatic calcification, alveolar microlithiasis, and radiation therapy. However, of those possibilities, only metastatic calcification would explain the findings in both the kidneys and the lungs.

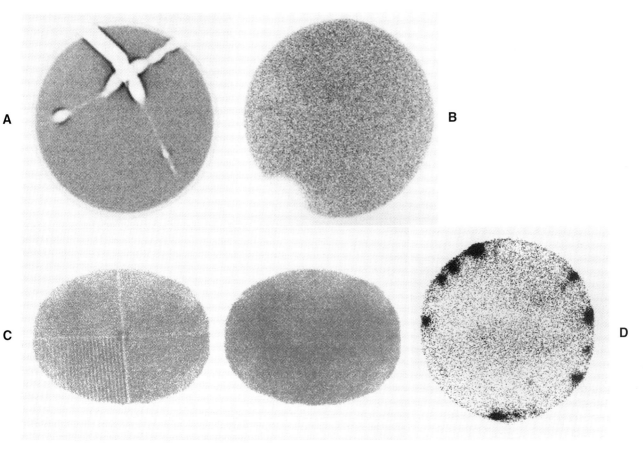

Provide the probable cause and give your recommendations for the abnormal gamma camera quality control floods.

1. A.

2. B.

3. C. Overnight change.

4. D. Change since prior patient that day.

Quality Control: Gamma Camera Floods

1. Cracked crystal (buy a new crystal).

2. Nonfunctioning photomultiplier tube (call service).

3. Distorted (not circular) and nonuniform image. Electronic tuning required. The power went off overnight. Call the service representative.

4. Contamination of crystal with radiopharmaceutical. (Clean camera or allow radiotracer to decay 10 half-lives.)

References

Alderson PO, Coleman RE, Grove RB, editors, et al: *Nuclear radiology* (syllabus, third series), Chicago, Ill, 1983, American College of Radiology, pp 18-31.

Patton JA: Quality assurance. In Sandler MP, Coleman RE, Wackers FJTh, et al, editors: *Diagnostic nuclear medicine,* ed 3, Baltimore, 1996, Williams & Wilkins, pp 18-31.

Cross-Reference

Nuclear Medicine: THE REQUISITES, ed 2, pp 27-30.

Comment

The gamma camera consists of a sodium iodine crystal optically coupled to an array of photomultiplier tubes. Gamma rays enter the crystal, undergo photoelectric and Compton interactions, and are absorbed. The gamma camera's response should be uniform across the field. However, the response is inherently nonuniform because of spatial distortions, systemic errors in location determination, variation in light transit efficiency, and so on. Digital microprocessors correct for this inherent nonuniformity. The output of the photomultiplier tubes are thereby adjusted to yield maximum uniformity.

Gamma camera quality control floods are performed on a daily basis each morning before patient studies. The method used varies. Daily floods are obtained either by placing a ^{99m}Tc source at a standard distance (3 to 5 feet) from the camera (usually hanging from above) with the collimator off (intrinsic flood). Alternatively, with the collimator on (extrinsic flood), the flood source is placed directly on the camera. ^{57}Co (122 keV, half-life 270 days) fixed in Plexiglas often is used or alternatively ^{99m}Tc is mixed in water and placed in a fillable Plexiglas disk.

The flood image from a well-tuned gamma camera with working photomultiplier tubes and uniformity correction circuitry should have a uniform appearance. The flood image evaluates the crystal, photomultiplier tubes, preamplifiers, pulse height analyzer, position electronics, and display system. The four-quadrant lead bar phantom (image C) is used to evaluate linearity and spatial resolution; weekly assessment is adequate. The bar phantom is placed between the source and the collimator.

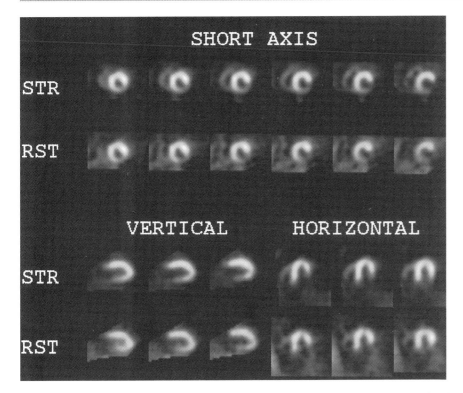

A 50-year-old patient with diabetes achieved 4.0 METS (metabolic equivalent) and 60% of maximum age-predicted heart rate (MPHR) on the exercise treadmill stress test.

1. When should the exercise treadmill stress test be discontinued?

2. Describe the myocardial stress and rest perfusion SPECT image findings.

3. Provide the differential diagnosis and likely involved vessel(s).

4. Discuss any other factor important to the interpretation of the scan.

Cardiovascular System: Inferior Lateral Wall Infarction

1. If the patient develops severe anginal chest pain, a decrease in blood pressure, frequent premature ventricular contractions (PVCs), or ST-T wave elevation suggestive of acute infarct. Also if the patient can walk no further on the treadmill because of general fatigue, leg pain, or dyspnea.

2. Severe stress and rest fixed defect in the basal lateral, inferior, and inferolateral walls, sparing the apex.

3. Myocardial infarction or possibly hibernation. Circumflex artery.

4. The exercise stress level.

Reference

Mayo Clinic Cardiovascular Working Group on Stress Testing: Cardiovascular stress testing: a description of the various types of stress tests and indications for their use, *Mayo Clinic Proc* 71:43-52, 1996.

Cross-Reference

Nuclear Medicine: THE REQUISITES, ed 2, pp 73-75.

Comment

The final report should include the qualifier that the patient had a low exercise threshold (4 METS and 60% MPHR). Inadequate exercise can decrease the sensitivity of the examination for detecting ischemia. The principle underlying stress perfusion imaging is that the degree of cardiac work must be sufficient to unmask ischemia abnormalities. The adequacy of exercise and the amount of cardiac work is indicated by the blood pressure and heart rate response. A double product (heart rate $\times$ systolic blood pressure) of greater than 25,000 is an indicator of adequate exercise. Another is achieving greater than 85% of the age-adjusted MPHR (220 − patient's age). Indirect measures of oxygen consumption frequently are used because oxygen uptake parallels cardiac work. At rest a healthy subject consumes approximately 3.5 ml/kg/min or 1 MET. A good correlation exists among oxygen uptake, METS, and exercise duration on the standard Bruce exercise protocol. Selecting a specific stress technique depends on local expertise and on the strengths and limitations of the techniques as they relate to the patient. Because exercise provides valuable cardiopulmonary information, treadmill stress testing generally is preferred to pharmacological stress. The Bruce protocol is the most common exercise protocol. However, other exercise protocols are available that use different workload increments. Exercise testing is usually maximal, i.e., discontinued because of physical symptoms, or may be submaximal, when exercise is discontinued at a lower work load because of concerns of patient safety, e.g., after myocardial infarction.

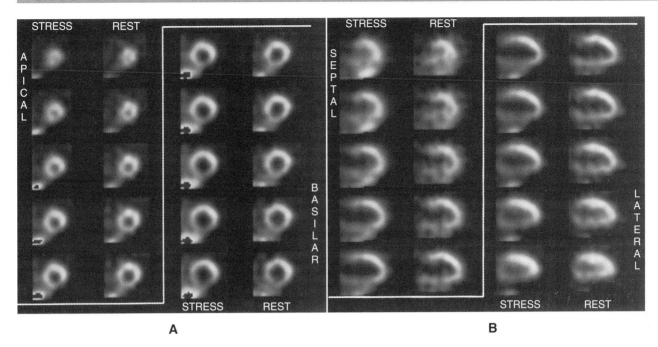

A

B

A 53-year-old man who had a recent myocardial infarction had a dipyridamole stress myocardial SPECT study before hospital discharge. SPECT short-axis *(A)* and vertical long-axis *(B)* images are shown.

1. Describe the SPECT findings.

2. Name the likely coronary artery or arteries involved.

3. Provide the differential diagnosis.

4. What prognostic information does the scan provide?

Cardiovascular System: Dipyridamole-Induced Reversible Inferior Wall Ischemia

1. A perfusion defect involving the entire inferior wall extending to the apex shows partial reversibility.

2. Right coronary artery.

3. Inferior wall ischemia with incomplete reversibility. The latter may represent scar (infarct) or hibernating myocardium.

4. The patient is at risk for a further cardiac event, either myocardial infarct or death.

Reference

Brown KA, Heller GV, Landin RS, et al: Early dipyridamole Tc-99m sestamibi SPECT imaging 2 to 4 days after acute myocardial infarction predicts in-hospital and postdischarge cardiac events: comparison with submaximal exercise imaging, *Circulation* 100:2060-2066, 1999.

Cross-Reference

Nuclear Medicine: THE REQUISITES, ed 2, pp 85, 392.

Comment

The SPECT images show reversibility, but a portion of the abnormality does not normalize. This raises the possibility that ischemic regions may coexist with areas of fibrosis or even hibernating myocardium, i.e., viable, but dysfunctional myocardium with reduced blood flow. The amount of viable myocardium could be further evaluated with metabolic imaging using FDG, a ^{201}Tl rest-rest study, or gated SPECT sestamibi images. Although FDG-PET is considered the gold standard, the other techniques can provide a good indication of myocardial viability.

The normal male pattern of myocardial perfusion shows decreased inferior wall uptake, which is attributed to diaphragmatic attenuation, meaning attenuation by soft tissue and organs below the diaphragm. This appears as a fixed defect and cannot always be differentiated from an inferior wall infarct. A gated SPECT study showing wall motion and myocardial thickening would confirm that it is caused by attenuation and not infarct.

Myocardial perfusion scintigraphy can be performed safely early after myocardial infarction using submaximal exercise treadmill stress or vasodilators. Dipyridamole can risk stratify patients better than submaximal exercise treadmill. The SPECT scan provides prognostic information for this patient. Multiple studies have shown that any rest perfusion abnormality and any stress-induced perfusion abnormality are independent adverse prognostic indicators. This patient is at risk for an adverse in-event (e.g., myocardial infarct or death). Consideration of revascularization is warranted.

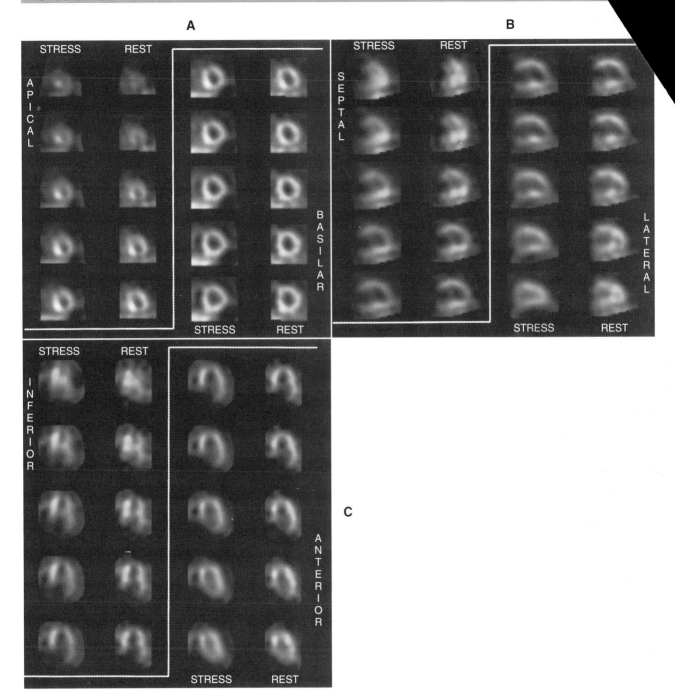

SPECT adenosine stress/rest myocardial perfusion images. SPECT short-axis *(A)*, vertical long-axis *(B)*, and horizontal long-axis *(C)* images are shown.

1. Describe the procedure for adenosine stress (a), adenosine's duration of action (b), and the procedure to deal with side effects of adenosine (c).

2. List contraindications to the use of intravenous adenosine.

3. Describe the SPECT findings and the diagnosis.

4. What are clinical indications for adenosine stress?

Adenosine Stress/
...teral Ischemia

...ously for 6 minutes
...es the radiotracer is
... continued for 3 more minutes.
...eared rapidly from the circulation
...conds). Return to baseline blood flow levels
...urs in 2 to 3 minutes after stopping the infusion. (c)
Stop the infusion.

2. Sinus node disease, second- or third-degree atrioventricular (AV) block, bronchospastic lung disease, adenosine allergy.

3. Small to moderately severe fixed defect at the apex on both stress and rest images consistent with infarct. Mildly improved perfusion of the anterior and lateral walls at rest compared with stress consistent with mild anterolateral ischemia.

4. Whenever adequate exercise stress is not possible.

Reference
Botvinick EH, editor: *Pharmacologic stress scintigraphy and associated topics* (Nuclear Medicine Self-Study Program III, Cardiology unit 2), Reston, Va, 1998, Society of Nuclear Medicine, pp 8-32.

Cross-Reference
Nuclear Medicine: THE REQUISITES, ed 2, pp 76-79, 85-86.

Comment
Adenosine, a potent coronary artery vasodilator, demonstrates regional disparity of coronary blood flow in patients with CAD. Partially occluded vessels cannot dilate to the same degree as normal vessels, thus producing nonuniform tracer distribution. The resulting images are similar to those obtained with exercise; however, the physiology is quite different. Exercise stress maximizes cardiac work to bring out ischemic regions of the heart. The accuracy of the two techniques is similar. Pharmacological stress is used in patients unable to exercise, e.g., those with claudication, severe arthritis, general fatigue, physical deconditioning, and so forth.

Theophylline-type drugs and caffeine block the effect of adenosine and dipyridamole and are thus prohibited before the study. Side effects of adenosine and dipyridamole are similar because both agents act through the stimulation of the adenosine receptors. Common side effects are chest pain, headache, and dizziness. The frequency of side effects is greater with adenosine, but their duration is short-lived and thus more easily controlled compared with dipyridamole. Conduction abnormalities may occur with adenosine: first-degree AV block in 10% of patients, transient second-degree block in 4%, and third-degree block in less than 1%. Again, because of its short duration of action, side effects are transient and generally not serious.

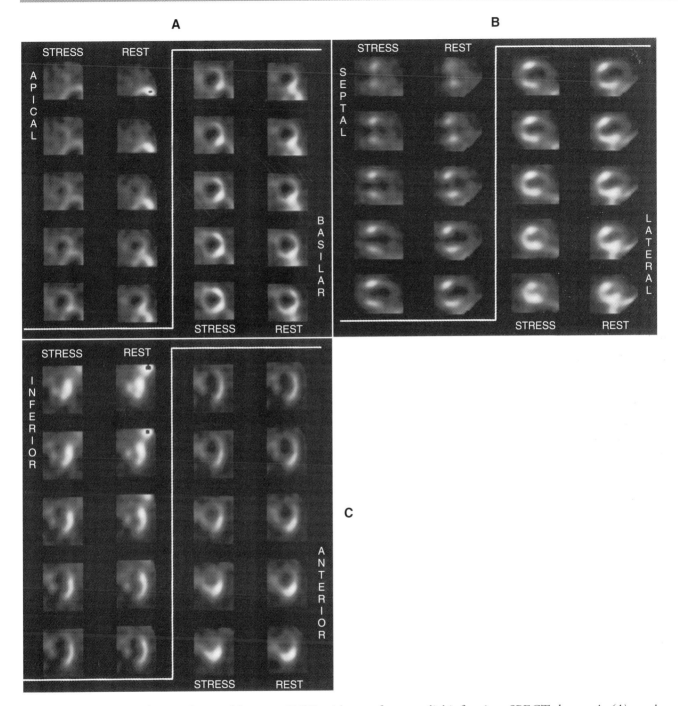

A
B
C

A 55-year-old man with CAD but no history or ECG evidence of myocardial infarction. SPECT short-axis *(A)*, vertical long-axis *(B)*, and horizontal long-axis *(C)* are shown.

1. Describe the findings on the SPECT.

2. Provide the differential diagnosis.

3. Describe the blood flow and functional state of hibernating myocardium.

4. Describe the blood flow and functional state of stunned myocardium.

C A S E 8 6

Cardiovascular System: Viability, Fixed LAD Defect

1. Extensive fixed defects involving the anterior wall, apex, septum, extending to the lateral wall.

2. Myocardial infarction versus hibernating myocardium

3. In hibernating myocardium, blood flow and function, e.g., contractility, are chronically reduced.

4. Blood flow is normal, recently restored after an acute occlusive state; function is reduced.

Reference

Botvinick EH, editor: *Cardiac PET imaging* (Nuclear Medicine Self-Study Program III, Cardiology unit 3), Reston, Va, 1998, Society of Nuclear Medicine, pp 32-49.

Cross-Reference

Nuclear Medicine: THE REQUISITES, ed 2, pp 89, 92.

Comment

Hibernating myocardium is chronically and severely ischemic tissue that is viable, but has fixed reduced perfusion and is non-functional on gated SPECT, echocardiography, or MRI. Hibernation may persist for a prolonged period, until progression to infarction, or preferably revascularization, occurs. Different radiopharmaceuticals can be used to evaluate for the presence of viable muscle. The nonischemic heart uses free fatty acids for its metabolism, whereas the ischemic heart uses glucose. Thus FDG, a glucose analogue, provides an ideal method for making this distinction. Methods using FDG include imaging with dedicated PET cameras, hybrid SPECT-PET coincidence systems, or even noncoincidence SPECT using high-energy collimators. Methods using single photon emitters include ^{201}Tl rest-rest imaging and gated SPECT using ^{99m}Tc-labeled perfusion agents to evaluate wall motion.

Stunned myocardium is viable myocardium in the immediate postocclusion phase and typically is seen after acute intervention to improve blood flow in the setting of impending infarction, e.g., patients who have recently received thrombolytic therapy or acute angioplasty. Normal or increased radiopharmaceutical uptake is seen; however, the stunned segment has decreased function. Depending on the severity and duration of the occlusive event, the area may return to normal or be permanently damaged. The period of stunning usually is short, generally a period of a few weeks. Stunning is not commonly seen on perfusion imaging because it is recommended that a myocardial perfusion study should not be performed until several weeks after angioplasty.

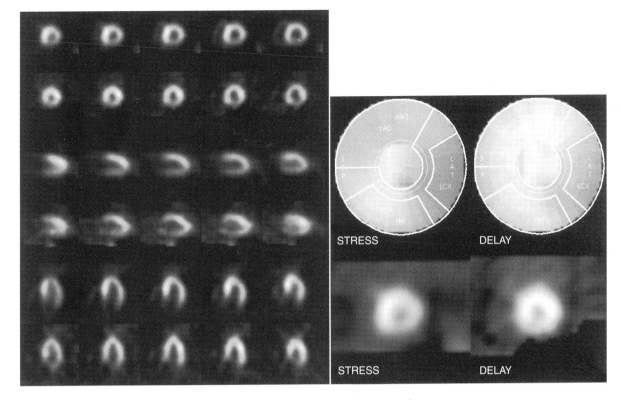

1. Describe the bull's-eye format for SPECT myocardial perfusion studies.

2. List possible errors that may occur when applying a bull's-eye quantitative analysis technique to myocardial perfusion SPECT.

3. Describe the findings and the likely culprit coronary artery or arteries. Does the bull's-eye plot confirm the image findings?

4. List the characteristics of perfusion scan abnormalities that should be included in any report.

Cardiovascular System: Bull's-Eye, Reporting Results

1. A polar plot is constructed by layering short-axis slices one on top of the other, with the apex forming the center and the base of the heart being the outermost portion.

2. Misregistration/misalignment, use of inappropriate reference database.

3. Stress: hypoperfusion of the anterior, lateral, and inferior walls. Rest, normalized perfusion of the anterior and lateral walls and incomplete normalization of the inferior wall. Most consistent with ischemia of the left circumflex and infarct of the right coronary artery. The bull's-eye confirms the image findings.

4. Include location and extent, severity, and reversibility for each perfusion abnormality. If gated SPECT is performed, include LVEF, wall motion, with or without wall thickening fractions. Note ancillary signs of significant CAD, e.g., increased ^{201}Tl lung activity, or stress-induced dilation of the left ventricle, if present.

References

Cooke CD, Faber TL, Areeda JS, et al: Advanced computer methods in cardiac SPECT. In DePuey G, Garcia EV, Berman DS, editors: *Cardiac SPECT imaging*, ed 2, Philadelphia, 2001, Lippincott Williams & Wilkins, pp 65-80.

Watson DD: Quantitative SPECT techniques, *Semin Nucl Med* 29:298-318, 1999.

Cross-Reference

Nuclear Medicine: THE REQUISITES, ed 2, pp 78-79.

Comment

Polar maps or bull's-eye displays were developed to illustrate the normalized stress and rest data of the entire left ventricle in a single picture. The display is produced by layering short-axis slices one on top of the other with the apex forming the center and the base of the heart the periphery. Circumferential count profiles from all slices are combined into a color-coded image, allowing for a quick and comprehensive overview. The points of each circumferential profile are assigned a color based on normalized count values. Abnormal areas can be identified at a glance. The bull's eye is most useful if it includes quantification of the degree of perfusion defects and percent change from rest to stress (not shown here). However, this requires a normal database for comparison, which is supplementary software available for purchase from commercial vendors. Reference normal databases should be generated in each institution's laboratory or another laboratory with similar equipment, technique, and patient population. As in all areas of nuclear medicine, quantitative data should be used only as an adjunct to image analysis and not interpreted in isolation. Now, three-dimensional quantitative displays also are available.

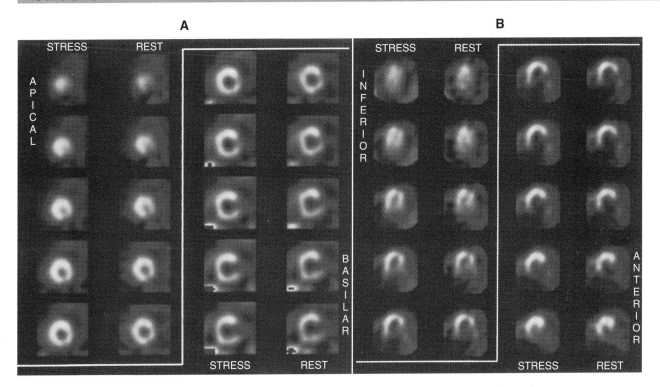

A patient had atrial fibrillation and high baseline resting heart rate. The patient exercised for only 3.5 minutes, achieved only 3.0 METS, but reached 100% of age-predicted maximum heart rate. SPECT short-axis *(A)* and horizontal long-axis perfusion images *(B)*.

1. Describe any perfusion abnormalities.

2. Describe any other findings.

3. What is the most likely culprit coronary artery?

4. Discuss the significance of failure to achieve adequate exercise.

Cardiovascular System: Inadequate Stress

1. Severe fixed defect involving the entire lateral wall.

2. Dilated left ventricular cavity at both stress and rest.

3. Left circumflex coronary artery.

4. False-negative studies for ischemia may result.

Reference

Yao SS, Rozanski A: Myocardial perfusion scintigraphy in conjunction with exercise and pharmacologic stress: prognostic applications in the clinical management of patients with coronary artery disease. In DePuey EG, Garcia EV, Berman DS, editors: *Cardiac SPECT imaging,* Philadelphia, 2001, Lippincott Williams & Wilkins, pp 263-296.

Cross-Reference

Nuclear Medicine: THE REQUISITES, ed 2, p 75.

Comment

Failure to achieve adequate exercise stress can result in false-negative studies for ischemia. Significant coronary stenoses involving less than 90% of vessel diameter may appear as normal regional perfusion under resting conditions. Because flow reserve across a fixed stenosis is limited, augmentation of blood flow by exercise or pharmacological intervention is necessary to unmask blood flow heterogeneity caused by coronary artery stenosis. Even if ischemia is demonstrated, it may be underestimated in extent or severity without adequate stress. Therefore the dictated report should include a qualification indicating that the patient reached a low exercise threshold, which could decrease the sensitivity of the examination for demonstration of ischemia. In this patient with rapid atrial fibrillation, the fact that he achieved greater than 85% of age-predicted maximum heart rate is not an indicator of adequate cardiac workload because it was increased at baseline. The low METS is consistent with low workload and short exercise duration.

Medications can result in a false-negative scan. β-Blockers can prevent the achievement of maximum heart rate during exercise. Nitrates or calcium channel blockers may mask or prevent cardiac ischemia. In some cases, it may not be feasible for the patient to stop the medications. At other times, medications are deliberately continued to assess the adequacy of drug therapy in blocking ischemia. In those circumstances, detection of CAD is not the goal, as these patients are already being treated medically for CAD.

Notes

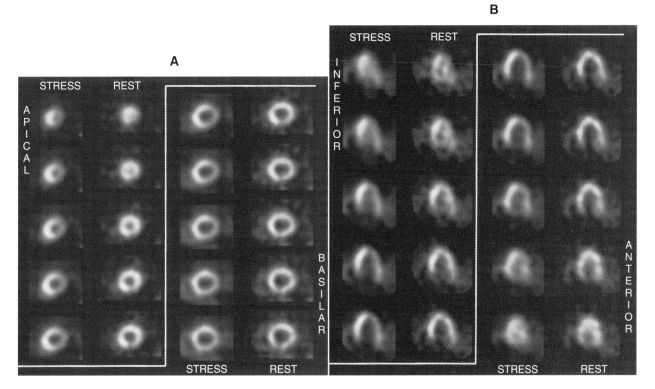

A 60-year-old patient with diabetes has severe chronic obstructive pulmonary disease (COPD) and uses a walker; he denies chest pain. Short-axis *(A)* and horizontal long-axis *(B)* SPECT myocardial perfusion images are presented.

1. What form of stress is indicated for this patient and why?

2. Describe the perfusion abnormalities.

3. What is the likely culprit coronary artery?

4. Explain the discrepancy between the findings and patient's lack of symptoms.

Cardiac: Silent Lateral Wall Ischemia

1. Dobutamine. The need of a walker precludes adequate exercise stress, and COPD is a contraindication to adenosine or dipyridamole use.

2. Moderately severe perfusion defect involving the entire lateral wall extending to the anterolateral, inferolateral regions, and apex on the stress images that nearly normalizes on the rest images. Incomplete reversibility of small portion of inferior wall.

3. Left circumflex coronary artery.

4. Silent myocardial ischemia.

Reference

Iskander S, Iskandrian AE: Risk assessment using single-photon emission computed tomographic technetium-99m sestamibi imaging, *J Am Coll Cardiol* 32:57-62, 1998.

Cross-Reference

Nuclear Medicine: THE REQUISITES, ed 2, pp 85-86.

Comment

Silent myocardial ischemia is defined as the presence of significant CAD without anginal symptoms. Thus coronary disease may go undetected until severe consequences have occurred, such as massive myocardial infarction, ischemic cardiomyopathy, or death. Patients with diabetes are at increased risk for silent ischemia as a result of autonomic neuropathy. Studies have shown that any perfusion abnormality or any stress-induced perfusion abnormality is an independent adverse prognostic indicator. Based on the scan findings, this patient is at risk for an adverse event (e.g., acute myocardial infarct, or death) in spite of the lack of anginal symptoms. Consideration of further revascularization is warranted.

In this case, coronary vasodilator stress with dipyridamole or adenosine is contraindicated because of the severe COPD because the drugs may induce bronchospasm. Dobutamine is a synthetic catecholamine that increases cardiac workload by increasing the heart rate and blood pressure. This patient is a typical candidate for dobutamine, i.e., one who cannot exercise and has bronchospastic pulmonary disease. Before stress, a patient should be checked for relative contraindications to dobutamine such as recent myocardial infarction or unstable angina, hemodynamically significant left ventricular outflow tract obstruction, atrial tachyarrhythmias, ventricular tachycardia, uncontrolled hypertension, aortic dissections, or large aneurysms.

Notes

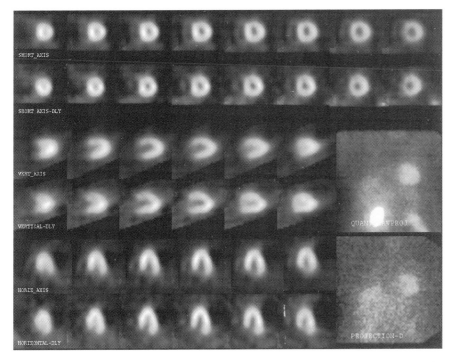

A 55-year-old woman with abnormal baseline ECG and left bundle branch block (LBBB) is sent for a stress dual-isotope SPECT study. LVEF and wall thickening by gated SPECT are normal.

1. Name the appropriate stress technique.

2. List stress methods that would be disadvantageous in this patient and state the reason.

3. Discuss the physiological advantage of adenosine or dipyridamole compared with other stress methods.

4. Describe the scintigraphic findings.

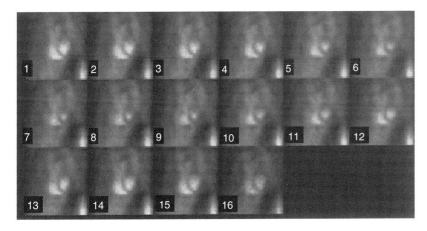

Gated radionuclide ventriculogram (RVG or MUGA) was performed.

1. Name the radiopharmaceutical used.

2. List methods for preparation of this radiopharmaceutical.

3. Describe the methodologies of radiolabeling.

4. List the advantages and disadvantages of the different labeling methods.

CASE 90

Cardiovascular System: LBBB

1. Dipyridamole or adenosine.

2. Exercise or dobutamine. Methods of stress that result in increased heart rate can be associated with false-positive findings of septal reversibility (identical to isolated septal ischemia) in patients with LBBB.

3. These agents do not result in an increase in heart rate.

4. The mild decreased activity in the anterior wall appears fixed and likely is caused by breast attenuation in light of the reported normal wall motion.

Reference

DePuey EG: Artifacts in SPECT myocardial perfusion imaging. In Gordon EG, Garcia EV, Berman DS, editors: *Cardiac SPECT imaging,* ed 2, Philadelphia, 2001, Lippincott Williams & Wilkins, pp 232-262.

Cross-Reference

Nuclear Medicine: THE REQUISITES, ed 2, pp 66-86.

Comment

Exercise-induced reversible perfusion defects involving the septum mimicking septal ischemia are seen in 30% to 90% of patients with LBBB. One theory postulates that the decrease in septal blood flow occurs because of asynchronous relaxation of the septum related to this conduction abnormality. Coronary blood flow occurs primarily during diastole; therefore flow to the septum is compromised by its asynchrony and by the shortening of diastole at high heart rates. At rest when the heart rate is not increased, no regional disparity in radiotracer activity is apparent, so the defect appears reversible. Perfusion defects caused by LBBB without coronary artery disease spare the apex and anterior wall.

Both exercise and dobutamine increase cardiac work by increasing myocardial oxygen demand as a result of increasing the heart rate and systolic blood pressure and contractility. Therefore these stress methods should not be used in patients with LBBB because the scan may be falsely positive for septal ischemia. However, regardless of the stress method, stress-induced perfusion abnormalities outside the septum have the same significance as in patients without LBBB and indicate coronary artery disease. Abnormal septal wall motion on gated images almost invariably is seen after CABG surgery as a result of disruption of the pericardium in the absence of LBBB.

Notes

CASE 91

Cardiovascular System: RBC Labeling for RVG/MUGA

1. ^{99m}Tc-labeled RBCs.

2. In vivo, modified in vivo, and in vitro methods.

3. In vivo: stannous pyrophosphate is administered intravenously, followed in 15 to 30 minutes by ^{99m}Tc pertechnetate. Modified in vitro: stannous pyrophosphate is administered intravenously and 15 to 30 minutes later, 3 to 5 ml of blood is withdrawn into an attached shielded syringe containing ^{99m}Tc pertechnetate and an anticoagulant, either acid-citrate-dextrose (ACD) or heparin. The blood is incubated for 10 minutes and periodically agitated, then infused. The syringe is left attached to the indwelling intravenous line during the procedure so that the entire system is closed. In vitro: blood is withdrawn and placed in a closed vial containing stannous chloride and sodium hypochlorite to oxidize excess extracellular stannous ion and prevent extracellular reduction of ^{99m}Tc pertechnetate. Labeling occurs when ^{99m}Tc pertechnetate is added, followed by a 20-minute incubation before reinjection of labeled cells.

4. The in vivo method is simplest and least costly, but has the lowest labeling efficiency. The in vitro kit method (UltraTag) has the highest labeling efficiency but requires more time, technologist effort, and cost.

Reference

Chilton HM, Callahan RJ, Thrall JH: Radiopharmaceuticals for cardiac imaging: myocardial infarction, perfusion, metabolism, and ventricular function (blood pool). In *Pharmaceuticals in medical imaging,* New York, 1990, Macmillan, pp 442-450.

Cross-Reference

Nuclear Medicine: THE REQUISITES, ed 2, pp 93-94.

Comment

With the in vivo approach, labeling efficiency ranges between 60% and 80%. The presence of free ^{99m}Tc pertechnetate contributes to increased background activity and erroneous calculation of the LVEF. With the modified in vivo technique, labeling efficiency is approximately 90%, and with the in vitro method, 95% to 98%. Various causes exist for poor RBC labeling. The most common are drug-drug interactions, e.g., with heparin, doxorubicin, methyldopa, hydralazine, iodinated contrast media, and quinidine. Other causes include circulating antibodies from prior transfusions, transplantation, and some antibiotics. Finally, insufficient or too great a dose of stannous ion, too short a "tinning" interval, and too short an incubation period for reduction of technetium (VII).

Notes

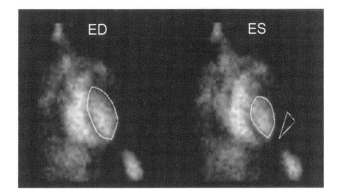

1. Describe and explain the processing performed on this equilibrium gated RVG or MUGA study.

2. How are the regions of interest (ROIs) selected?

3. List the nuclear medicine techniques by which left ventricular function can be assessed.

4. Provide the equation for determination of LVEF.

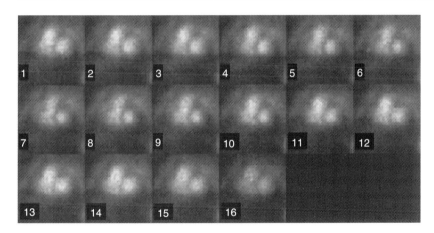

Radionuclide planar gated blood pool study. Sequential gated image frames are shown.

1. Estimate the left ventricular ejection fraction (LVEF) based on the submitted images and explain the decreased intensity of image No. 16.

2. Discuss the importance of patient positioning on calculation of the LVEF.

3. List factors that may result in reduced accuracy of the LVEF calculation.

4. Describe the effect on the LVEF if *(A)* no background is subtracted; *(B)* a background region is used that includes the spleen.

Cardiac: Calculation of LVEF for RVG (MUGA)

1. Left anterior oblique end-diastolic and end-systolic images show left ventricular and background (bkg) ROIs drawn on computer for calculation of the LVEF.

2. Acquisition in the left anterior oblique (LAO) view with greatest separation of the left and right ventricle. ROI for the left ventricle at end-systole, at end-diastole, and for adjacent background.

3. Equilibrium gated blood pool (RVG); first-pass radionuclide ventriculography; gated perfusion SPECT.

4. LVEF = end-diastolic counts − end-systolic counts/end-diastolic counts (corrected for bkg counts).

Reference

Borges-Neto S, Coleman RE: Radionuclide ventricular function analysis, *Radiol Clin North Am* 31:817-830, 1993.

Cross-Reference

Nuclear Medicine: THE REQUISITES, ed 2, pp 93-101, 103-104.

Comment

The most common technique to assess ventricular function without perfusion imaging is the equilibrium gated RVG or MUGA. The patient's heart rhythm is electrically gated. Each cardiac cycle is divided into at least 16 frames to maximize temporal resolution so that end-diastolic and end-systolic frames can be identified for LVEF quantification. To obtain sufficient counts for high-quality images, approximately 300 cardiac cycles are acquired after ^{99m}Tc RBC equilibration in the blood. The first-pass radionuclide angiocardiogram (RNA) method quantifies ventricular function during radiotracer bolus transit through the heart, approximately six cardiac cycles. These volume-based methods (radioactive counts are proportional to ventricular volume) are more accurate than geometric methods e.g., echocardiography or contrast ventriculography.

For calculation of LVEF, an ROI is drawn around the ventricle in end-diastole and end-systole. A background ROI is placed between the left ventricle and the spleen. Normal LVEF range from 55% to 75%. Many laboratories use 50% as the lower limit of normal. Calculation of right ventricular ejection fraction (RVEF) using the gated blood pool technique is subject to error caused by overlap of the atria and ventricles; first-pass RNA is superior because RVEF is calculated using only cycles that the bolus resides within the right ventricle. SPECT is potentially more accurate than the planar MUGA because selected ROIs minimize overlap of the atria and ventricles, but it is difficult to justify the extra procedure when planar imaging performs so well.

Notes

Cardiovascular System: RVG/MUGA Technique

1. LVEF appears normal (>55%). End-systolic at Frame 8. Frame 16 shows decreased intensity compared with other frames, resulting from variability in the patient's heart rate, e.g., frequent PVCs.

2. The left anterior oblique (LAO) position selected is that which provides the best separation of the left and right ventricles, approximately a 45-degree LAO view, but varies depending on the patient's anatomy (best septal view).

3. Patient-related factors: arrhythmia, inability to gait, suboptimal RBC labeling, e.g., concomitant drugs. Technique-related: poor LAO positioning, suboptimal RBC labeling; incorrect ROI for left ventricle or background.

4. *A,* Falsely low; *B,* falsely high.

References

Borer JS: Measurement of ventricular function and volume. In Zaret BL, Beller GA, editors: *Nuclear cardiology,* St Louis, 1999, Mosby, pp 201-215.

Borges-Neto S, Coleman RE: Radionuclide ventricular function analysis, *Radiol Clin North Am* 31:817-830, 1993.

Cross-Reference

Nuclear Medicine: THE REQUISITES, ed 2, pp 93-101.

Comment

The images represent the frames into which the R-R interval was divided using simultaneous cardiac gating. By visual estimation the LVEF appears normal (calculated to be 65%). The radionuclide equilibrium gated blood pool and first-pass techniques are accurate methods for measuring the LVEF because calculation is based on volume changes and not geometric assumptions of cardiac shape as are contrast ventriculography and echocardiography. A limitation of the gated blood pool technique is cardiac arrhythmia. The LVEF becomes less reliable when the R-R interval is highly irregular. When ventricular premature beats occur in more than one of every six beats, quantification must be suspect. Overestimation of background activity falsely elevates the LVEF, and underestimation of background activity depresses the LVEF. The error in LVEF that results from mild arrhythmia is not significant because most of the beat length variability occurs at the end of the cycle. When the R-R interval varies, fewer counts are shown in the terminal frames. The drop-off in the intensity may appear as a flicker when viewing the gated images in cinematic display.

Notes

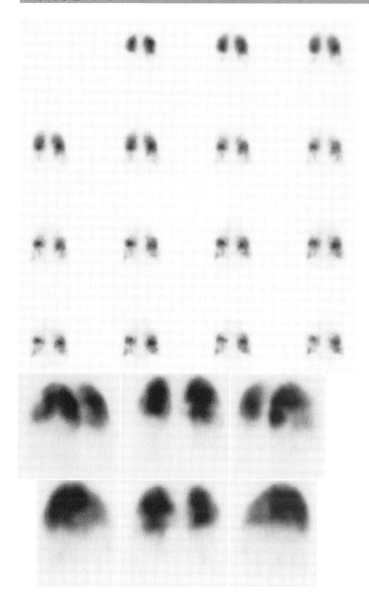

A 35-year-old man with increasing dyspnea was referred for ventilation-perfusion (V/Q) study. The chest film was clear of infiltrate, mass, or pleural disease.

1. Name the three phases of a ^{133}Xe ventilation scan.

2. Describe the phases.

3. Describe the findings on the ventilation and perfusion scans.

4. Provide an interpretation and offer a diagnosis for the underlying disease.

CASE 94

Pulmonary System: Emphysema Caused by α_1-Antitrypsin Deficiency

1. Single breath or wash-in, equilibrium, and washout phases.

2. Single breath: patient breathes in and holds a single maximum deep inspiration while a 100,000-count image is acquired. Equilibrium: patient breathes a mixture of air and xenon while serial images are obtained every 60 to 90 seconds for 3 minutes. Washout: patient breathes room air and exhales xenon while serial images are obtained.

3. Ventilation: nonuniform in the upper lung zones bilaterally. Initially near absent at the bases. As upper lobes wash out, xenon fills and is retained in both bases indicating severe air trapping. Perfusion: heterogeneous to both upper lung zones that match the early ventilation images. The extensive perfusion abnormalities in both lower lung zones are matched with areas of washout air trapping.

4. Low probability for pulmonary embolism, α_1-antitrypsin deficiency.

Reference

Armstrong P, Wilson AG, Dee P, et al: *Images of diseases of the chest,* ed 3, St Louis, 2000, Mosby, p 932.

Cross-Reference

Nuclear Medicine: THE REQUISITES, ed 2, pp 147-148, 154-157.

Comment

^{133}Xe, an inert gas, demonstrates the abnormal physiology of obstructive airway disease. Initially, decreased and delayed xenon wash-in is followed by slow washout or trapping of gas. The wash-in phase distribution corresponds to ^{99m}Tc aerosol particle images. The advantage of ^{133}Xe is that the washout phase is very sensitive for obstructive airway disease. Disadvantages of ^{133}Xe are that images can be obtained only in one view (two if two-headed camera). The study is best done before the perfusion study because of the low ^{133}Xe energy photopeak (80 keV). Emphysema is a lung disease characterized pathologically by abnormal permanent enlargement of air spaces distal to the terminal bronchial accompanied by destruction of the walls without obvious fibrosis. Panlobular emphysema is associated with α_1-antitrypsin deficiency, although it may occur in smokers and elderly patients. Upper lobe air trapping is seen with the more common chronic obstructive pulmonary disease. Lower lobe air trapping is suggestive of α_1-antitrypsin deficiency. α_1-Antitrypsin is a serum protein that inhibits lysosomal proteases released during inflammatory reactions and prevents their damaging effects. Patients with reduced levels of α_1-antitrypsin are at risk for emphysema. Smoking further increases this risk.

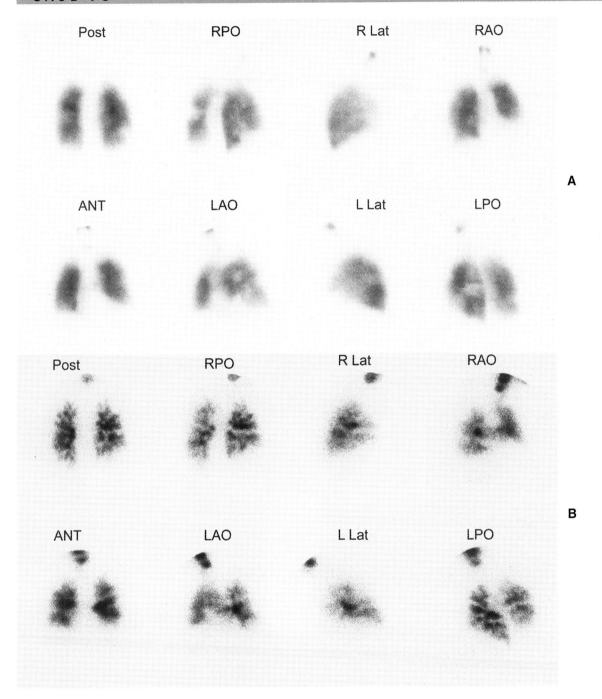

A 64-year-old man has recent onset of shortness of breath. The chest x-ray was clear.

1. Describe the image findings *(A,* perfusion; *B,* ventilation) and give an interpretation.

2. What is the ventilation study radiopharmaceutical, and what is its mechanism of distribution? What are the likely reasons for their appearance on this study?

3. Is the ventilation or perfusion study usually performed first and why?

4. What is another commonly used ventilation radiopharmaceutical that could be used, and what are the advantages and disadvantages?

Pulmonary System: ^{99m}Tc DTPA Ventilation Study with Aerosol Clumping

1. Multiple perfusion defects in upper and lower lung fields. Many appear segmental, e.g., the lateral basal of the right lower lobe, superior segment of the left lower lobe. Ventilation study shows extensive diffuse "clumping" within the airways throughout both lung fields making determination of matching or mismatching difficult. The study was interpreted as intermediate probability since the ventilation study could not be interpreted; however, the segmental perfusion defect pattern is suspicious for embolus.

2. ^{99m}Tc DTPA aerosol particles (0.1 to 0.5 μm in size) normally distribute on first impact within the alveoli. With airway turbulence, e.g., asthma or COPD, particles impact proximally within bronchi and appear as focal hot spots.

3. ^{99m}Tc DTPA aerosol ventilation study usually is performed first. The patient breathes in less than 1 mCi at tidal volume until an adequate count rate is obtained (3,000 counts/sec). The sixfold larger ^{99m}Tc MAA perfusion dose (5-mCi) overwhelms the retained ventilation dose, allowing for two consecutive ^{99m}Tc studies.

4. ^{133}Xe, an inert gas, is advantageous for patients with COPD and asthma. Delayed filling and clearance (air trapping) in regions of obstructive disease can be seen. Disadvantage: only posterior views are possible because of rapid exhalation.

Reference

Trujillo NP, Pratt JP, Tahisani S, et al: DTPA aerosol in ventilation/perfusion scintigraphy for diagnosing pulmonary embolism, *J Nucl Med* 38:1781-1783, 1997.

Cross-Reference

Nuclear Medicine: THE REQUISITES, ed 2, pp 146-162.

Comment

^{133}Xe mimics air exchange within the lung. Xenon's disadvantages are its low energy (81 keV) and therefore low resolution and rapid temporal changes in distribution, allowing only posterior views, unless a two-headed camera is used. ^{127}Xe's higher photopeaks allow for postperfusion images; however, it is expensive and not available generally. Good airflow and a negative-pressure room are required, otherwise xenon, a heavy gas, layers out on the floor. A xenon "trap" is required to absorb and retain exhaled gas. ^{81m}Kr (^{81}Rb with 190 keV) allows postperfusion imaging, but it is expensive and generally not available. ^{99m}Tc "technegas" consists of very small carbon particles that do not settle out in the lung. It is used in many parts of the world but not approved by the U.S. Food and Drug Administration.

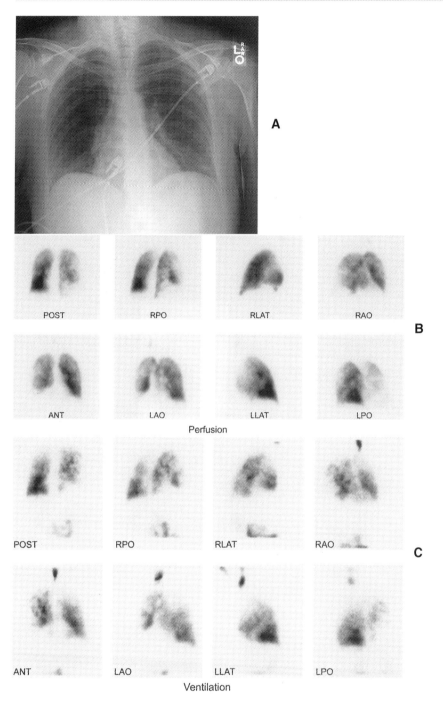

A

B

POST   RPO   RLAT   RAO

ANT   LAO   LLAT   LPO

Perfusion

C

POST   RPO   RLAT   RAO

ANT   LAO   LLAT   LPO

Ventilation

A 54-year-old man with known cardiopulmonary disease complains of increasing dyspnea. *A,* Chest radiograph; *B,* perfusion scan; *C,* ventilation scan.

1. What are the scintigraphic findings and interpretation?

2. What is the likelihood of pulmonary embolus in this patient?

3. What is the likelihood of pulmonary embolus in a patient with a normal scan?

4. How are perfusion defects classified as to size?

Pulmonary System: Low-Probability Ventilation-Perfusion Scan

1. Bilateral inhomogeneous distribution. Matched perfusion and ventilation abnormalities throughout the upper and lower lobes, especially in the right lower lobe basal segments. Minimal atelectasis in the lower lobes on chest x-ray. Low probability for pulmonary embolus.

2. Less than 20%.

3. Less than 1%.

4. Large (segmental): greater than 75% of a segment.
   Moderate (subsegmental): 25% to 75% of a segment.
   Small (small subsegmental): less than 25% of a segment.

References

Worsley DF, Alavi A: Radionuclide imaging of acute pulmonary embolism, *Radiol Clin North Am* 39:1035-1052, 2001.

Stein PD, Gottshalk A: Review of criteria appropriate for a very low probability of pulmonary embolism on ventilation-perfusion lung scans: a position paper, *Radiographics* 20:99-105, 2000.

Cross-Reference
Nuclear Medicine: THE REQUISITES, ed 2, pp 145-161.

Comment

One of the new findings of the Prospective Investigation of the Pulmonary Embolism Diagnosis (PIOPED) study was that a V/Q study showing extensively decreased perfusion in a lung field with matching ventilation should be interpreted as low probability as long as some perfusion exists to that lung field. Before the PIOPED study, this pattern was called indeterminate. Another finding was that if the referring clinician has a high clinical suspicion for pulmonary embolus, but the scan is low probability, the likelihood of proven pulmonary embolus increases to 40%. Conditions commonly associated with V/Q-matched abnormalities include COPD, bronchiectasis, alveolar pulmonary edema and pleural effusion, asthma, mucus plugs, and tumor.

Criteria have been proposed to define a very low-probability category, i.e., less than 10%. They include nonsegmental perfusion defects, matched defects in two or three zones in a single lung only, and the stripe sign. The stripe sign refers to activity seen along the pleural surface of a segment that otherwise appears hypoperfused. The stripe sign lessens the likelihood of pulmonary embolus for that lung region because perfusion defects caused by vascular occlusion should extend to the pleural surface.

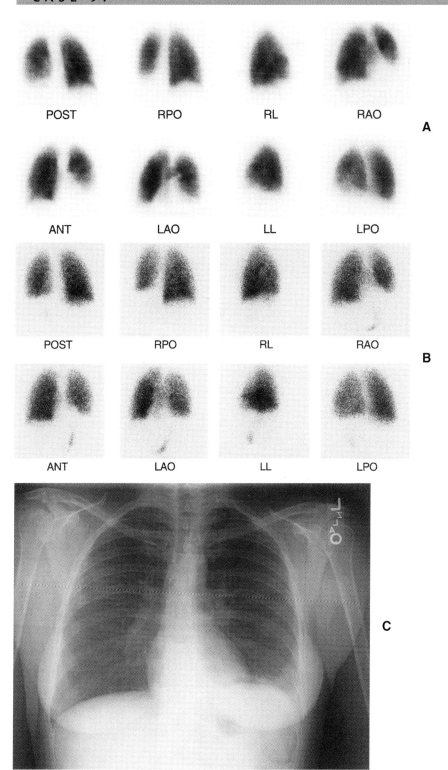

A 29-year-old pregnant woman has a history of asthma and recent onset of dyspnea.

1. Is any patient preparation indicated?
2. Would the patient's pregnancy change the V/Q protocol?
3. Describe the perfusion (A) and ventilation (B) images and radiograph findings (C).
4. Give your interpretation of the study.

Pulmonary System: Intermediate Probability and Pregnancy

1. Bronchodilator therapy before V/Q study as an asthmatic therapeutic trial.

2. Pulmonary emboli are life threatening to the patient and fetus. The radiation dose to the patient and fetus is low (less than 2 rads). The benefit/risk ratio is high. No change in procedure is required. In young, nonsmoking patients without cardiopulmonary disease, one might reduce the dose, conduct only a perfusion study, or both.

3. Hypoperfusion of the left lower lobe, except the superior segment. Better ventilation than perfusion with mismatching, in the anterior basal and part of the lateral basal segments. No ventilation in the posterior basal and part of the lateral basal. Costophrenic angle loss seen in left lateral and LPO views. Radiograph: atelectasis/infiltrate with elevation of the left diaphragm.

4. Intermediate probability for pulmonary embolus. One large/one moderate segmental mismatch and one large and one moderate segmental match corresponding to the x-ray atelectasis/infiltrate.

Reference
Worsley DF, Alavi A: Radionuclide imaging of acute pulmonary embolism, *Radiol Clin North America* 39:1035-1052, 2001.

Cross-Reference
Nuclear Medicine: THE REQUISITES, ed 2, pp 128-129.

Comment
A normal V/Q scan excludes the diagnosis of pulmonary embolus. Patients with low-probability scans and a low clinical likelihood do not require anticoagulation or further evaluation. Patients with low-probability scans, but an intermediate or high clinical likelihood of disease, should have lower extremity venous studies. If results are negative, anticoagulation or angiography is unnecessary. If positive, the patient requires treatment. Patients with an intermediate-probability V/Q scan require a noninvasive venous study of the lower extremities. If positive, treatment is indicated. If negative, CT angiography or pulmonary angiography is indicated. Patients with a high-probability scan and high likelihood of disease require treatment. Those with a low or intermediate likelihood need noninvasive evaluation. Understanding of the appropriate use of CT for evaluation of pulmonary embolus is evolving. At present, CT angiography is considered sensitive and specific for diagnosing central pulmonary emboli, but insensitive for diagnosing subsegmental emboli. The safety of withholding anticoagulant treatment in patients with negative CT results is uncertain. Further prospective studies to evaluate the sensitivity and specificity of CT angiography are required.

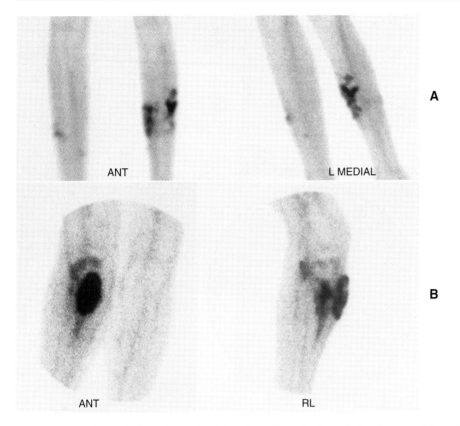

ANT L MEDIAL **A**

ANT RL **B**

Two patients (*A* and *B*) with similar histories of a soft tissue infection overlying the tibia. ^{99m}Tc HM-PAO leukocyte studies were ordered to confirm or exclude underlying osteomyelitis.

1. Would a bone scan be useful as the initial study in these cases?

2. When would a bone marrow study with ^{99m}Tc sulfur colloid be useful in this clinical setting?

3. Would an ^{111}In oxine leukocyte study or ^{67}Ga study be preferable?

4. Describe the findings. What are the diagnoses?

Infection and Inflammation: ^{99m}Tc HM-PAO Leukocytes and Osteomyelitis

1. A negative bone scan rules out osteomyelitis with a high degree of certainty.

2. A bone marrow study can improve the specificity of a leukocyte study if there is displaced normal marrow (orthopedic hardware). This is most helpful in the hips and knees.

3. ^{111}In leukocytes can make the same diagnosis. The superior imaging resolution of ^{99m}Tc HM-PAO often better differentiates soft tissue and bone infection. ^{67}Ga is less specific because increased uptake occurs with bone remodeling from any cause.

4. Patient *A:* soft tissue uptake. No bone uptake rules out osteomyelitis; consistent with cellulitis. Patient *B:* soft tissue and bone localization consistent with osteomyelitis.

References

Elgazzar AH, Abdel-Dayem M: Imaging skeletal infections: evolving considerations. In Freeman LM, editor: *Nuclear medicine annual 1999,* Philadelphia, 1999, Lippincott Williams & Wilkins, pp 157-192.

Palestro CJ, Torres MA: Radionuclide imaging in orthopedic infections, *Semin Nucl Med* 27:334-435, 1997.

Cross-Reference

Nuclear Medicine: THE REQUISITES, ed 2, pp 184-189.

Comment

The most common cause for osteomyelitis in adults is direct extension from a soft tissue infection. Although hematogenous spread occurs in adults, it is seen more commonly in children. Long bone metaphyses commonly are affected in children because of the relatively slow blood flow in metaphyseal sinusoidal veins and the paucity of phagocytes. Adult hematogenous acute osteomyelitis rarely involves the long bones. In adults, osteomyelitis is often the result of direct introduction of bacteria from soft tissue wounds, compound fractures, contamination of bone during surgery.

A negative three-phase bone scan rules out osteomyelitis with a high degree of accuracy in adults without previous fracture, infection, or orthopedic hardware. A ^{99m}Tc sulfur colloid bone marrow study is most useful for evaluating proximal marrow filled bones, e.g., hip or knee prosthesis or orthopedic hardware causing marrow displacement. ^{111}In oxine and ^{99m}Tc HM-PAO leukocytes have similar accuracy for diagnosis of osteomyelitis. Image quality is better with ^{99m}Tc HM-PAO and the radiation dose is lower, which is an advantage in children. However, both have a high false-negative rate for osteomyelitis of the spine; thus ^{67}Ga may be preferable in those cases. However, ^{67}Ga may be positive in the presence of bone remodeling.

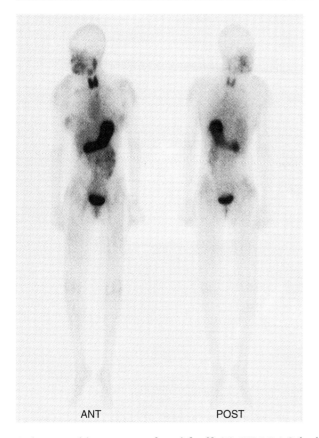

ANT   POST

A 49-year-old man was referred for ^{99m}Tc HM-PAO leukocyte study to locate the source of *Staphylococcus aureus* sepsis.

1. What are the scintigraphic findings?
2. What is your interpretation of the study?
3. What are the most common causes for false-positive radiolabeled leukocyte studies?
4. What is the optimal imaging period for ^{67}Ga, ^{111}In oxine leukocytes, ^{99m}Tc HM-PAO leukocytes for infection imaging?

Infection and Inflammation: ^{99m}Tc HM-PAO Leukocytes–free ^{99m}Tc pertechnetate

1. Activity in the salivary glands, thyroid, stomach, bowel, and bladder.

2. Free ^{99m}Tc pertechnetate. Nondiagnostic study.

3. Gastrointestinal bleeding, swallowed leukocytes from oropharyngeal, esophageal, or lung inflammation/infection, accessory spleen, uninfected postoperative surgical wounds, intestinal stomas, and catheter sites.

3. ^{67}Ga, 48 hours; ^{111}In oxine leukocytes, 24 hours; ^{99m}Tc HM-PAO leukocytes, 1 to 4 hours.

Reference

Datz FL, Taylor AT: Cell labeling: techniques and clinical utility. In Freeman and Johnson's clinical radionuclide imaging, ed 3, update, New York, 1986, Grune & Stratton, pp 1785-1847.

Cross-Reference

Nuclear Medicine: THE REQUISITES, ed 2, pp 177-190.

Comment

Free ^{99m}Tc pertechnetate is caused by poor cell labeling. It is more commonly seen with bone scintigraphy. Poor cell labeling results in a suboptimal scan, thus limiting infection detection because of the reduced number of labeled leukocytes, poor count density where it matters, and intraabdominal clearance of pertechnetate, which complicates detection of intraabdominal infection. Quality control of radiolabeled leukocytes before injection is limited to microscopic examination of the leukocytes and determining labeling percent efficiency since the radiolabeled cells must be injected promptly to ensure cell viability. Leukocyte viability is difficult to evaluate but critical to diagnostic accuracy. Morphological characteristics are checked microscopically. However, the ultimate test of viability is in vivo function. Little blood pool is normally seen on leukocyte studies. The presence of increased blood pool indicates a high portion of the label is on the red cells, platelets, or both. Prolonged lung uptake indicates cellular damage. Usually the spleen has highest uptake. If the spleen/liver ratio is reversed, this suggests cell damage. Because both organs normally have high uptake, this is not a sensitive parameter of cell viability.

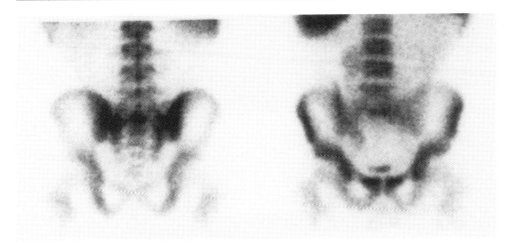

A 25-year-old man has fever and abdominal pain. ^{99m}Tc HM-PAO–labeled leukocyte images.

1. Which leukocytes are labeled with the two radiopharmaceuticals used for leukocyte scans?

2. What is the explanation for the prominent skeletal uptake?

3. What is the optimal imaging time for ^{111}In oxine–labeled leukocytes and ^{99m}Tc HM-PAO leukocytes?

4. Give an image interpretation and diagnosis in this case.

Infection and Inflammation: Intraabdominal Abscess

1. ^{99m}Tc HM-PAO binds only to neutrophils. ^{111}In oxine binds to mixed leukocytes.

2. Normal bone marrow distribution of the radiolabeled leukocytes.

3. Abdominal imaging: ^{99m}Tc HM-PAO images are acquired at 1 to 2 hours because hepatobiliary, intestinal, and renal clearance occurs subsequently, complicating interpretation. Extremity imaging: 2 to 6 hours. ^{111}In leukocytes: 24 hours. Four-hour imaging for inflammatory bowel disease because sloughing of intestinal mucosa leukocytes may occur and 24-hour may be misleading.

4. Infection in the right lower quadrant overlying the sacroiliac joint in the anterior view and lateral right of the spine. The patient had a perforated appendix.

References

Colak T, Gungor F, Ozugur S, et al: Value of 99m Tc-HMPAO labeled white blood cell scintigraphy in acute appendicitis patients with an equivocal clinical presentation, *Eur J Nucl Med* 28:575-580, 2001.

Stahlberg D, Veress B, Mare K, et al: Leukocyte migration in acute colonic inflammatory bowel disease: comparison of histological assessment and Tc-99m HMPAO labeled leukocyte scan, *Am J Gastroenterol* 92:283-288, 1997.

Cross-Reference
Nuclear Medicine: THE REQUISITES, ed 2, pp 184-190.

Comment
^{99m}Tc HM-PAO initially was used for cerebral perfusion imaging. Its lipophilicity allows it to cross the blood brain barrier and become fixed intracellularly. This property is used to transport the ^{99m}Tc into leukocytes. ^{99m}Tc HM-PAO and ^{111}In oxine label RBCs, platelets, and leukocytes. However, cells other than leukocytes are removed during the labeling process. Except for renal and biliary clearance, the distribution of HM-PAO leukocytes is similar to that of ^{111}In oxine-labeled leukocytes. Greatest uptake is in the spleen, followed by liver and bone marrow. The spleen has the highest radiation dose, 15 to 20 rads with ^{111}In oxine and 2 rads with ^{99m}Tc HM-PAO. Thus ^{99m}Tc HM-PAO is the preferred agent in children. Additional advantages of ^{99m}Tc HM-PAO is its better image resolution. A disadvantage of all radiolabeled cells is the minimum 2-hour preparation time and the problem of blood-borne disease. ^{99m}Tc leukocytes are used for patients with inflammatory bowel disease as an alternative to repeat endoscopy or contrast studies. Good correlation exists between the amount and site of uptake of radiolabeled leukocytes compared with endoscopy and radiological localization for patients with ulcerative colitis and Crohn's disease (granulomatous or regional enteritis).

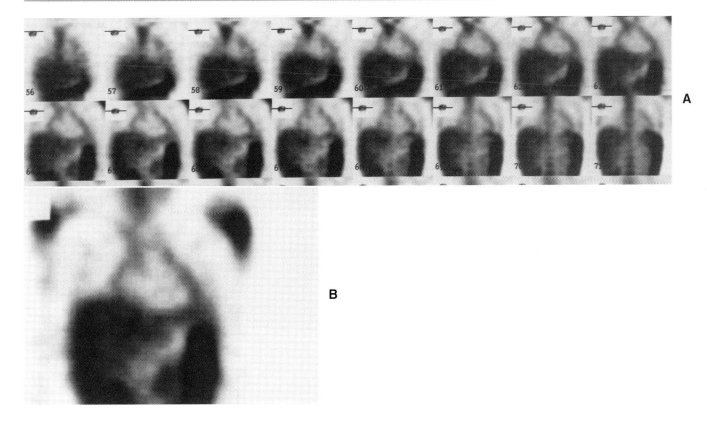

An 8-year-old girl with juvenile rheumatoid arthritis and persistent fever after resolution of recent pneumonia. She has no current symptoms of arthritis.

1. Describe the findings on ^{67}Ga sequential coronal SPECT chest images *(A)* and a selected enlarged image *(B)*. Image intensity is high. What is the differential diagnosis?

2. What is the advantage of ^{67}Ga over indium- or technetium-labeled leukocytes for fever of unknown origin?

3. What is the target organ (highest radiation absorbed dose) for ^{67}Ga?

4. Which pulmonary infections or inflammatory diseases show increased ^{67}Ga uptake?

Infection and Inflammation: Pericarditis—⁶⁷Ga

1. Abnormal uptake in myocardium, pericardium, or both consistent with pericarditis or myocarditis. The patient developed a pericardial friction rub the day after the ⁶⁷Ga scan. Incidental note of normal liver uptake and transverse and left colon clearance.

2. ⁶⁷Ga shows uptake not only with inflammation and infection, but also in tumors that can sometimes be the cause of persistent fever, e.g., lymphoma.

3. Large bowel, approximately 4.5 rads.

4. Most pulmonary inflammatory and infectious diseases. Uptake is nonspecific, although the pattern of uptake and the clinical setting, e.g., AIDS, may be helpful in determining the differential diagnosis.

References

Desai SP, Yuille DL: The unsuspected complications of bacterial endocarditis imaged by gallium-67 scanning, *J Nucl Med* 34:955-957, 1993.

Shulkin BL, Wahl RL: SPECT imaging of myocarditis, *Clin Nucl Med* 12:841-842, 1987.

Cross-Reference

Nuclear Medicine: THE REQUISITES, ed 2, pp 171-175.

Comment

In cardiovascular disease, ⁶⁷Ga has been used to detect infection of synthetic vascular grafts, mycotic aneurysms, myocarditis, and pericarditis. Distinction between the latter two can be difficult because of limited resolution. Sensitivity for endocarditis is poor. ⁶⁷Ga has a larger role in evaluating the cause and effectiveness of therapy of pulmonary inflammatory and infectious disease, e.g., sarcoidosis, *Pneumocystis carinii,* bleomycin toxicity, interstitial lung disease.

Because ⁶⁷Ga is excreted by the colon, the radiopharmaceutical generally is not used to evaluate for intraabdominal infection. Bowel cleansing with laxatives is used to better visualize the abdomen, but delayed imaging is often necessary. ¹¹¹In oxine leukocytes are preferable for abdominal infection because there is no colonic clearance. ⁹⁹ᵐTc HM-PAO byproducts are cleared through the biliary and renal system, rendering it also suboptimal for intraabdominal infection. Imaging before 2 hours after reinjection can prevent this problem. The usual adult dose of ⁶⁷Ga is 5 mCi. Higher does (7 to 10 mCi) are used for tumor imaging with SPECT. With small children, ⁶⁷Ga is not an ideal imaging agent and often results in suboptimal images because of the low administered dose, poor crystal sensitivity for ⁶⁷Ga because of its multiple high photopeaks (185, 300, 394 keV), and the need for a medium-energy collimator.

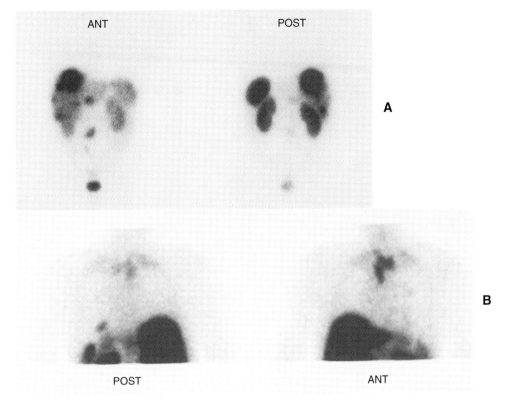

A, 70-year-old man with recent onset of flushing, diarrhea, elevated 5-hydroxyindoleacetic acid (5-HIAA), and a diagnosis of carcinoid syndrome. *B,* 56-year-old patient with past history of medullary carcinoma of the thyroid and recent increase in serum calcitonin levels.

1. Provide the mechanism of uptake of ^{111}In pentetreotide (OctreoScan).

2. List the category of tumors for which this radiopharmaceutical is particularly useful.

3. Describe the image findings on these two studies: *A* (abdominal/pelvis view) and *B* (chest views), and give your interpretation.

4. Name the organs that normally have greatest uptake of the radiopharmaceutical.

Oncology: Neuroectodermal Tumors

1. Peptide analogue of somatostatin and octreotide. Binds to tumors with somatostatin receptors.

2. Neuroendocrine tumors.

3. *A,* Multiple metastases to both lobes of the liver. Two large foci and one small focus of uptake consistent with paraaortic tumor adenopathy. Possible small tumor in right hilum (confirmed by later CT). *B,* Prominent irregular uptake in the anterior mediastinum and focal uptake in the left lower lung posteriorly.

4. Kidneys and spleen.

References

Krenning EP, Kwekkeboom DJ, Bakker WH, et al: Somatostatin receptor scintigraphy with [111-in-DTPA-Dphe-1] and [123 I-Tyr-3]-octreotide: the Rotterdam experience with more than 1000 patients, *Eur J Nucl Med* 20:716-731, 1993.

Gibril F, Reynolds JC, Lubensky IA, et al: Ability of somatostatin receptor scintigraphy to identify patients with gastric carcinoids: a prospective study, *J Nucl Med* 41:1646-1656, 2000.

Cross-Reference

Nuclear Medicine: THE REQUISITES, ed 2, pp 223-225.

Comment

Neuroendocrine tumors (APUDomas) are derived from neural crest cells. They can synthesize amines from precursors and produce peptides that act as hormones and neurotransmitters. Many neuroendocrine tumors can be difficult to detect on conventional imaging because of their small size. All have increased somatostatin receptors to varying degrees, and many have a high tumor uptake ratio on [111]In OctreoScan. SPECT can help detect small tumors and improve localization compared with planar scans.

Sensitivity for tumor detection varies depending on the neuroendocrine tumor: gastrinoma (95%), carcinoid (>80%), glucagonoma (>70%), medullary carcinoma of the thyroid (>50%), pheochromocytoma and neuroblastoma (>90%). Other nonrelated tumors with somatostatin receptors with uptake include small cell lung cancer, lymphoma, and breast cancer. Seventy percent of these tumors take up the [111]In OctreoScan. Uptake also occurs in astrocytomas, meningiomas, and thymomas. Therapeutic analogues labeled with beta-emitters are being investigated.

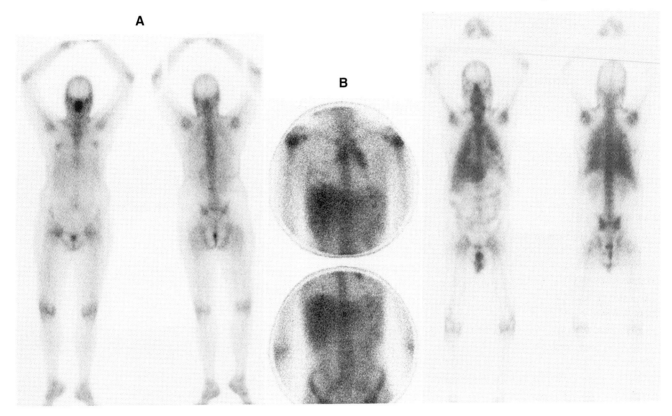

A

B

C

Three patients in images *A, B,* and *C* have whole body ^{67}Ga scans.

1. What is the normal distribution of ^{67}Ga?

2. Which studies show postchemotherapy changes? What are the findings?

3. What are other causes of ^{67}Ga lung uptake?

4. Which study shows an altered distribution of the radiopharmaceutical? Causes?

Oncology: Postchemotherapy ^{67}Ga Findings

1. Greatest to least uptake: liver, bone/bone marrow, spleen, kidney (excretion pathway), salivary and lacrimal glands.

2. *B,* Thymus uptake is not an uncommon nonpathological finding after chemotherapy. *C,* Diffuse pulmonary uptake is consistent with pulmonary toxicity, e.g., bleomycin-induced lung disease.

3. Gallium-avid tumor, inflammation, and infection.

4. *A,* Decreased hepatic and marrow uptake. Causes: recent MRI gadolinium contrast study, very recent chemotherapy, or iron saturation, e.g., multiple transfusions.

Reference

Front D, Bar-Shalom R, Israel O: Role of gallium-67 and other radiopharmaceuticals in the management of patients with lymphoma. In Freeman LM, editor: *Nuclear medicine annual 1998,* Philadelphia, 1998, Lippincott-Raven, pp 247-264.

Cross-Reference

Nuclear Medicine: THE REQUISITES, ed 2, pp 194-195.

Comment

The kidney excretes 25% of the administered dose in the first 24 hours. The kidneys may be seen at 24 to 48 hours but usually not at 72 hours. The colon is the major route of clearance, but clearance is slow with 75% of the administered dose remaining at 48 hours.

Because iron competes with ^{67}Ga for binding to transferrin, iron overload syndromes, e.g., repeated transfusions, can saturate receptors and result in decreased hepatic and marrow uptake and increased renal uptake. Extensive hepatic metastases from a non–gallium-avid tumor, hepatic insufficiency, and vincristine given within 24 hours of injection can also reduce hepatic uptake. ^{67}Ga injection should not be performed for 2 weeks after chemotherapy to minimize these potential problems.

The most common chemotherapeutic agents that cause pulmonary toxicity and lung uptake are bleomycin, cytoxan, and busulfan. Amiodarone, a cardiac drug, can cause a similar problem. Diffuse pulmonary uptake can also be the result of lymphangitic spread within the lung, but this is rarely homogenous. Inflammatory and infectious causes also can result in pulmonary uptake, particularly in immunocompromised patients. Thymus uptake is common in children after chemotherapy. It usually can be differentiated from adenopathy in conjunction with CT.

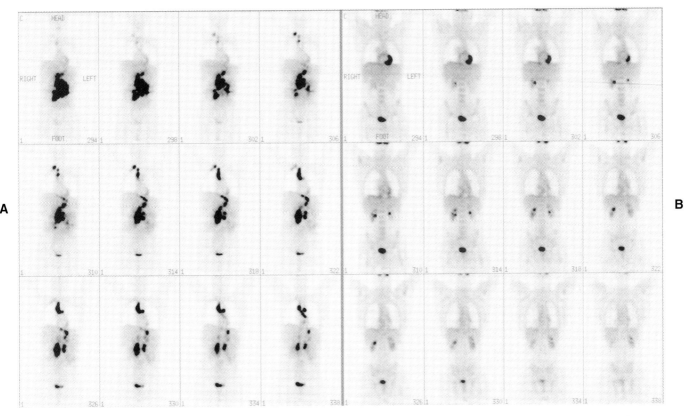

A patient with malignant B-cell lymphoma. Initial FDG-PET study *(A)* shows tumor above and below the diaphragm. Postchemotherapy CT shows a residual abdominal mass. Posttherapy FDG-PET *(B)*.

1. Is remission complete or partial based on the CT and subsequent PET study?
2. What are the limitations of CT for staging and restaging of disease in patients with lymphoma?
3. List imaging limitations of ^{67}Ga.
4. What are the advantages of ^{18}F FDG-PET compared with ^{67}Ga?

Oncology: ^{18}F FDG-PET—Lymphoma

1. The CT scan is indeterminate, but FDG-PET demonstrates a complete response.

2. CT assessment of tumor response is based on a decrease in the size of the mass or complete resolution. However, posttherapy residual masses are common and CT cannot differentiate residual tumor from posttherapy fibrosis and necrosis.

3. Multiple high-energy photopeaks: 185, 300, 394 resulting in poor image resolution; frequent need for delayed imaging (48 to 72 hours and sometimes 5 to 7 days) to allow for bowel clearance.

4. Study completed 2 hours after injection. FDG-PET target-to-background ratio is higher and image quality superior to ^{67}Ga. Usually little bowel activity with FDG. Data are limited, but consensus is that FDG is superior to ^{67}Ga.

References

Delbeke D, Martin WH: Positron emission tomography imaging in oncology, *Radiol Clin North Am* 39:883-918, 2001.

Moog F, Bangerter M, Diedrichs CG, et al: Extranodal malignant lymphoma; detection with FDG PET versus CT, *Radiology* 206:475-481, 1998.

Cross-Reference

Nuclear Medicine: THE REQUISITES, ed 2, p 213.

Comment

Of malignant lymphomas, 15% are caused by Hodgkin's disease and of T-cell origin; the remaining 85% are non-Hodgkin's lymphoma of B-cell origin. The incidence of malignant non-Hodgkin's lymphoma is increasing and now is the sixth most common malignancy. Staging is critical for determining appropriate therapy. Restaging is required to determine the effectiveness of therapy and the need for further appropriate treatment. CT and ^{67}Ga have been used for staging purposes. ^{67}Ga is equal to CT for initial staging and superior to CT in restaging and evaluating response to therapy. ^{67}Ga is valuable in determining whether a residual chest or abdominal mass after chemotherapy or radiation therapy is persistent tumor or merely necrosis and fibrosis. Although studies are limited comparing ^{67}Ga and FDG-PET, patients and physicians who have experience with both invariably have a strong preference for FDG-PET. Image quality is superior, the tumor-to-background ratio is higher, imaging is complete 2 hours after injection, and bowel activity rarely is a problem.

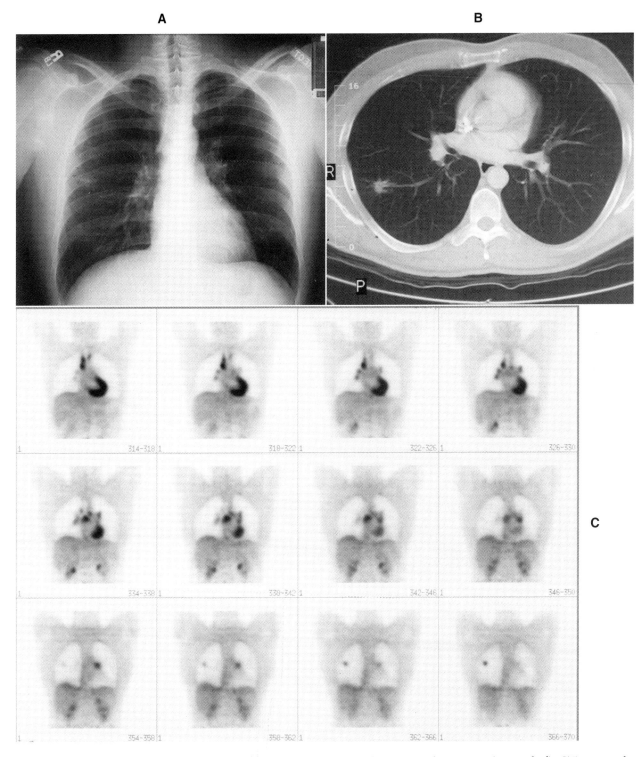

A 33-year-old male smoker has a poorly defined right mid-lung density on chest x-ray *(A, marked)*. CT reported a 1.5-cm lesion with infiltrative margins in the superior segment of the RLL *(B)* but no other abnormality.

1. Describe the ^{18}F FDG-PET scan findings *(C)*. Sequential coronal slices are shown.

2. How has this PET scan affected the patient's preoperative staging?

3. What is the overall accuracy of CT and MR for preoperative staging of lung cancer?

4. What is the overall accuracy of ^{18}F FDG-PET for preoperative lung cancer staging?

Oncology: ¹⁸F FDG-PET—Lung Cancer Staging

1. Focal increased uptake corresponding to the nodule on CT (frames 358-370). In addition, abnormal uptake is seen in the right and left paratracheal regions, the right and left hilum, and the mediastinum, all consistent with tumor adenopathy.

2. ¹⁸F FDG-PET has preoperatively upstaged the patient, who is no longer a surgical candidate.

3. Approximately 65%.

4. Approximately 85%.

References

Marom EM, McAdams HP, Erasmus JJ, et al: Staging non-small lung cancer with whole-body PET, *Radiology* 212:803-809, 1999.

Pieterman RM, Van Putten JWG, Meuzelaar JJ, et al: Preoperative staging of non-small-cell lung cancer with positron-emission tomography, *N Engl J Med* 343:254-260, 2000.

Cross-Reference

Nuclear Medicine: THE REQUISITES, ed 2, pp 209-211.

Comment

Lung cancer is the leading cause of cancer mortality for men and women in the United States, accounting for 25% to 30% of cancer deaths. At the time of presentation, 30% to 50% of patients have metastatic disease. Preoperatively, only 20% to 30% of lung cancers are considered resectable. The accuracy of conventional preoperative staging of non–small cell lung cancer is poor. At surgery, almost 10% of patients are discovered to have unresectable disease. Within the first year after surgery, 14% of patients die after their lung cancer was resected due to incorrect preoperative staging. CT and MR have poor accuracy for preoperative staging of lung cancer because the diagnosis of tumor adenopathy is based on nodal size. However, approximately 24% of metastases are found in normal size lymph nodes. Also inflammatory nodes often are enlarged. FDG-PET's unique metabolic information allows diagnosis of tumor adenopathy in nonenlarged nodes and exclusion of tumor in enlarged inflammatory nodes.

Many studies now have reported consistent accuracy of FDG-PET for the staging of lung cancer. PET is clearly superior to conventional imaging. In 2000, the *New England Journal of Medicine* reported the sensitivity and specificity of FDG-PET to be 91% and 86%, respectively, compared with 75% and 66% for CT. PET upstaged 42% of patients and downstaged 20%. A study from Duke University reported that the sensitivity and specificity for FDG-PET in separating surgical from nonsurgical disease (N3) was 92% and 93% compared with conventional imaging (CT, MR) of 25% and 98%. State-of-the-art preoperative non–small cell lung cancer staging requires FDG-PET.

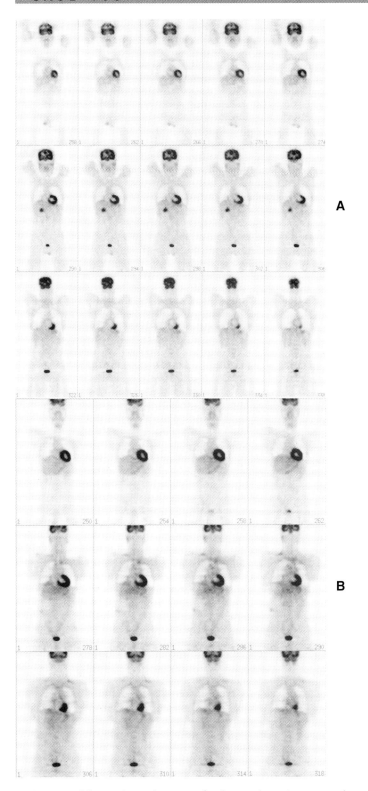

A

B

A 69-year-old man has a history of colorectal carcinoma and surgical resection. The carcinoembryonic antigen (CEA) level is increasing and the CT scan shows a new 2.3-cm lesion in the right lobe of the liver.

1. FDG-PET scan *(A)* was then obtained. What are the findings?

2. Why was the FDG-PET scan ordered?

3. What are clinical indications for FDG-PET in colorectal carcinoma?

4. FDG-PET scan *(B)* was performed 6 months after resection of the liver lesion. Describe the findings.

195

Notes

Oncology: ^{18}F FDG-PET—Colorectal Cancer Metastatic to Liver

1. Increased uptake consistent with tumor in the liver corresponding to the reported CT mass. No other liver lesions or metastases are seen elsewhere in the whole body scan.

2. Surgical resection is planned. The preoperative FDG-PET scan is used to determine the presence of any other metastases in the liver or elsewhere in the body that might change the surgical approach or make the patient inoperable.

3. (1) Increasing serum CEA levels with normal conventional imaging, (2) equivocal lesion with conventional imaging, and (3) preoperative staging before curative resection.

4. Negative scan. No evidence of tumor.

References

Delbeke D, Vitola JV, Sandler MP, et al: Staging recurrent metastatic colorectal carcinoma with PET, *J Nucl Med* 38:1196-1201, 1997.

Valk PE, Abella-Columna, Haseman MK, et al: Whole-body PET imaging with F-18 FDG in management of recurrent colorectal carcinoma, *Arch Surg* 134:503-511, 1999.

Cross-Reference

Nuclear Medicine: THE REQUISITES, ed 2, pp 211-213.

Comment

Colorectal cancer is the second most common cause of cancer death in the United States. The liver is the most common site of colorectal metastases, although local recurrence is not uncommon. Many patients die with metastases exclusively to the liver. Although resection of the hepatic metastasis is potentially curative, it is associated with significant morbidity and mortality. Resectability depends on the number of metastases and their location. In the past, only 25% of patients with partial hepatic resection were cured because of the presence of occult, often extrahepatic, metastases. Extrahepatic metastases usually are a contraindication to surgery.

Serum CEA elevation is only 50% sensitive and 85% specific for metastases. Of course, it provides no information on location. The sensitivity of CT for detection of liver metastases is surprisingly low. Multiple studies have confirmed the superiority of PET over CT for staging of recurrent colorectal cancer. A recent large study of 155 patients with recurrent colorectal cancer found a sensitivity and specificity for CT of 69% and 96% and for PET, 93% and 98%. FDG-PET had a clinical effect in more than 30% of patients, often eliminating unnecessary surgery. Studies of cost-effectiveness have shown that the addition of FDG-PET to the preoperative evaluation decreases the overall cost of caring for patients with recurrent colorectal cancer.

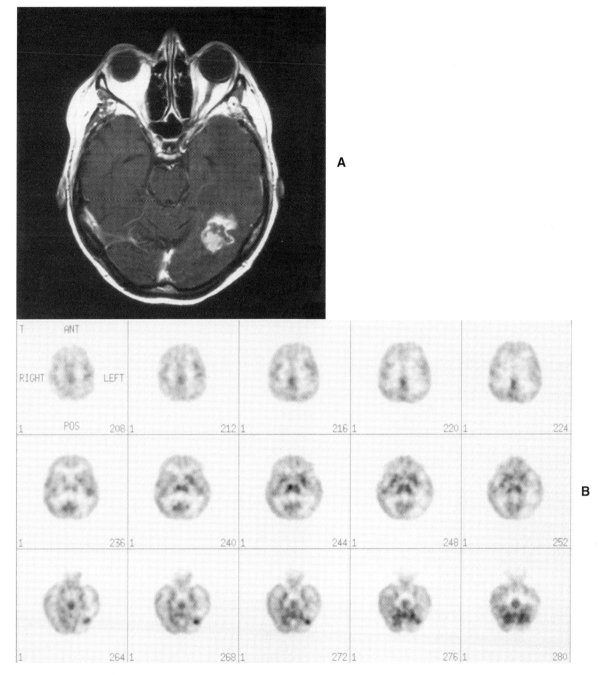

A 54-year-old woman with bronchogenic carcinoma metastatic to the brain recently underwent stereotactic radio-surgery for a lesion in the left temporoparietal region. MRI could not differentiate posttherapy changes from viable tumor *(A)*.

1. Give the relative accuracy of FDG-PET versus CT or MRI for diagnosing malignant tumor in the brain.
2. What is the relative accuracy of FDG-PET versus CT/MRI for differentiating recurrent or persistent tumor from postradiation necrosis?
3. Describe the image findings and interpret the transaxial images *(B)* of FDG-PET of the brain.
4. List single photon radiotracers used for brain imaging and describe the expected findings.

Oncology: ^{18}F FDG-PET—Bronchogenic Cancer Metastatic to Brain

1. CT and MRI are more sensitive for tumor detection. Normal brain uses only glucose for metabolism and has higher uptake than any other organ. This results in high background that can make tumor detection difficult.

2. FDG-PET is more accurate than CT or MRI for determining whether posttherapy changes are the result of residual/recurrent tumor or radiation necrosis.

3. Focal increased uptake in the left temporoparietal region that correlates with the lesion on MRI. This is consistent with viable residual or recurrent tumor.

4. ^{201}Tl and ^{99m}Tc sestamibi have increased uptake in tumors. Tumors usually are cold on ^{99m}Tc HM-PAO and ECD.

References

Hagge RJ, Wong TZ, Coleman RE: Positron emission tomography: brain tumors and lung cancer, *Radiol Clin North Am* 39:871-882, 2001.

Griffeth LK, Rich KM, Dehdasti F, et al: Brain metastases from non-central nervous system tumors: evaluation with PET, *Radiology* 186:37-44, 1993.

Cross-Reference
Nuclear Medicine: THE REQUISITES, ed 2, pp 301-305.

Comment
FDG-PET detection of metastatic tumors to the brain has been reported to be more variable than primary brain tumors. It is less sensitive for initial staging for brain metastasis than CT/MRI. Therefore imaging of the brain is not routine at most centers when performing whole body PET imaging. The brain has the highest uptake of FDG of any organ and thus serves as a high background, making detection of increased uptake in tumors more difficult.

After therapy, CT and MRI often cannot differentiate posttherapy, necrotic or fibrotic masses from viable residual or recurrent tumor. Surgical biopsy is not always possible and poses associated morbidity. FDG-PET can be useful as in this case. Uptake indicates viable tumor, and the lack of uptake signifies effective therapy. FDG-PET also is proving useful for radiation therapy planning. Fusion of FDG-PET and MR or CT studies can help direct the radiation beam to the residual tumor within a heterogenous tumor mass.

Notes

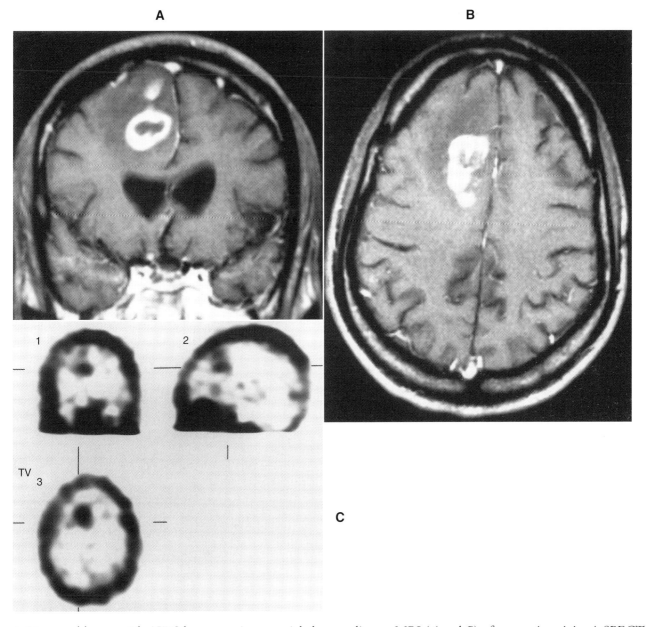

A 35-year-old-man with AIDS has a new intracranial abnormality on MRI (*A* and *B*) of uncertain origin. A SPECT study (C1, coronal; C2, sagittal; C3, transverse) was ordered to assist in the differential diagnosis.

1. What is the radiopharmaceutical?
2. What is the differential diagnosis before the SPECT study?
3. What is the likely diagnosis after the radionuclide study?
4. What is the accuracy of the radionuclide method?

Oncology: ^{201}Tl—Intracranial Lymphoma

1. ^{201}Tl was used. ^{99m}Tc sestamibi also can be used; however, it is taken up by the choroid plexus and could pose diagnostic problems in some cases.

2. Tumor, particularly lymphoma, versus infection, usually toxoplasmosis, or other opportunistic infections, e.g., cytomegalic inclusion virus, herpes simplex, *Cryptococcus.*

3. Malignant lymphoma.

4. Approximately 90% sensitivity for tumor. False-positive rate of less than 10%.

References

O'Malley JP, Ziessman HA, Kumar PN, et al: Diagnosis of intracranial lymphoma in patients with AIDS: value of 201-Tl single-photon emission computed tomography, *AJR Am J Roentgenol* 163:417-421, 1994.

Hoffman JM, Waskin HA, Shifter T, et al: FDG-PET in differentiating lymphoma from non-malignant CNS lesions in patients with AIDS, *J Nucl Med* 34:567-575, 1993.

Cross-Reference

Nuclear Medicine: THE REQUISITES, ed 2, pp 314-316.

Comment

Toxoplasma gondii is the most common cause of focal encephalitis in patients with AIDS. However, intracranial lymphoma is increasing in incidence and is the second most common cause; it is a very aggressive and often lethal disease. CT and MR are not reliable for distinguishing between tumor and infectious causes. Both may appear as ring-enhancing lesions on MRI. Often patients are treated empirically for toxoplasmosis, and biopsy is performed only if therapy yields no response. However, a clinical response may take at the minimum several days and as long as many weeks. Drug toxicity is high. Prompt therapy of these aggressive tumors would be optimal. ^{201}Tl also can be used to evaluate for radiation necrosis versus viable tumor in patients with treated brain tumors and equivocal or suspicious MRIs.

Tumors usually are metabolically more active than infection. ^{201}Tl is taken up in many benign and malignant tumors. The resolution is not high in brain tumor imaging with ^{201}Tl, but the target-to-background ratio is very high, allowing straightforward diagnosis. Tumors have high uptake, whereas infection usually has poor uptake. Uncommonly, uptake is seen with inflammatory disease. SPECT is mandatory.

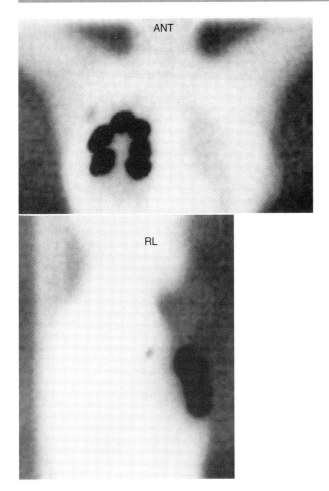

A 49-year-old woman was referred for breast lymphoscintigraphy after recent biopsy of a right breast mass and the diagnosis of breast cancer.

1. What is the implication of axillary node involvement in breast cancer?

2. What is a sentinel node?

3. What is the purpose of sentinel node biopsy?

4. What is the radiopharmaceutical used, and how is the study performed?

Oncology: Breast Cancer Lymphoscintigraphy

1. The 5-year survival rate for breast cancer decreases with axillary node involvement. Adjuvant chemotherapy is indicated.

2. A sentinel node is the first node drained by the lymphatics in a nodal basin.

3. If the sentinel node biopsy is tumor negative, no axillary dissection is needed. If positive, axillary dissection is performed.

4. The pharmaceutical often used is filtered ^{99m}Tc sulfur colloid. It is injected around the lesion or biopsy site. Imaging usually is performed. At surgery a gamma probe is used to help locate the sentinel node.

References

Krag D, Weaver D, Ashikaga T, et al: The sentinel lymph node in breast cancer: a multicenter validation study, *N Engl J Med* 339:941-974, 1998.

Alazraki NP, Styblo T, Grant SF, et al: Sentinel node staging of early breast cancer using lymphoscintigraphy and the intraoperative gamma detecting probe, *Radiol Clin North Am* 3:947-956, 2001.

Cross-Reference

Nuclear Medicine: THE REQUISITES, ed 2, pp 226-227.

Comment

In breast cancer the presence of axillary adenopathy and number of nodes involved is important for prognosis. Clinical evaluation of the axilla for abnormal nodes is not predictive; almost 40% of patients have metastases to axillary nodes that are not detected clinically. More than 80% of women who undergo axillary node dissection have at least one postoperative complication, most commonly, lymphedema.

The rationale for lymphoscintigraphy is that the status of the sentinel node predicts whether nodal metastases are present. Skip lesions are very rare. Many studies have shown high accuracy for lymphoscintigraphy. Blue dye often is also used at surgery to identify and the sentinel lymph node. Timing is critical because the dye moves quickly and can flood the field. Increasingly, surgeons use both blue dye and lymphoscintigraphy for best results. Surgeons now use a gamma probe in the operating room to help locate the sentinel node.

Filtered ^{99m}Tc sulfur colloid is used in the United States. The larger particles that tend not to be taken up by lymphatics are filtered out. Injections usually are made subdermally and subcutaneously at multiple sites around the lesion or biopsy site. Approximately 100 μCi is injected. Imaging usually is completed within an hour. Lateral and anterior views are needed to localize the sentinel node.

Breast lymphoscintigraphy is not yet the standard of care; a multicenter trial is ongoing.

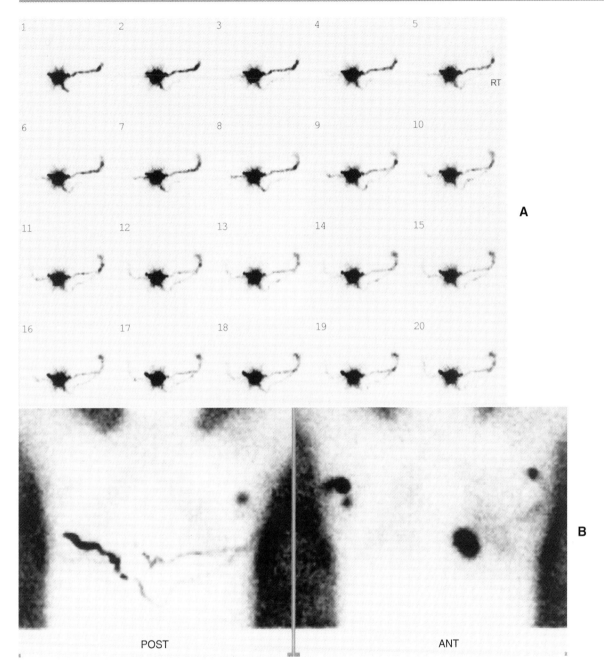

Sentinel node lymphoscintigraphy was performed for malignant melanoma in the mid-left posterior thorax. One-minute posterior images *(A)* are followed by anterior and posterior static images with a cobalt transmission source placed behind the patient for body contour *(B)*. A lead shield was placed over the injection site on the static posterior images (appears cold).

1. What is the radiopharmaceutical commonly used and what is the rationale for its use?

2. Describe the study findings.

3. What is the normal drainage of a mid posterior chest or flank lesion?

4. How are patients with melanoma selected for lymphoscintigraphy?

Oncology: Melanoma Lymphoscintigraphy

1. Filtered ^{99m}Tc sulfur colloid particles, 0.1 to 0.22 μm in size, are injected intradermally, taken up by the lymphatics, and demonstrate lymphatic channels and nodes.

2. One-minute dynamic images: drainage to the right axilla through two separate lymphatic channels, also drains to the left axilla. Nodal uptake in the right axilla is seen on the static posterior view. The anterior view shows two right sentinel nodes and one on the left.

3. Drainage is unpredictable, and may drain to either axillary or to inguinal regions.

4. Prognosis is determined by lesion depth. Those less than 0.76 mm are low risk and rarely metastasize; those deeper than 4 mm often metastasize. Patients with intermediate-thickness lesions are referred for lymphoscintigraphy and sentinel node biopsy.

References

Kraznow AZ, Hellman RS: Lymphoscintigraphy revisited: 1999. In Freeman LM, editor: *Nuclear medicine annual 1999,* Philadelphia, 1999, Lippincott Williams & Wilkins, pp 17-98.

Berman CG, Choi J, Hersh MR, et al: Melanoma lymphoscintigraphy and lymphatic mapping, *Semin Nucl Med* 30:49-55, 2000.

Cross-Reference

Nuclear Medicine: THE REQUISITES, ed 2, pp 226-227.

Comment

As skin melanoma lesions progress, they move deeper into the dermis. Spread from the primary tumor to local lymph nodes occurs before systemic metastases. The current approach is to locate the first lymph node, the sentinel node, that drains the nodal basin. This sentinel node is located on the lymphoscintigram and marked on the patient's skin preoperatively. At the time of surgery, a gamma probe is used to aid in the localization of the sentinel node that is then removed for pathological examination. Many surgeons simultaneously use blue dye. The combination of the two gives best results. If the node is positive for tumor, the other nodes in that basin also are resected. If the node is negative, no further dissection is performed. Because no effective therapy for melanoma exists once it has become widely metastatic, this aggressive surgical approach is increasingly used.

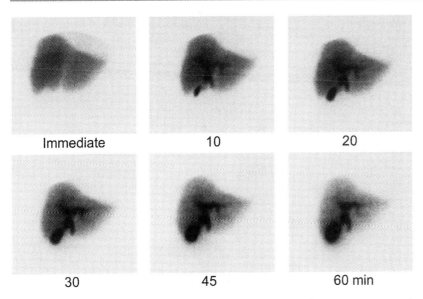

Immediate   10   20

30   45   60 min

A 43-year-old woman was hospitalized with abdominal pain, nausea, and vomiting that started 24 hours before cholescintigraphy.

1. What are the cholescintigraphic findings?

2. What clinical information would be helpful to correctly interpret the study?

3. What is the differential diagnosis?

4. What would you do next?

Hepatobiliary System: Delayed Biliary-to-Bowel Transit

1. Normal gallbladder filling and secretion into biliary ducts; however, no clearance of radiotracer from the common duct or biliary-to-bowel transit by 60 minutes.

2. Is the patient receiving narcotics? Was sincalide (CCK) given before the study?

3. Partial common duct obstruction, functional obstruction caused by sincalide administered before the study, recent narcotic administration, or normal variation.

4. Obtain delayed images or give CCK. The latter would give the answer more promptly.

Reference

Ziessman HA, Zeman RK, Akin EA: Cholescintigraphy: correlation with other hepatobiliary imaging modalities. In Sandler MP, Coleman RE, Wackers FJTh, et al: *Diagnostic nuclear medicine,* ed 4, Baltimore, 2002, Lippincott Williams & Wilkins.

Cross-Reference

Nuclear Medicine: THE REQUISITES, ed 2, pp 242-243.

Comment

In this case, partial common duct obstruction must be excluded. Note that with high-grade obstruction, cholescintigraphy shows hepatic uptake without secretion into the biliary tract because of the high back-pressure. However, with partial common duct obstruction the ^{99m}Tc iminodiacetic acid (IDA) is secreted into the biliary tract but clears poorly from the biliary ducts into the bowel.

Other causes of delayed biliary-to-bowel transit should be considered in addition to obstruction; possible causes are listed above. In this case, sincalide (Kinevac), the terminal octapeptide of CCK, was infused before the study to empty the gallbladder because the patient had no oral intake for more than 24 hours. This is a common reason for delayed biliary-to-bowel transit. As the gallbladder relaxes after sincalide-stimulated contraction, a negative intravesical filling pressure causes bile to preferentially flow to the gallbladder rather than to the common duct. Delayed biliary-to-bowel transit is seen with chronic cholecystitis and has been reported in up to 20% of normal subjects. Obtaining 2- to 4-hour delayed images or sincalide infusion can confirm or exclude partial common duct obstruction. The 2.5-minute half-life of sincalide allows for repeat administration. In a nonobstructed duct, CCK relaxes the sphincter of Oddi and results in prompt biliary-to-bowel transit. Sincalide has a major advantage over delayed imaging in that the answer is known within 30 minutes.

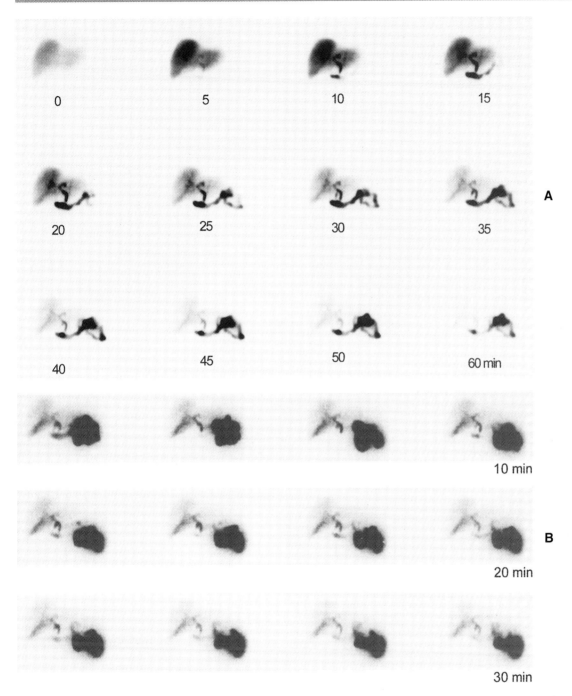

A, 60-minute cholescintigraphy. B, Additional 30-minute images after administration of morphine.

A 63-year-old woman has been hospitalized for 9 days with multiple serious medical problems and is receiving hyper-alimentation. Now acute abdominal pain has developed. She has been referred for cholescintigraphy to rule out acute cholecystitis. *A,* 60-minute cholescintigraphy. *B,* Additional 30-minute images after administration of morphine.

1. What is the relative accuracy of cholescintigraphy in this patient's clinical setting?

2. Describe the cholescintigraphic findings.

3. What is the clinical significance of these findings?

4. What pathological condition is likely?

Hepatobiliary System: RIM Sign

1. Increased incidence of false-positive study results in patients who have been fasting more than 24 hours, those receiving hyperalimentation, or those with concomitant serious illness.

2. Nonvisualization of the gallbladder after 60 minutes. After morphine administration no filling of the gallbladder occurs. Increased uptake is seen in the region of the gallbladder fossa, which persists after most of the liver has washed out (RIM sign).

3. Nonvisualization of the gallbladder after morphine administration is consistent with acute cholecystitis, but the specificity is reduced somewhat in this clinical setting (hyperalimentation). The RIM sign is very specific for acute cholecystitis and confirms the diagnosis.

4. The RIM sign indicates severe acute cholecystitis, which is associated with an increased incidence of gallbladder gangrene and perforation.

References

Brachman MB, Tanasescu DE, Ramanna L, et al: Acute gangrenous cholecystitis: radionuclide diagnosis, *Radiology* 151:209-221, 1984.

Meekin GK, Ziessman HA, Klappenbach RS: Prognostic value and pathophysiologic significance of the rim sign in cholescintigraphy, *J Nucl Med* 28:1679-1682, 1987.

Cross-Reference

Nuclear Medicine: THE REQUISITES, ed 2, p 239.

Comment

With severe acute cholecystitis, gallbladder inflammation may spread from the inflamed gallbladder wall to the adjacent hepatic parenchyma. Surgeons sometimes see an inflammatory exudate with adherence of the gallbladder to the adjacent liver. Cholescintigraphy often shows increased blood flow to the inflamed pericholecystic liver region and/or increased uptake and persistence of the IDA radiotracer (RIM sign). Persistence of this activity is attributed to a reduced hepatocyte ability to clear the tracer and possible local obstruction of bile canaliculi as a result of inflammatory edema. The RIM sign has been reported in 25% to 60% of patients with acute cholecystitis. Thus its sensitivity for acute cholecystitis is poor. However, its specificity is very high. The pathophysiological progression of acute cholecystitis is cystic duct obstruction first, then mucosal edema, polymorphonuclear cell infiltration, finally hemorrhage and necrosis, and if left untreated, gangrene and perforation. The RIM sign suggests that the patient's disease has progressed far along this spectrum of disease. The high specificity of this sign increases the clinician's confidence that the patient has acute cholecystitis, even if the patient has an increased likelihood for a false-positive study, e.g., prolonged fasting, hyperalimentation, concomitant serious illness.

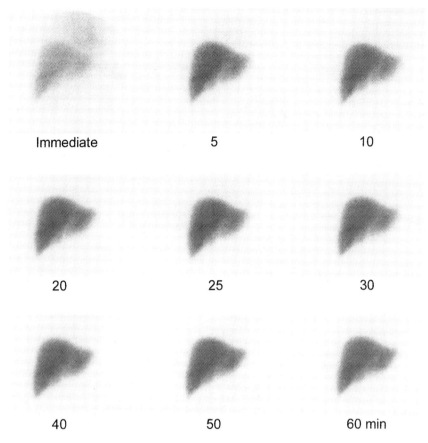

Immediate   5   10

20   25   30

40   50   60 min

A 50-year-old woman has acute onset of abdominal pain of 4 hours' duration. Ultrasonography results are normal.

1. What are the cholescintigraphic findings and the diagnosis?
2. Differentiate the terms *surgical jaundice, biliary obstruction,* and *bile duct dilation.*
3. Differentiate the ^{99m}Tc IDA findings of high- and low-grade biliary obstruction.
4. How do the cholescintigraphic findings of hepatic insufficiency differ from this case?

Hepatobiliary System: High-Grade Biliary Obstruction

1. Prompt hepatic uptake, no excretion into the biliary tract, consistent with high-grade common duct obstruction. Cholestatic jaundice, e.g., drug reaction, may look similar.

2. Obstruction may occur without jaundice. Jaundice is a late manifestation. Obstruction does not always result in ductal dilation. Dilation can be present without obstruction.

3. High-grade: hepatic uptake, no biliary clearance. Low-grade: secretion into biliary ducts, delayed clearance from the biliary ducts, and delayed biliary-to-bowel transit.

4. Hepatic insufficiency: delayed liver uptake and delayed hepatic and background clearance, often delayed biliary-to-bowel transit.

Reference

Ziessman HA, Zeman RK, Akin EA: Cholescintigraphy: correlation with other hepatobiliary imaging modalities. In Sandler MP, Coleman RE, Wackers FJTh, et al: *Diagnostic nuclear medicine,* ed 4, Baltimore, 2002, Lippincott Williams & Wilkins.

Cross-Reference

Nuclear Medicine: THE REQUISITES, ed 2, pp 241-243.

Comment

In early biliary obstruction the serum alkaline phosphatase concentration often is elevated before hyperbilirubinemia. The degree of bile duct dilation varies but is directly related to the duration, degree, and cause of obstruction. Dilation is most prevalent in long-standing obstruction, especially when caused by malignancy. Patients with early, low-grade, or intermittent biliary obstruction may not have dilated ducts. Benign causes of obstruction are less likely to cause significant dilation of the biliary tract. In some cases, ductal dilation may be restricted by edema and scarring as a result of infection or cirrhosis. Once dilated, biliary ducts often remain so even after the stone has passed or surgery has relieved the obstruction. Thus discordance often exists between the physiological scintigraphic results and the morphological images of ultrasonography and CT.

The pathophysiological sequence of events in high-grade biliary obstruction progresses in a predictable manner: obstruction, increased intraductal pressure, reduced bile flow, biliary duct dilation, increased cellular permeability, and finally fibrogenesis leading to cirrhosis. Dilation may not become evident until 24 to 72 hours after the initiating event. Although ultrasonography usually is the first imaging study in the setting of biliary obstruction, cholescintigraphy is indicated when ducts are not dilated. Alternatively, cholescintigraphy is necessary to diagnose or exclude obstruction in patients with previous biliary dilation and suspected acute obstruction.

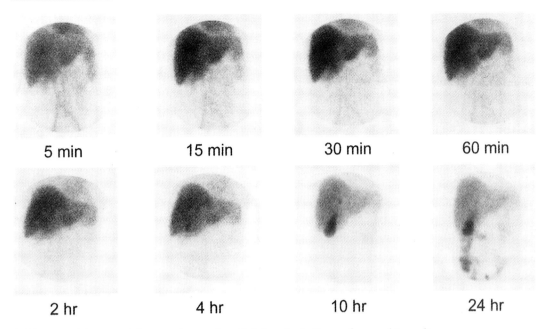

5 min   15 min   30 min   60 min

2 hr   4 hr   10 hr   24 hr

A 50-year-old man with several months of abdominal discomfort and jaundice.

1. Describe the cholescintigraphic findings.
2. What is the differential diagnosis at 60 minutes?
3. How have delayed images helped make the diagnosis?
4. What are the possible FDA-approved radiopharmaceuticals and their alternative route of excretion?

Hepatobiliary System: Hepatic Insufficiency

1. Poor hepatic function: delayed blood pool (heart and great vessels) and background clearance, no secretion into biliary ducts at 60 minutes. Delayed images show very late filling of the gallbladder and biliary-to-bowel transit by 24 hours.

2. Hepatic insufficiency, biliary obstruction with secondary hepatic insufficiency.

3. Delayed images show no radiotracer retention within the biliary ducts and biliary-to-bowel transit, ruling out obstruction.

4. ^{99m}Tc mebrofenin or bromotriethyl minodiacetic acid (IDA; Choletec) or ^{99m}Tc disofenin or DISIDA (Hepatolite). Renal excretion.

Reference

Ziessman HA, Zeman RK, Akin EA: Cholescintigraphy: correlation with other hepatobiliary imaging modalities. In Sandler MP, Coleman RE, Wackers FJTh, et al: *Diagnostic nuclear medicine,* ed 4, Baltimore, 2002, Lippincott Williams & Wilkins.

Cross-Reference

Nuclear Medicine: THE REQUISITES, ed 2, pp 234, 241-242.

Comment

With recent onset of high-grade biliary obstruction, hepatic function usually remains good. With time, secondary hepatic insufficiency may ensue. If radiotracer fills the biliary system and transits the common duct without evidence of retention, the cause is not obstruction. With partial obstruction, there is retention of activity proximal to the site of obstruction. There may or may not be biliary-to-bowel transit.

The differential diagnosis of primary parenchymal liver disease is long. It may be a self-limiting disease, e.g., acute viral hepatitis, alcoholic hepatitis, drug-induced, or chronic and progressive disease, e.g., cirrhosis, chronic active hepatitis. Imaging can differentiate parenchymal disease from diseases that require surgical intervention, e.g., biliary obstruction. In this case the liver does not appear shrunken as in end-stage cirrhosis. This patient probably has acute or subacute hepatic disease. Patients with hepatic insufficiency do not have abdominal pain, although they may have abdominal discomfort from hepatosplenomegaly and ascites.

With normal hepatic function, less than 9% of ^{99m}Tc disofenin is excreted through the kidneys compared with less than 1% for ^{99m}Tc mebrofenin. With increasing hepatic dysfunction, more of the radiotracer is excreted through the kidneys. ^{99m}Tc mebrofenin is preferable to disofenin with hepatic insufficiency because of its greater hepatic extraction (98% versus 88%).

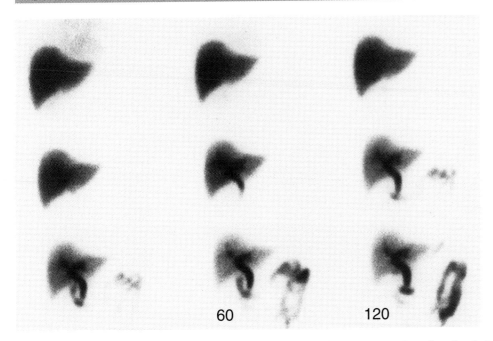

60   120

A 39-year-old woman with abdominal pain; history of cholecystectomy. Results of real-time ultrasonography are normal.

1. Describe the cholescintigraphic findings.

2. Give the differential diagnosis at 60 minutes.

3. Give the diagnosis at 120 minutes.

4. What is an alternative method for making the diagnosis?

Hepatobiliary System: Acute Cholecystitis and Biliary Obstruction

1. Nonfilling of the gallbladder, prominent retained activity in the common duct at 60 minutes, with definite biliary-to-bowel clearance. Continuing biliary-to-bowel transit at 120 minutes, however, increased retention in the common duct. Minor enterogastric reflux.

2. Partial biliary obstruction, hyptonic sphincter of Oddi (normal variation, CCK given before the study, chronic cholecystitis.

3. Very suspicious for partial common duct obstruction.

4. Administer CCK.

References

Ziessman HA: Cholecystokinin cholescintigraphy: clinical indications and proper methodology, *Radiol Clin North Am* 39: 997-1007, 2001.

Ziessman, HA, Zeman RK, Akin EA: Cholescintigraphy: correlation with other hepatobiliary imaging modalities. In Sandler MP, Coleman RE, Wackers FJTh, et al, editors: *Diagnostic nuclear medicine,* ed 4, Philadelphia 2002, Lippincott Williams & Wilkins.

Cross-Reference
Nuclear Medicine: THE REQUISITES, ed 2, pp 235-236, 241-243.

Comment
The ultrasonographic criterion for the diagnosis of biliary obstruction is intrahepatic and extrahepatic biliary dilation. Overall accuracy for common bile duct obstruction is high; however, patients with early, low-grade, or intermittent biliary obstruction may not have dilated ducts. In these cases a discrepancy exists between the results of functional cholescintigraphy and anatomical imaging procedures. With partial biliary obstruction, cholescintigraphy shows delayed clearance of the common duct. Delayed biliary clearance from the common duct at 60 minutes can have various causes, including chronic cholecystitis, precholescintigraphy administration of CCK for prolonged fasting, or normal variation. However, no clearance on 2- to 4-hour delayed imaging or after CCK infusion is consistent with a partial biliary obstruction. CCK relaxes the sphincter of Oddi. Without biliary obstruction, bile clearance from the common duct occurs promptly. The lack of clearance is consistent with obstruction. Although delayed biliary-to-bowel transit is characteristic of biliary obstruction, it is not uncommon for some transit of radiotracer into the intestines to be seen at 60 minutes with partial obstruction, as in this case. The lack of common bile duct clearance is the most sensitive finding.

Biliary obstruction may coexist in patients with acute cholecystitis as a result of the passage of small stones into the common bile duct or Mirizzi syndrome, i.e., edema of the common hepatic duct. This case is such an example. Thus ERCP is needed before cholecystectomy.

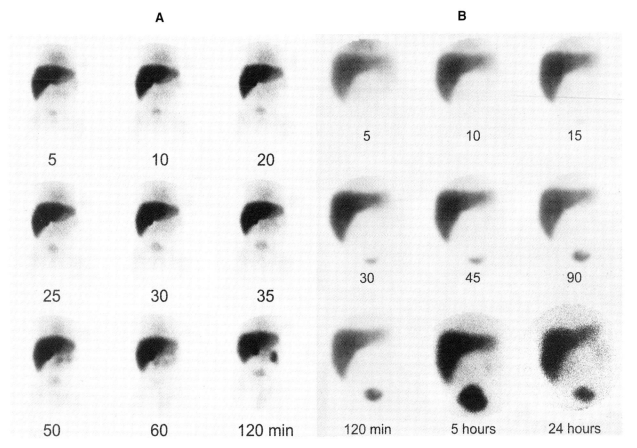

A

B

Both patients are 4 weeks old (*A* and *B*). They have hyperbilirubinemia and were referred to rule out biliary atresia.

1. What patient preparation is required before the cholescintigraphic study?
2. What is the differential diagnosis of hyperbilirubinemia in this age group?
3. What are the scintigraphic findings on these studies and your interpretations?
4. What is the accuracy of cholescintigraphy to diagnose biliary atresia?

Hepatobiliary System: Biliary Atresia

1. Phenobarbital, 5 mg/kg/day for 3 to 5 days before the study.

2. Inflammatory, infectious, and metabolic causes for neonatal hepatitis and biliary atresia.

3. *A,* Delayed blood pool clearance (note heart) as a result of hepatic insufficiency. Biliary clearance at 50 minutes and increasing through 120 minutes. Note the medial edge of the gallbladder (image intensity set high to see bowel activity). *B,* Good liver function. No secretion into biliary ducts during the initial 120 minutes or at 5 and 24 hours. Case *B* is consistent with biliary atresia, case *A* with neonatal hepatitis.

4. Sensitivity 97%, specificity 82%.

Reference

Treves ST, Jones AG, Markisz BA: Liver and spleen. In *Pediatric nuclear medicine,* ed 2, New York, 1994, Springer-Verlag, pp 471-474.

Cross-Reference

Nuclear Medicine: THE REQUISITES, ed 2, p 243.

Comment

Neonatal hepatitis can be difficult to differentiate clinically from biliary atresia because they have similar clinical, biochemical, and histological findings. Early diagnosis is critical because surgery is most successful during the first 3 months of life. The pathological process of biliary atresia is that of a progressive sclerosing cholangitis of the extrahepatic biliary system. Major biliary ducts are partially or totally absent. Periportal fibrosis and intrahepatic proliferation of small bile ducts are characteristic. Cirrhosis develops unless surgically corrected, e.g., Kasai procedure (hepatoportoenterostomy). The extrahepatic damaged ducts are removed and a direct connection is made between the liver and intestines.

Numerous liver diseases mimic biliary atresia. Referred to as neonatal hepatitis, they include infectious agents (cytomegalic virus, hepatitis A and B, rubella, toxoplasma) and metabolic defects (α1-antitrypsin deficiency, inborn errors of metabolism). With neonatal hepatitis the biliary system is patent, but ^{99m}Tc IDA uptake and clearance is delayed as a result of hepatic insufficiency. Biliary-to-bowel transit is variable but should be seen by 24 hours. Patients are pretreated with phenobarbital to maximize the test sensitivity by activating liver excretory enzymes. The serum phenobarbital should be in the therapeutic range. The lack of biliary-to-bowel transit by 24 hours strongly suggests biliary atresia, although a repeat study a few days to a week later sometimes is performed to ensure the correct diagnosis has been made. Definitive diagnosis is made by transhepatic cholangiography, laparotomy, or laparoscopy.

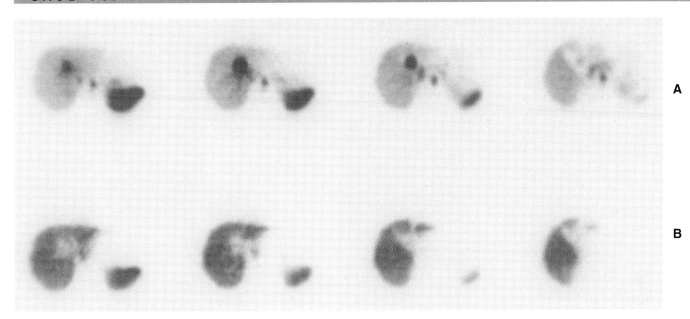

A 46-year-old woman had two different SPECT radionuclide liver studies (*A* and *B*). Comparable selected transaxial slices are shown for the two studies.

1. Name the two radiopharmaceuticals used.
2. What are the scintigraphic findings?
3. What is the differential diagnosis of scan *B* alone?
4. What is the diagnosis in this patient?

Hepatobiliary System: Cavernous Hemangioma of the Liver

1. *A,* ^{99m}Tc-labeled RBC liver study. *B,* ^{99m}Tc sulfur colloid study.

2. Increased uptake on the ^{99m}Tc-labeled RBC study in the same region where a defect (photopenic region) is seen on the ^{99m}Tc sulfur colloid study.

3. Any benign or malignant mass lesion of the liver.

4. Cavernous hemangioma of the liver.

References

Birnbaum BA, Weignreb JC, Meigibow AJ, et al: Definitive diagnosis of hepatic hamartomas: MR imaging versus Tc-99m labeled red blood cell SPECT, *Radiology* 176:95-101, 1990.

Ziessman HA, Silverman PM, Patterson J, et al: Improved detection of small cavernous hemangiomas of the liver with high-resolution three-headed SPECT, *J Nucl Med* 32:2086-2091, 1991.

Cross-Reference
Nuclear Medicine: THE REQUISITES, ed 2, pp 250-253.

Comment

The three-phase planar ^{99m}Tc-labeled RBC study has been used to diagnose cavernous hemangiomas for many years. Classically, blood flow is normal, blood pool has decreased uptake, and 2-hour delayed images show increased uptake. The positive findings have a very high positive predictive value. Few false-positive results have been reported in more than 20 years of use. Its only limitation is its sensitivity for detection of small hemangiomas. SPECT is now used routinely because it provides high-contrast, cross-sectional images. Many studies have shown that SPECT has superior sensitivity compared with planar imaging for detection of hemangiomas that are small, centrally located, multiple, or located near areas of increased uptake such as the heart, spleen, kidneys, and major vessels. ^{99m}Tc sulfur colloid was used in this case for anatomical correlation. CT is more commonly used for that purpose.

MRI and single-headed SPECT have been reported to have similar diagnostic accuracy for detection of hemangiomas, down to a size of 2 cm. Multiheaded SPECT cameras can detect almost all lesions greater than 1.4 cm in size and can detect smaller lesions as small as 0.5 cm, although with a lower sensitivity. MRI has a diagnostic advantage for smaller lesions, particularly those adjacent to major vessels.

A   B

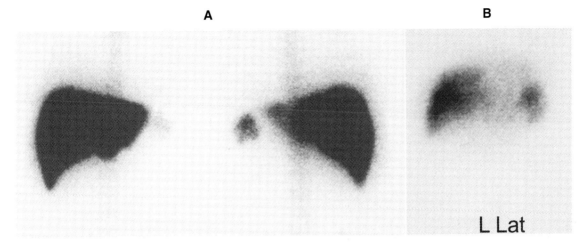

L Lat

This patient has a history of idiopathic thrombocytopenic purpura and prior splenectomy, and now has clinical evidence of recurrent disease. Anterior, posterior *(A),* and left lateral view of a radionuclide scan *(B)* with the intensity set high.

1. What is the radiopharmaceutical?

2. What is the likely purpose of the study?

3. Could other studies be used to make the same diagnosis?

4. How would you interpret the study?

Hepatobiliary System: Splenic Remnant

1. ^{99m}Tc sulfur colloid.

2. To detect a splenic remnant, splenosis, or accessory splenic tissue.

3. Heat or chemically damaged ^{99m}Tc RBC study.

4. Positive for the presence of a splenic remnant.

References

Stewart CA, Sakimura IT, Siegel ME: Scintigraphic demonstration of splenosis, *Clin Nucl Med* 11:161-164, 1986.

Spencer RP: Spleen imaging. In Sandler MP, Coleman RE, Wackers FJTh, et al, editors: *Diagnostic nuclear medicine,* ed 3, Baltimore, 1996, Williams & Wilkins.

Cross-Reference

Nuclear Medicine: THE REQUISITES, ed 2, p 259.

Comment

Splenic imaging has a long history in nuclear medicine. This case shows the use of a ^{99m}Tc sulfur colloid liver spleen scan to detect a splenic remnant in a patient with prior splenectomy. This can be identified as a ^{99m}Tc sulfur colloid study because of uptake by reticuloendothelial cells in splenic tissue, as well as liver (Kupffer cells) and bone marrow. A potential disadvantage of ^{99m}Tc sulfur colloid is that if the splenic tissue is adjacent to the liver, it may be difficult to detect because of the considerable hepatic uptake. SPECT can be helpful.

The classic method to detect functioning splenic tissue is by using heat-denatured or chemically damaged RBCs previously radiolabeled with ^{99m}Tc. This results in splenic uptake with no or little liver uptake. Splenic tissue can also be seen with ^{111}In leukocyte or platelet scans, but they are not used clinically for this indication. The labeling of white blood cells or platelets is more technically demanding, and the administered dose of ^{99m}Tc is much higher than ^{111}In, resulting in superior images for the former and higher dosimetry for the latter. The image quality of this ^{99m}Tc sulfur colloid study seems to be poor but is appropriate because the intensity is set high enough that the splenic remnant can be seen.

Notes

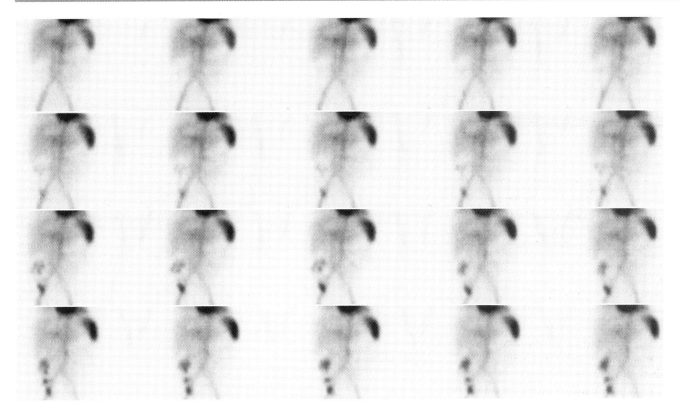

Bright red blood per rectum. No prior history.

1. What radionuclide study is this? Describe the scintigraphic findings.
2. Provide an accurate location for the findings.
3. Name another method of image review that should be used.
4. Provide the differential diagnosis.

Gastrointestinal System: Gastrointestinal Bleeding as a Result of Angiodysplasia

1. ^{99m}Tc-labeled erythrocyte study. Abnormal focal uptake appearing simultaneously at two sites in the right abdomen, increasing in intensity and changing in pattern with time.

2. Cecum and ascending colon.

3. Review images on a computer monitor in cinematic mode.

4. Acute bleeding due to angiodysplasia, diverticula, neoplasm, inflammatory bowel disease, and ischemia.

Reference

Halpert RD, Feczko PJ: *The requisites: gastrointestinal radiology*, ed 2, St Louis, 1999, Mosby, pp 312-314.

Cross-Reference

Nuclear Medicine: THE REQUISITES, ed 2, pp 280-287.

Comment

The radionuclide bleeding scan can determine whether bleeding is active and locate the approximate site of bleeding. In this patient it is difficult to be certain from the images if there are one or two bleeding sites. Review of the images in a cinematic mode often is diagnostically helpful because of the rapid framing rate, usually 1 min/frame. In this case, cine review suggested two bleeding sites that were subsequently confirmed on contrast angiography. ^{99m}Tc RBC scintigraphy is considered the most sensitive method for detecting active gastrointestinal hemorrhage. It provides a longer observation window than ^{99m}Tc sulfur colloid scintigraphy or other techniques, e.g., angiography, colonoscopy. A major advantage of scintigraphy is that intermittent bleeding can be identified, although correct localization of the site of bleeding requires frequent or even continuous imaging. Otherwise, abnormal labeled cells may be seen within the bowel indicating interval bleeding, but the bleeding site may not be evident because of the intraluminal movement of the activity in either an antegrade or retrograde fashion.

Angiodysplasia is a vascular anomaly of the submucosa or mucosa, often multiple, greater than 0.5 cm in diameter, and predominantly found in the right colon. It accounts for 80% of the vascular anomalies of the colon and may coexist with other causes of bleeding. In autopsy series, lesions have been found in 2% of asymptomatic elderly patients. On angiography the angiodysplasia appears as a tangle of small vessels. Early filling of draining veins may be demonstrated, but extravasation of contrast is not commonly seen.

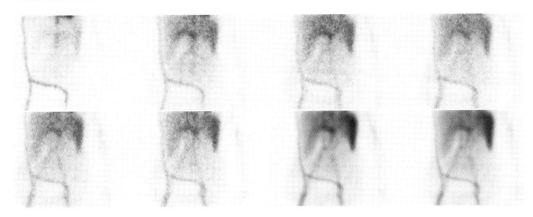

Recent bright red blood per rectum and low hematocrit.

1. Based on the history, what nuclear scans would be appropriate?

2. What information from the history is critical to determine the appropriate time to perform the examination?

3. Name the radiopharmaceutical used for this examination.

4. Describe the scintigraphic findings (first six images are blood flow, last two are delayed statics).

Gastrointestinal System: ^{99m}Tc RBC Scan— Axillobifemoral Bypass Graft

1. ^{99m}Tc-labeled red blood cells or ^{99m}Tc sulfur colloid.

2. Evidence of current or recent gastrointestinal bleeding.

3. ^{99m}Tc-labeled RBCs.

4. The vascular flow and delayed static images show no active gastrointestinal bleeding. Labeled red cells are shown in a tubular shape in the right abdomen that connects after a Y bifurcation to the two iliac vessels as a result of an axillobifemoral vascular bypass graft. The patient has prominent splenomegaly.

References

Weist PW, Hartshorne MF: Atlas of gastrointestinal bleeding (RBC) scintigraphy. In Ziessman HA, Van Nostrand D, editors: *Selected atlas of gastrointestinal scintigraphy,* New York, 1992, Springer-Verlag, pp 35-74.

Craig KC, Skillmann JJ: Clinical aspects of peripheral vascular disease. In Kim D, editor: *Peripheral vascular imaging and intervention,* St Louis, 1992, Mosby, p 59.

Cross-Reference

Nuclear Medicine: THE REQUISITES, ed 2, pp 280-287.

Comment

As is true throughout radiology, distinguishing what is normal from abnormal is the fundamental challenge. At times the presence of altered anatomy increases the challenge. In this case the tubular structure in the right abdomen is easily explained if consideration is given to the fact that native vascular structures and surgically altered vessels or grafts are demonstrated. Similarly, aneurysmal dilatation or prominent varices can complicate interpretation. By relying on simple but essential criteria for determining a positive scan, the skilled interpreter can avoid false-positive study results. Paraphrasing Weist and Hartshorne, a scan is positive if the activity (1) comes out of nowhere, (2) gets hotter and varies in intensity, and (3) moves away through the bowel. This case clearly does not meet these criteria.

Like the axillobifemoral graft, extraanatomical grafts including femorofemoral and axillofemoral grafts are procedures generally reserved for patients who cannot tolerate intraabdominal procedures and aortic cross-clamping or have undergone previous procedures that failed. The 5-year patency rate for axillobifemoral grafts is less than that for aortobifemoral grafts.

A

B

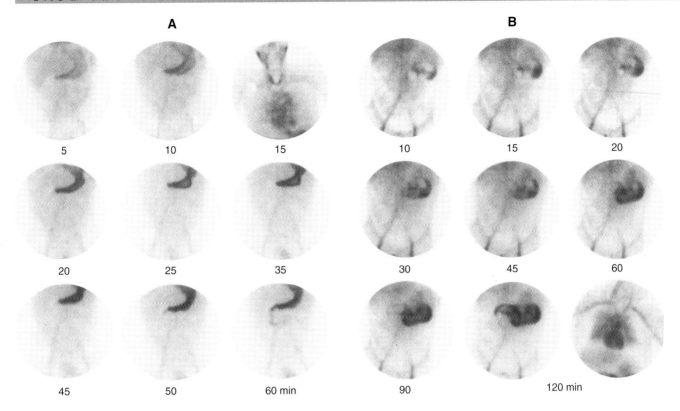

5   10   15   10   15   20

20   25   35   30   45   60

45   50   60 min   90   120 min

Two patients (*A* and *B*) were referred for a radionuclide gastrointestinal bleeding study.

1. What is the radiopharmaceutical used in these studies?

2. Describe the image findings in both studies.

3. Interpret the two studies.

4. Which method of radiolabeling of RBCs has the highest labeling efficiency?

Gastrointestinal System: ^{99m}Tc RBC–Free Pertechnetate versus Gastric Bleeding

1. ^{99m}Tc pertechnetate labeled to RBCs.

2. In both studies the stomach visualizes promptly. The chest and neck image shows thyroid and salivary uptake in study *A* (15-minute image) but not in study *B* (120-minute image).

3. *A,* Free ^{99m}Tc pertechnetate. Negative for gastrointestinal bleeding. *B,* Active bleeding originating from the stomach.

4. In vitro.

References

Srivasta SC, Straub RF: Blood cell labeling with ^{99m}Tc: progress and perspectives, *Semin Nucl Med* 20:41-51, 1990.

Ziessman HA: The gastrointestinal tract. In Harbert JC, Eckelman WC, Neumann RD, editors: *Nuclear medicine, diagnosis and therapy,* New York, 1996, Thieme, pp 617-627.

Cross-Reference

Nuclear Medicine: THE REQUISITES, ed 2, pp 280-287.

Comment

Although the radionuclide bleeding study is ordered to evaluate lower gastrointestinal bleeding, upper tract bleeding sites may be detected. High radiolabeling efficiency is critical for optimum studies and correct interpretation because free ^{99m}Tc pertechnetate is taken up and secreted by gastric mucosa and subsequently moves through the small and large bowel. Gastric bleeding can be differentiated from free pertechnetate by detecting evidence of free pertechnetate uptake in the stomach, thyroid, and salivary glands. The neck and chest view provides this information. In vivo labeling efficiency also can be estimated by the heart blood pool distribution relative to background, e.g., labeling efficiency is higher in case *B* than *A*.

Three methods for radiolabeling of the patient's RBCs have been used over the years. The in vivo method is simplest. Stannous pyrophosphate is intravenously injected first followed 15 minutes later by ^{99m}Tc pertechnetate. The tin allows the ^{99m}Tc pertechnetate to bind to the beta chain of hemoglobin. This binding occurs in vivo with a labeling efficiency of 75% to 80%. The method is adequate for radionuclide ventriculography but not for gastrointestinal bleeding studies. Thus the modified in vivo method was developed. Stannous pyrophosphate is first intravenously injected, then blood is withdrawn into a syringe containing ^{99m}Tc sodium pertechnetate; labeling occurs in the syringe over 10 minutes and then the blood is reinfused. Labeling efficiency is 85% to 90%. The in vitro method is performed totally outside the body and is now available in a simple kit form (UltraTag). It has a 98% labeling efficiency and is the method of choice.

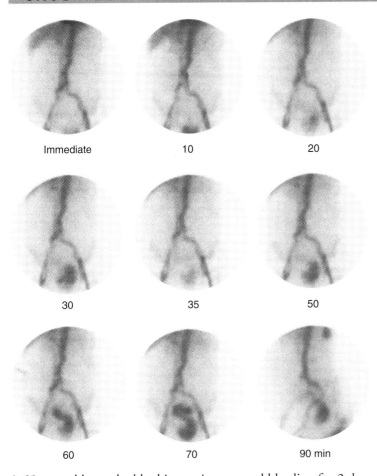

Immediate   10   20

30   35   50

60   70   90 min

A 65-year-old man had had intermittent rectal bleeding for 2 days.

1. Describe the scintigraphic findings during this 90-minute study.

2. What is the purpose of the oblique/lateral pelvic view (last image) in this case?

3. What is your interpretation of the study?

4. What are the criteria for diagnosing and localizing a bleeding site?

Gastrointestinal System: Rectal Bleeding

1. Abnormal activity accumulates early in the lower midline pelvis. The appearance is changing over time and seems to decrease and then increase again.

2. To differentiate activity in the rectum from bladder and penis, in this patient the activity is seen in the rectum.

3. Positive for gastrointestinal bleeding is not the answer. Localization is critical. The 90-minute lateral view confirms that this is rectal bleeding.

4. New activity, increases in amount over time, and moves intraluminally.

References

Wiest PW, Harshoren MF: Atlas of gastrointestinal bleeding (RBC) scintigraphy. In Ziessman HA, Van Nostrand HL, editors: *Selected atlases of gastrointestinal scintigraphy,* New York, 1992, Springer-Verlag, pp 35-73.

Suzman MS, Talmor M, Jennis R, et al: Accurate localization and surgical management of active gastrointestinal hemorrhage with Tc-labeled erythrocyte scintigraphy, *Ann Surg* 224:29-36, 1996.

Cross-Reference

Nuclear Medicine: THE REQUISITES, ed 2, pp 280-287.

Comment

Radionuclide gastrointestinal bleeding studies have greater than 90% accuracy for localization of bleeding sites in the setting of acute bleeding. However, when the study is ordered after all other evaluations are negative and the bleeding has slowed or stopped, the accuracy is poorer. Similarly, the accuracy is not high for slow chronic bleeding.

Interpretive pitfalls should be considered to provide the referring physician with accurate localization information. This case study demonstrates one. Using anterior views only, a bleeding site in the rectum often cannot be differentiated from activity in the bladder or possibly penis blood pool. Lateral images are required. Delayed imaging also can be a potential pitfall. Activity in the left colon at 18 to 24 hours yields no additional information and can be misleading. Blood moves very rapidly and delayed activity could have come from anywhere proximal to that site. Delayed images should be acquired dynamically over a 30- to 60-minute period to determine if and where new active bleeding is occurring. Rapid rate computer acquisition (1 minute per frame) is recommended. Cinematic display can aid in the identification of the bleeding site.

Other common pitfalls are caused by activity in the genitourinary tract and vascular structures. Many are fixed abnormalities, e.g., aneurysms, varices, hemangioma, ectopic kidney. Others are more problematic, e.g., urinary tract activity, ectopic kidneys. Frequent image acquisition and cinematic display is critical.

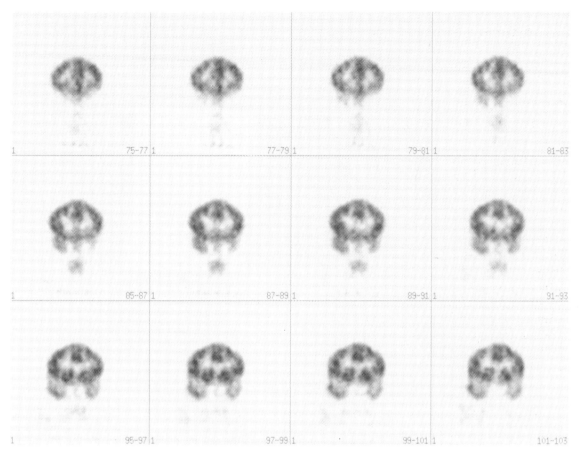

A patient has a seizure disorder unresponsive to medical therapy and is being considered for surgical treatment.

1. Describe the image finding on these coronal ^{18}F FDG-PET slices.
2. What is the differential diagnosis of this image finding if no history was available?
3. What is the probable seizure focus site?
4. What is the utility of PET or SPECT in seizure disorders?

Central Nervous System: Seizure Disorder

1. Decreased metabolism in the left temporal lobe.

2. Temporal lobe infarct, benign mass or low-grade tumor, postradiation therapy changes, interictal left temporal lobe seizure focus.

3. Interictal seizure focus in the left temporal lobe.

4. Confirmation of the location of the seizure focus in a candidate for temporal lobectomy. Study is an alternative to surgical depth electrode placement.

References

Chugani HT: The use of positron emission tomography in the clinical assessment of epilepsy, *Semin Nucl Med* 22:247-253, 1992.

Van Heertum RL, Drocea C, Ichise M, et al: SPECT and PET in the evaluation of neurologic disease, *Radiol Clin North Am* 39:1007-1034.

Cross-Reference

Nuclear Medicine: THE REQUISITES, ed 2, pp 313-314.

Comment

Patients with complex partial seizures uncontrolled by medications may be candidates for temporal lobectomy. Excision of the seizure focus, pathologically medial temporal sclerosis, can eliminate seizures or produce an improvement in pharmacological control in 80% of patients. The success of surgical intervention requires accurate localization preoperatively. CT and MR have poor sensitivity for seizure focus detection. Electroencephalography (EEG) is not always diagnostic or may show bilateral abnormalities and in any case requires confirmation. Surgical placement of intracranial EEG depth electrodes, the traditional confirmatory method, is invasive and has risk. Cerebral FDG-PET or perfusion SPECT findings that are concordant with the history and EEG are an accepted alternative to invasive intracranial monitoring procedures.

An interictal seizure focus is seen on FDG-PET or SPECT perfusion agents as decreased uptake. An ictal seizure focus shows increased perfusion with ^{99m}Tc HM-PAO or ECD SPECT. The sensitivity for interictal detection is approximately 65% to 75%. Data suggest that PET is slightly more accurate. Accuracy of 90% is reported with ictal SPECT studies. However, ictal studies are technically and logistically more demanding, requiring patient hospitalization with EEG monitoring. The radiopharmaceutical must be near the bedside and injected at the time of the seizure. SPECT has a definite advantage for ictal studies because of its radiopharmaceutical properties, e.g., the injection can be given during the seizure, while imaging can be delayed because the radiopharmaceutical fixes intracellularly. The short half-life of FDG-PET (110 minutes) does not allow for delayed image acquisition.

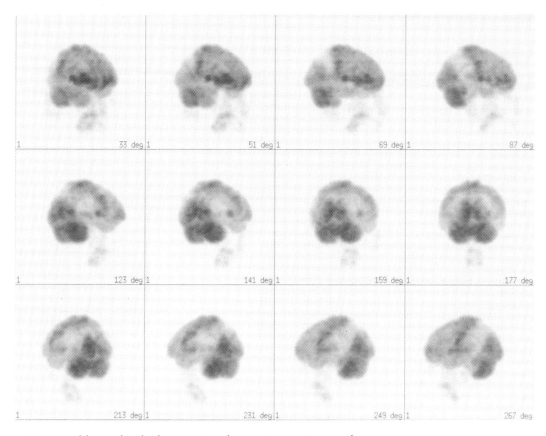

A 55-year-old man has had worsening dementia over 10 months.

1. Give a clinical differential diagnosis for dementia.

2. How can SPECT or PET aid in this differential diagnosis?

3. Describe the ^{18}F FDG-PET findings on the reconstructed three-dimensional volume display.

4. What is the diagnosis and with what degree of certainty?

Central Nervous System: Alzheimer's Disease

1. Multiinfarct, Alzheimer's disease, AIDS-related, substance abuse, alcoholism, Parkinson's, Pick's, Creutzfeldt-Jacob disease, depression, metabolic.

2. Diagnostic patterns using ^{99m}Tc HM-PAO/ECD SPECT and FDG-PET: multiinfarct dementia, Alzheimer's disease, frontal lobe dementias, e.g., Pick's disease.

3. Hypometabolism (decreased FDG uptake) of the posterior parietal and temporal lobes bilaterally and to a lesser extent the frontal lobes. Note persistent metabolism of sensorimotor cortex.

4. Alzheimer's disease; greater than 80% certainty.

References

Van Heertum RL, Drocea C, Ichise M, et al: Single photon emission of CT and positron emission tomography in the evaluation of neurologic disease, *Radiol Clin North Am* 39:1007-1034, 2001.

Hoffman JM, Welsh-Bohmer KA, Hanson M, et al: FDG PET imaging in patients with pathologically verified dementia, *Nucl Med* 41:1920-1928, 2000.

Cross-Reference

Nuclear Medicine: THE REQUISITES, ed 2, pp 311-312.

Comment

The diagnosis of Alzheimer's disease can be difficult to clinically differentiate from other causes of dementia. Although presenile dementia occurs in middle-aged patients, the largest group of patients are elderly, with an incidence of greater than 50% for those older than 80 years of age. Histopathological changes include abnormal tangles of nerve fibers and degenerative neuritic plaques in the posterior parietotemporal cortex. Frontal lobe involvement occurs with severe disease. The patterns on SPECT and PET are similar, although caused by different mechanisms. FDG uptake represents glucose metabolism, whereas HM-PAO/ECD uptake reflects regional cerebral blood flow. The single-photon radiopharmaceuticals are lipophilic and cross the blood-brain barrier. HM-PAO is converted to a hydrophilic complex and ECD to a negatively charged complex; both are trapped intracellularly and cannot diffuse out. The typical scintigraphic pattern in Alzheimer's disease is bilateral hypoperfusion/hypometabolism of the posterior parietal and temporal lobes, sometimes asymmetrical, sparing the occipital and sensorimotor cortex and subcortical gray matter. Frontal lobe hypofunction is seen with advanced disease. A similar distribution can be seen in late Parkinson's dementia and in patients with diffuse Lewy body disease, a degenerative dementia now more widely recognized. The main features are visual hallucinations, fluctuating cognitive decline, and parkinsonian symptoms. Often these patients also have occipital involvement.

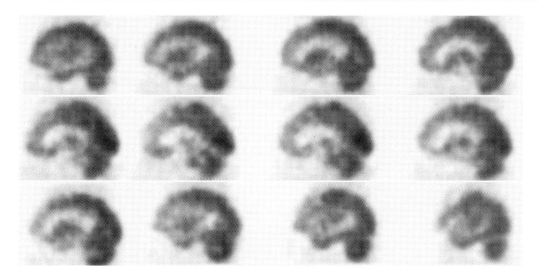

A 55-year-old man has increasing dementia. Recently he had a normal MRI. Sagittal SPECT sections are submitted.

1. List the most common causes of dementia in the elderly.
2. Describe the mechanism of uptake of the radiopharmaceutical used.
3. What causes of dementia are associated with characteristic SPECT perfusion patterns?
4. Describe the findings and the most likely diagnosis.

Central Nervous System: Pick's Disease

1. Alzheimer's disease, multiinfarct, late-stage Parkinson's disease, metabolic, drug-related, depression.

2. The lipophilic ^{99m}Tc HM-PAO or ECD agents cross the intact blood-brain barrier and have rapid intracellular uptake in proportion to cerebral blood flow. They are fixed intracellularly. Subsequent imaging provide a "snapshot" of the blood flow pattern at the time of the injection.

3. Alzheimer's, multiinfarct dementia, Pick's disease.

4. Decreased blood flow in the frontal cortex bilaterally as a result of frontal lobe dementia, e.g., Pick's disease.

References

Sakamoto IK, Sasaki M, et al: Cerebral glucose metabolism in patients with frontotemporal dementia, *J Nucl Med* 39:1875-1878, 1998.

Grossman RI, Yousem DM: *Neuroradiology: the requisites,* St Louis, 1994, Mosby, pp 229-231.

Cross-Reference

Nuclear Medicine: THE REQUISITES, ed 2, pp 306, 311-312.

Comment

Pick's disease is a neurodegenerative disorder that results in altered cognition and personality changes. Symptoms may include memory loss, confusion, cognitive and speech dysfunction, apathy, and abulia. No treatment exists for Pick's disease, and progressive deterioration occurs over months or years. Functional brain imaging using a ^{99m}Tc brain perfusion agent, HM-PAO or ECD, or a metabolic agent, ^{18}F FDG, can reveal decreased function before anatomical changes have occurred. As in Alzheimer's disease, associated atrophy may occur late in the disease, but the distribution is different. In contrast to Alzheimer's disease that typically involves both posterior parieto-temporal regions, Pick's disease affects the anterior frontal and anterior temporal lobes and spares the posterior cortex. Multiinfarct dementia is characterized by multiple asymmetrical defects in the cortex and deep gray matter.

Notes

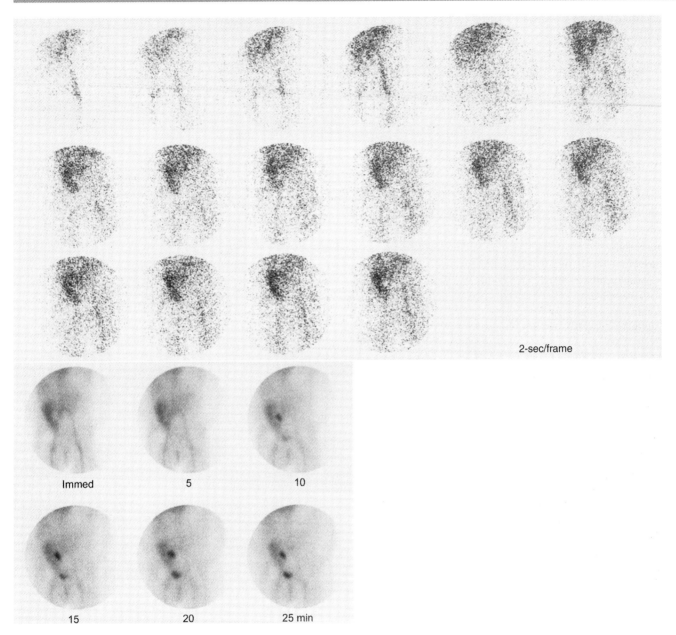

2-sec/frame

Immed   5   10

15   20   25 min

A 25-year-old woman had a kidney transplant 7 days earlier.

1. What are the scintigraphic findings of this ^{99m}Tc MAG3 study?

2. What is the most likely diagnosis?

3. What are the usual associated clinical symptoms and findings?

4. How is the final diagnosis established?

Genitourinary System: Acute Renal Transplant Rejection

1. Very decreased and delayed blood flow and poor transplant function.

2. Acute rejection.

3. Fever, transplant tenderness and enlargement, decreased urinary output, and rising serum creatinine level.

4. Biopsy.

Reference

Choyke PL, Becker JA, Ziessman HA: Imaging the transplanted kidney. In Pollack HM, McClennan BL, editors: *Clinical urology,* ed 2, Philadelphia, 2000, WB Saunders, pp 3091-3118.

Cross-Reference

Nuclear Medicine: THE REQUISITES, ed 2, pp 348-354.

Comment

Acute allograft rejection is a clinical diagnosis. The patients have typical symptoms and findings as described above. Imaging studies are performed to ensure adequate blood flow (viability) and to rule out obstruction. The diagnosis usually is made by biopsy. Renal scintigraphy can be used to follow the clinical course to confirm response to therapy and viability.

The typical scintigraphic findings of acute rejection are decreased blood flow and poor function. Although acute rejection of the renal allograft often begins 5 to 7 days after transplantation, it may occur weeks or months later. Accelerated acute rejection begins the first week after transplantation in patients who have had previous transplants or have received multiple blood transfusions before transplantation, which have sensitized their immune systems. Acute rejection usually is reversible with appropriate therapy, steroids, and immunotherapy. Conversely, chronic rejection progresses slowly over months and years and is unresponsive to therapy.

Acute rejection is a cell-mediated process. Sensitized lymphocytes migrate to the graft and destroy the cells of the graft without the participation of humoral antibodies. Chronic rejection is mediated by an antibody-induced injury to the endothelial and interstitial cells, which suggests a humoral mechanism. Histological changes include arterial narrowing, which progresses to eventual complete obliteration of the lumen, and glomerular lesions.

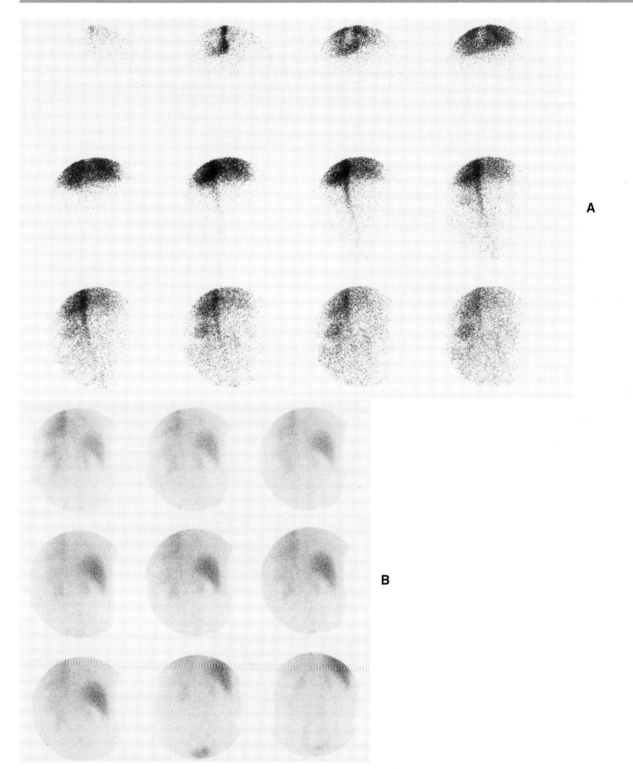

A 59-year-old man admitted to the hospital with pneumonia, elevated serum creatinine level, and no known renal disease.

1. In what projection are renal studies acquired? Name the structures seen on the flow study *(A)*.

2. What are the findings on the postflow dynamic 30-minute study *(B)?* What is the diagnosis?

3. What three general causes of renal failure can the radionuclide study help diagnose?

4. Name the appropriate radiopharmaceutical in this clinical setting?

Genitourinary System: Renal Insufficiency— Small Kidneys, Poor Function

1. Posterior. Right ventricle, lungs, left ventricle, aorta, spleen (not left kidney). The kidneys are very poorly visualized on this flow study, consistent with poor blood flow.

2. Bilaterally small kidneys. Extremely poor renal function. Clearance into the bladder. Diagnosis of chronic renal insufficiency secondary to parenchymal disease.

3. The radionuclide renogram can differentiate prerenal, intrarenal (parenchymal), and postrenal causes.

4. ^{99m}Tc MAG3.

Reference

Choyke PL, Ziessman HA: Imaging of renal failure. In Pollack HM, McClennan BL, editors: *Clinical urography,* ed 2, Philadelphia, 2000, WB Saunders, pp 3053-3058.

Cross-Reference

Nuclear Medicine: THE REQUISITES, ed 2, p 336.

Comment

Although the specific cause cannot always be ascertained with renal scintigraphy, the study can often differentiate prerenal, parenchymal, or postrenal causes of renal insufficiency. Parenchymal causes often can be further clarified as acute or chronic, e.g., small, normal, or enlarged kidneys. Unilateral versus bilateral disease can be noted and a quantitative estimate of relative renal function can be provided. A normal serum creatinine level can be maintained with a single, normal-functioning kidney. Thus an elevated serum creatinine level suggests bilateral dysfunction. Renal scintigraphy is particularly helpful for noninvasive evaluation of the adequacy of blood flow and diagnosis or exclusion of urinary obstruction. In the past, glomerulonephritis was the most common cause of chronic renal failure. Today the leading causes are diabetes mellitus and hypertension.

^{99m}Tc MAG3 is the preferred agent in renal insufficiency because of its high renal extraction; it is secreted by the renal tubules that provide more than 80% of total renal function. The 60% extraction of ^{99m}Tc MAG3 is an advantage compared with the 20% extraction of ^{99m}Tc DTPA. Blood flow to the kidneys, as in this study, often appears to be decreased in severe renal insufficiency. In this case the small kidney size makes it difficult to see the early arterial flow to the kidneys. With nephrectomy or poor renal blood flow the spleen may be misinterpreted as the left kidney. Obstruction is ruled out because activity has reached the bladder without any holdup in the renal collecting system.

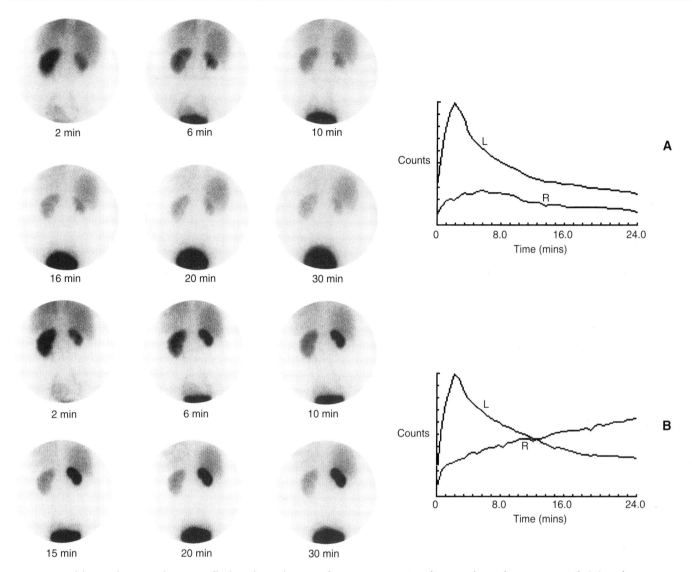

A 30-year-old man has poorly controlled and accelerating hypertension. Baseline study without captopril *(A)* and ^{99m}Tc MAG3 renal studies with captopril *(B)* are shown.

1. What is the rationale and physiological mechanism for the captopril renal study?

2. What are the scintigraphic and time-activity curve findings and diagnosis?

3. Could ^{131}I hippuran or ^{99m}Tc DPTA have been used instead?

4. What is the accuracy of captopril renography?

Genitourinary System: Captopril Renography

1. With renal artery stenosis, glomerular perfusion decreases and glomerular filtration rate (GFR) drops. Renin released from the juxtaglomerular apparatus converts angiotensin I to angiotensin II. Angiotensin II causes vasoconstriction of the glomerular efferent arterioles, raising filtration pressure and maintaining GFR. An angiotensin-converting enzyme (ACE) inhibitor, e.g., captopril, blocks conversion of angiotensin I to II, resulting in a decrease in GFR.

2. The right kidney is small but with good function. With captopril cortical retention persists, consistent with renin-dependent renovascular hypertension of the right kidney. This is confirmed by the renal cortical time-activity curves.

3. Yes. The accuracy of ^{131}I hippuran, ^{99m}Tc DTPA, and ^{99m}Tc MAG3 are similar.

4. Sensitivity, 90%; specificity, 95%. Sensitivity is less for detection of renin-dependent hypertension if the patient has been taking an ACE inhibitor chronically or has renal insufficiency.

References

Fine EJ: Diuretic renography and angiotensin converting enzyme inhibitor renography, *Radiol Clin North Am* 39:979-996, 2001.

Taylor A: Radionuclide renography: a personal approach, *Semin Nucl Med* 29:102-127, 1999.

Cross-Reference

Nuclear Medicine: THE REQUISITES, ed 2, pp 336-340.

Comment

Renal artery stenosis refers to anatomical narrowing. Renovascular hypertension is the pathophysiological result in some patients. Many patients with stenosis do not have renin-dependent hypertension and their hypertension will not be cured by surgical or angioplastic intervention. Captopril renography is a functional test that allows selection of patients with renovascular hypertension who will likely respond to therapy aimed at the stenosis. Intravenous enalapril can be used as an alternative to oral captopril; the advantage is a shorter test with no need to wait for enteric absorption, as with captopril. The ACE inhibitor and baseline study can be performed the same day. Diagnosis depends on seeing cortical function and deriving accurate time-activity curves. Both could be obscured or erroneous in the presence of renal pelvocalyceal retention; thus a diuretic can be given with the radiotracer. The MAG3 finding in renin-dependent renovascular hypertension is persistent cortical retention as a result of delayed urine flow in the renal tubules on the affected side, as seen in this case. The delay in uptake, seen with ^{99m}Tc DTPA and ^{131}I hippuran, may not be seen with MAG3. Bilateral renovascular hypertension is rare. When it occurs, it frequently is asymmetrical. A symmetric response would suggest other factors, e.g., dehydration.

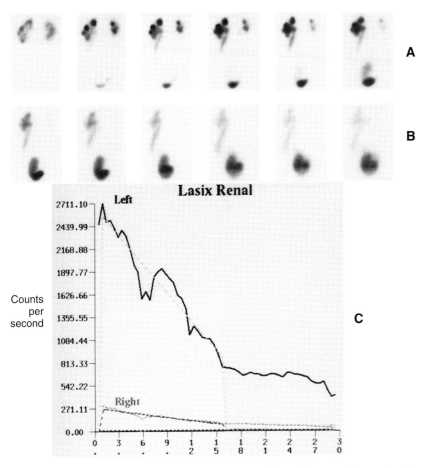

A 7-year-old with hydronephrosis demonstrated on ultrasound examination. No prior history.

1. Based on the history, list the preferred radiopharmaceutical(s) for this study.

2. Would a renal cortical agent be appropriate?

3. Describe the initial findings *(A)* and following diuretic administration (*B* and *C*).

4. List the differential diagnosis and most likely diagnosis.

Primary Megaureter

1. ^{99m}Tc MAG3 or ^{99m}Tc DTPA.

2. No, both ^{99m}Tc dimercaptosuccinic acid (DMSA) or ^{99m}Tc glucoheptonate fix to the renal cortex.

3. Left kidney excretes promptly into collecting system with retention in prominent pelvis and ureter. Prominent dilation distally. After diuretic: prompt clearance of the left collecting system by visual and quantitative assessment. Normal right kidney.

4. Dilated nonobstructed left ureter. Possible causes: vesicoureteral reflux, corrected ureteral vesicle junction obstruction, and primary megaureter; the latter is more likely based on the prominent dilatation of the distal ureter.

References

Blickman H: *Pediatric radiology: the requisites,* ed 2, St Louis, 1998, Mosby, pp 164-166.

Halpert RD, Feczko PJ: *Genitourinary radiology: the requisites,* ed 2, St Louis, 1999, Mosby, pp 177-178.

Cross-Reference

Nuclear Medicine: THE REQUISITES, ed 2, pp 340-348.

Comment

Primary megaureter is unilateral in 75% of patients and usually is discovered incidentally. It often is associated with urinary tract infection or urolithiasis. Because ureteral reflux is a possible cause of ureteral dilatation, contrast or radionuclide voiding cystourethrogram should be performed to distinguish the entities. Generally, primary megaureter leads to a massive dilatation of the lower third of the ureter. However, the entire ureter may become dilated, although the calyces generally maintain a normal appearance. Occasionally it is associated with another congenital abnormality, megacalycosis, where the calices are increased in number. Megacalyces are often squared, which can be mistaken for obstruction. Therefore when megaureter and megacalycosis coexist, it is important to distinguish this from chronic ureteral obstruction by analyzing the number of calices and their shape on iodinated contrast studies.

^{99m}Tc MAG 3, a tubular agent, has a higher renal extraction fraction (60%) than ^{99m}Tc DTPA (20%), a glomerular agent. MAG3 is thus the preferable agent in patients with renal insufficiency. Timing of diuretic infusion varies. It is often administered as the pelvis fills (15 to 20 minutes). Another common method acquires a second acquisition after the initial routine renogram, imaging for an additional 20 minutes on computer. Recently investigators reported that the diuretic can be administered before or simultaneously with radiopharmaceutical administration. All these techniques work well when the methodology is standardized.

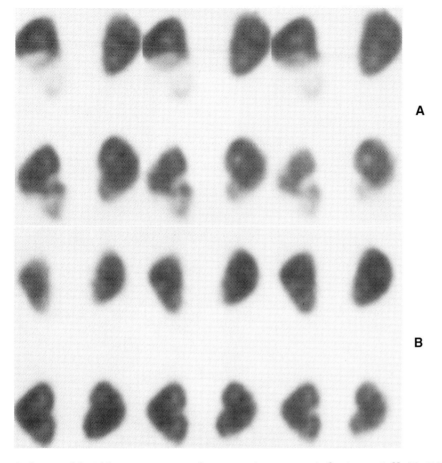

A 6-year-old girl has recurrent and recent urinary tract infections. *A,* ^{99m}Tc DMSA SPECT renal study. *B,* A repeat study 6 months later (comparable coronal slices).

1. What is the mechanism of uptake of ^{99m}Tc DMSA?

2. What are the most common indications for a ^{99m}Tc DMSA study?

3. What are the scintigraphic SPECT findings and what is the diagnosis? What would have been the diagnosis if the second study *(B)* looked similar to the first study *(A)?*

4. What is the clinical importance of differentiating upper and lower tract infection?

Genitourinary System: Pyelonephritis and ^{99m}Tc DMSA

1. Forty percent of ^{99m}Tc DMSA binds and fixes to functioning proximal cortical renal tubules.

2. Diagnosis of pyelonephritis or cortical scarring.

3. Decreased uptake in the lower half of the right kidney on initial imaging *(A)*. Repeat SPECT show normalization of uptake. *A*, Pyelonephritis; *B*, renal cortical scarring.

4. ^{99m}Tc DMSA in the early stages of infection is the best predictor of renal sequelae. Identification of pyelonephritis will increase the duration of antibiotic therapy.

References

Piepsz A, Blaufox I, Granerus GG, et al: Consensus on renal cortical scintigraphy in children with urinary tract infection, *Semin Nucl Med* 29:160-174, 1999.

Rossleigh MA: Renal cortical scintigraphy and diuresis renography in infants and children, *J Nucl Med* 42:91-95, 2001.

Cross-Reference

Nuclear Medicine: THE REQUISITES, ed 2, pp 328-333, 351-354.

Comment

^{99m}Tc DMSA is the most sensitive imaging modality for detection of renal infection or scarring. The advantage of ^{99m}Tc DMSA renal scintigraphy over ^{99m}Tc MAG 3 is that DMSA allows high-resolution cortical images without the presence of overlying collecting system activity. Only 25% of DMSA is cleared by the bladder, and delayed imaging allows adequate time for urinary clearance except with obstruction or severe vesicoureteral reflux. SPECT reportedly has slightly higher sensitivity than planar imaging and planar imaging has higher specificity; however, the differences are not great. DMSA is taken up solely by functioning renal tubular cells and thus cannot differentiate renal scarring from tumor, abscess, or cysts. It has been used in the past to differentiate a renal mass from functional congenitally enlarged column of Bertin (pseudotumor).

With planar imaging a pinhole or converging collimator is used, particularly for children, for magnification and improved resolution. Good SPECT usually requires sedation of younger children. Single defects resulting in localized deformity of the renal outlines (volume loss) are likely the result of scarring and show no improvement on subsequent studies. Large regions of decreased uptake in the upper or lower pole without deformity of the outlines and with indistinct edges (no volume loss) are likely to improve when infection resolves. A follow-up study to differentiate infection from scar should be conducted 3 to 6 months later, allowing time for adequate antibiotic therapy and infection resolution.

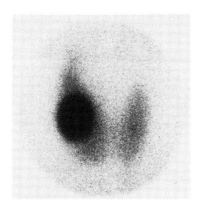 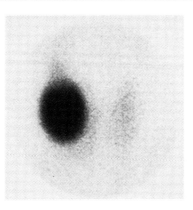 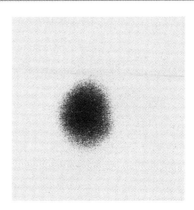

A 39-year-old woman has a 3-year history of hyperthyroidism. ^{123}I thyroid scans were performed each year, shown from left to right.

1. Describe the scintigraphic findings.
2. Give the diagnosis.
3. What treatment options are appropriate for this patient?
4. What would you expect the radioactive iodine thyroid uptake to be?

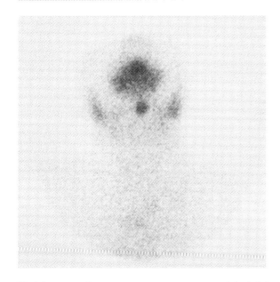

^{99m}Tc pertechnetate scan in a 3-year-old child with a sublingual mass. Patient is euthyroid.

1. What is the mechanism of ^{99m}Tc pertechnetate and ^{123}I sodium iodide uptake?
2. What is the advantage of ^{99m}Tc pertechnetate over ^{123}I in this patient?
3. Describe the scintigraphic findings.
4. What is the diagnosis?

CASE 131

Endocrine System: Toxic Autonomous Thyroid Nodule

1. Hot nodule in the mid-right lobe of the thyroid, with increasing suppression of the remaining gland at each successive year.

2. Toxic autonomous thyroid nodule.

3. Surgery and radioactive ^{131}I are the usual methods of treatment. Therapy with propylthiouracil (PTU) or methimazole (Tapazole) sometimes is used as initial treatment.

4. The radioactive iodine uptake may be moderately elevated, but it often is in the normal range. Normal 24-hour uptake is 10% to 30%.

Reference

Freitas JE: Therapeutic options in the management of toxic and nontoxic nodular goiter, *Semin Nucl Med* 30:88-97, 2000.

Cross-Reference

Nuclear Medicine: THE REQUISITES, ed 2, pp 372-374.

Comment

The patient in this case had subclinical hyperthyroidism at the time of the first two scans (low thyroid-stimulating hormone [TSH]), normal thyroxine (T_4). Because she had no symptoms, she would not accept surgery or radioactive iodine therapy until she developed symptoms (third scan). Nodules larger than 2.5 cm finally usually produce clinical symptoms. A "hot nodule" is defined as a palpable or sonographically confirmed nodule with increased activity on a ^{123}I scan and definite suppression of the remaining gland. The increased T_4/T_3 (T_3, triiodothyronine) suppresses TSH and prevents ^{123}I uptake in the nonautonomous portion of the gland. Occasionally a region on a thyroid scan may appear focally hot but the remainder of the gland is not suppressed. This can be caused by a small autonomous nodule producing insufficient T_4/T_3 to suppress TSH or be due to hyperplastic nonautonomous tissue with relatively better function than other portions of the gland, e.g., in resolving thyroiditis.

The advantage of ^{131}I therapy for toxic nodule disease is that it is taken up preferentially by the nodule, with very little taken up by the normal suppressed gland. After therapy the hyperfunctioning nodule becomes nonfunctional and the remaining gland, no longer suppressed, usually functions normally. Typically 20 to 25 mCi of ^{131}I is given for therapy because autonomous nodules are more resistant to therapy than Graves' disease. After treatment of a single hot nodule, hypothyroidism is very uncommon, in contrast to Graves' disease, because the remaining gland receives little beta radiation.

Notes

CASE 132

Endocrine System: Lingual Thyroid

1. ^{99m}Tc pertechnetate is taken up (trapped) by thyroid follicular cells like iodine but not organified. ^{123}I is taken up and organified.

2. Lower radiation exposure to the pediatric patient.

3. Focal uptake at the base of the tongue. Normal in submandibular glands and mouth. No thyroid in neck.

4. Lingual thyroid.

References

Kalan A, Tariq M: Lingual thyroid: clinical evaluation and comprehensive management, *Ear Nose Throat J* 78:340-349, 1999.

Winslow CP, Weisberger EC: Lingual thyroid and neoplastic change: a review of the literature and description of a case, *Otolaryngol Head Neck Surg* 117:S100-102, 1997.

Cross-Reference

Nuclear Medicine: THE REQUISITES, ed 2, p 376.

Comment

Lingual thyroid is the term applied to a mass of ectopic thyroid tissue located at the base of the tongue midline. This is a rare anomaly resulting from failure of the embryonic gland anlage to descend, occurring between 3 and 7 weeks of embryological development. Thyroid tissue may be located in any position along this thyroglossal tract. The lingual thyroid is the only functioning thyroid tissue in 70% of cases. Hypothyroidism occurs in up to 33% of patients because the ectopic tissue often is hypofunctional. Other symptoms include dysphagia, dysphonia, dyspnea, and hemorrhage. Rare thyroid carcinomas may arise.

Lingual thyroids have two primary clinical pictures. One group consists of infants and young children whose hypothyroidism is detected on routine screening. The differential diagnosis of congenital hypothyroidism includes an absent gland, an ectopic gland (usually lingual), or an inborn error of metabolism causing goiter. These patients often fail to thrive and have mental retardation if thyroid hormone replacement is not initiated early in life. The second group is seen after the onset of dysphagia and oropharyngeal obstruction before or during puberty.

^{99m}Tc pertechnetate scans avoid the need for diagnostic biopsy with the attendant risks of intractable hemorrhage and acute thyrotoxicosis. Suppression with thyroid hormone often is the treatment of choice, although surgery sometimes is necessary for symptomatic patients.

Notes

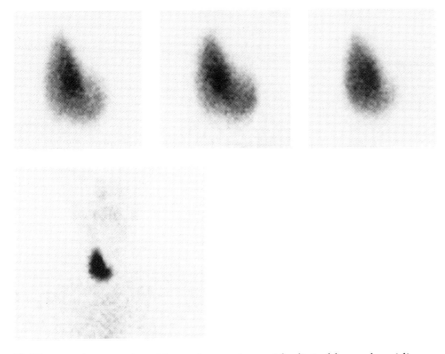

^{99m}Tc pertechnetate thyroid scan in a patient with clinical hyperthyroidism.

1. Describe the scintigraphic findings.
2. Describe the scan evidence that supports the reported hyperthyroidism.
3. What is the differential diagnosis regarding the left lobe?
4. The right lobe is two times normal size by examination. The left lobe is not palpable, no nodules are felt, and no scars are present. What is the most likely diagnosis?

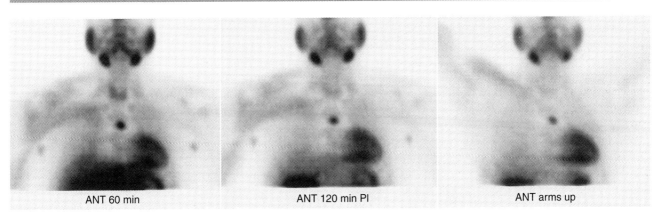

ANT 60 min   ANT 120 min PI   ANT arms up

A 45-year-old man had surgery for hyperparathyroidism that has persisted postoperatively.

1. What is the radiopharmaceutical and study?
2. Describe the scintigraphic findings.
3. What is the differential diagnosis for these findings?
4. What is the likely diagnosis in this clinical setting?

Endocrine System: Thyroid Left Lobe Agenesis—Graves' Disease

1. Uniform uptake in a bulbous-appearing right lobe, without focal areas of increased or decreased uptake. No activity in the expected location of the left lobe or elsewhere in the neck or upper chest.

2. The uniform activity in the right lobe is more intense than in the salivary glands, indirect evidence of an elevated uptake in the absence of intrinsic salivary gland disease.

3. Surgical excision, replacement by hypofunctioning adenoma or carcinoma, suppression by autonomously functioning adenoma on the right, agenesis of the left lobe with Graves' disease of the solitary right lobe.

4. Graves' disease with agenesis of the left lobe.

Reference

Som PM, Curtain HD: *Head and neck imaging,* ed 3, St Louis, 1996, Mosby, pp 757-761.

Cross-Reference

Nuclear Medicine: THE REQUISITES, ed 2, pp 370-371.

Comment

Common causes of hyperthyroidism include Graves' disease (diffuse toxic goiter), toxic multinodular gland, solitary toxic adenoma, and subacute and painless thyroiditis. Less common are iatrogenic ingestion of thyroid hormone, iodine-induced hyperthyroidism, e.g., secondary to contrast, and ectopic disease, e.g., struma ovarii.

Thyroid development begins early in embryonic life between the second and third weeks and is completed by the eleventh week. Embryological descent occurs, which can leave remnants of thyroid tissue anywhere along the course of the thyroglossal duct. During descent interaction with the developing brachial pouches occurs, which may explain the occasional existence of ectopic thyroid tissue in the larynx, esophagus, lateral neck, mediastinum, and pericardium. Morphological features and size of the normal adult thyroid vary. Asymmetry is common. Agenesis can be complete or unilateral. Hemiagenesis is more common on the left.

^{99m}Tc is most often used in children for thyroid imaging because of its low radiation dose and good image quality due to its higher administered dose (adult dose of ^{123}I is 300 μCi compared with 3 to 5 mCi ^{99m}Tc). ^{99m}Tc is trapped by thyroid follicular cells by the same mechanism as ^{123}I; however, it is not organified. ^{99m}Tc uptake can be quantified at 15 to 20 minutes after injection (normal, 0.3% to 3%); iodine uptakes are better standardized.

Notes

Endocrine System: Mediastinal Parathyroid Adenoma

1. Parathyroid scan with ^{99m}Tc sestamibi or ^{99m}Tc tetrofosmin. (Image quality would be inferior with ^{201}Tl.)

2. Focal persistent uptake in the mediastinum, normal salivary, liver, cardiac uptake. Apparent axillary uptake resolves with arms elevated, thus is caused by skin folds.

3. Various benign or malignant neoplasms.

4. Mediastinal parathyroid adenoma.

References

Lossef SV, Ziessman HA, Alijani MR, et al: Multiple hyperfunctioning mediastinal parathyroid glands in a patient with tertiary hyperparathyroidism, *AJR Am J Roentgenol* 161:285-286, 1993.

Iyer RB, Whitman GJ, Aysegul S: Parathyroid adenoma of the mediastinum, *Am J Radiol* 173:94, 1999.

Cross-Reference

Nuclear Medicine: THE REQUISITES, ed 2, pp 384-387.

Comment

Parathyroid adenomas usually are solitary. The parathyroid glands are derived from the pharyngeal pouches. Most persons have four glands, two superior and two inferior ones located close to the thyroid. Ectopic parathyroid adenomas in the anterior mediastinum are derived from the inferior glands that descend with the thymus. Only 3% of parathyroid adenomas are found in the mediastinum. Rare reports exist of more than one parathyroid adenoma found in the mediastinum.

This patient had prior resection of a parathyroid adenoma in the neck. However, the serum calcium and serum parathormone levels remained elevated indicating persistent disease. Mediastinal parathyroid adenomas usually are easily seen on ^{99m}Tc sestamibi scans because of the lack of thyroid background, a problem in the neck. Although special techniques such as computer subtraction of the thyroid or delayed differential washout relative to the thyroid are very helpful in the neck, they are not necessary in the chest. Rarely SPECT can be helpful. Occasionally adenomas are found high in the neck; thus oblique imaging encompassing the upper neck can be helpful. ^{99m}Tc sestamibi and tetrofosmin are nonspecific tumor-imaging agents taken up by a variety of benign and malignant neoplasms. However, in the setting of persistent hyperparathyroidism after neck dissection, focal uptake in the mediastinum is likely to be the culprit parathyroid adenoma.

Notes

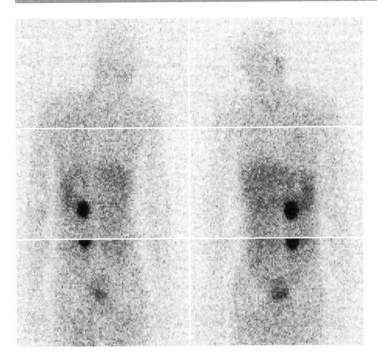

A 47-year-old woman with recent onset of severe hypertension and elevated catecholamine levels.

1. What is the radiopharmaceutical?

2. What is the radiopharmaceutical's mechanism of uptake?

3. What is the accuracy of this study for locating the site of disease? What is the disease?

4. What other diseases take up this radiopharmaceutical?

Endocrine System: MIBG—Pheochromocytoma

1. [131]I meta-iodo-benzyl-guanidine (MIBG).

2. Localization occurs through the norepinephrine reuptake mechanism. It localizes in catecholamine storage vesicles in presynaptic adrenergic nerve endings and the cells of the adrenal medulla.

3. Sensitivity, 90%; specificity, 95% for detection of pheochromocytomas.

4. Various neuroendocrine tumors take up the radiopharmaceutical: neuroblastoma (90%), carcinoid (50%), and medullary carcinoma of the thyroid (25%).

Reference

Gross MD, Shulin BL, Shapiro B, et al: Adrenal scintigraphy and therapy of neuroendocrine tumors with radioiodinated metaiodobenzylguanidine. In Sandler MP, Coleman RE, Wackers FJTh, et al, editors: *Diagnostic nuclear medicine,* ed 3, Baltimore, 1996, Williams & Wilkins, pp 1023-1045.

Cross-Reference

Nuclear Medicine: THE REQUISITES, ed 2, pp 383-384.

Comment

MIBG has a molecular structure similar to the neurotransmitter catecholamine hormone, norepinephrine, and the ganglionic blocking drug, guanethidine. Numerous drugs may interfere with uptake of ^{131}I MIBG and they must be discontinued before the study. These include reserpine, tricyclic antidepressants, and labetalol, both an alpha- and beta-blocker. The patient's thyroid must be blocked with Lugol's solution or SSKI to prevent free radioiodine uptake. Imaging is usually performed at 24, 48, and 72 hours after injection, which allows time for further uptake and background clearance. [123]I MIBG has advantages over ^{131}I MIBG, with better image resolution and the potential for SPECT; however, it is not approved for clinical use.

[131]I MIBG is not a screening test for pheochromocytoma. The diagnosis must first be made clinically with elevated catecholamine levels in the blood or urine. The role of MIBG is in the localization of the tumor. The majority of pheochromocytomas are single, sporadic, and localized in the adrenal gland. [131]I MIBG can be particularly valuable for localizing the 10% of pheochromocytomas that are extraadrenal and occur at various locations from the base of the skull to the pelvis where frequently they are not detected by conventional imaging. Ten percent of pheochromocytomas are multifocal and 10% malignant. The most common sites of metastases are the skeleton, lymph nodes, lung, and peritoneum.

Notes

Challenge Cases

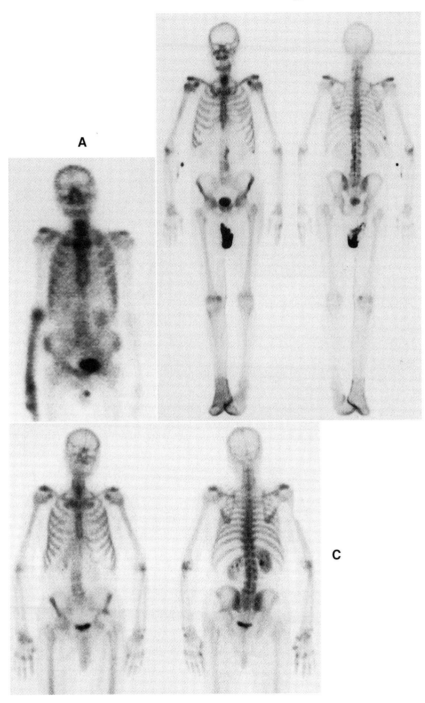

B

A

C

Bone scans *A*, *B*, and *C*.

1. Describe the bone scan findings.

2. Interpret the studies.

3. Name the physical principle that is involved in *C*.

4. Name the most likely type of material involved in *C*.

Skeletal System: Arterial Injection, Boot Artifact, Photopenic Attenuation Artifact

1. *A,* Increased uptake in the right upper extremity from elbow through hands. *B,* Uptake outside bone in both feet and ankles, right greater than left. Urinary contamination of scrotum. *C,* Photopenia of a portion of the right mid-humerus on the posterior view only. Lumbar scoliosis. Left hip prosthesis.

2. *A,* Intraarterial injection. *B,* Urinary contamination of socks (boot artifact). *C,* Attenuation artifact of right humerus.

3. Attenuation of photons.

4. Metal.

References

Chandra R: *Introductory physics of nuclear medicine,* ed 4, Philadelphia, 1992, Lea & Febiger, pp 136, 175-176.

Ryo UY, Alavi A, Collier BD, et al: *Atlas of nuclear medicine artifacts and variants,* ed 2, Chicago, Ill, 1990, Year Book.

Cross-Reference

Nuclear Medicine: THE REQUISITES, ed 2, pp 13-15, 113-116.

Comment

Given that the majority of bone abnormalities appear as "hot" lesions, through experience, radiologists are conditioned to "look for" and therefore "see" lesions that demonstrate increased activity. Photopenic lesions on bone scans can be overlooked easily if one does not specifically check to see that all the expected structures are demonstrated. In case *C,* once the finding is "seen" and noted not to be present on the anterior view, artifacts can be considered. Because the finding is photopenic with normal bone uptake in this region on the anterior view, some material must be between the bone and the posterior detector to account for the reduction in photons reaching the detector. Attenuation is removal of photons from a radiation flux because of absorption. The materials that block or absorb gamma rays are the same as those that block x-rays; therefore metal is the most likely, although barium and calcium also cause attenuation. The technologist confirmed that a metal strip left by maintenance personnel had been found on the imaging table when the patient left. The most common cold artifacts are metal on clothing, coins in the pocket, and metal medallions on the chest.

An intraarterial injection is very uncommon and occurs inadvertently. Technologist hesitate to admit it, but the pattern is characteristic and tells the story. The "boot" artifact is a more common finding and is seen in patients incontinent of urine. Invariably other evidence of urinary contamination is seen on the scan, as in this patient.

A   B

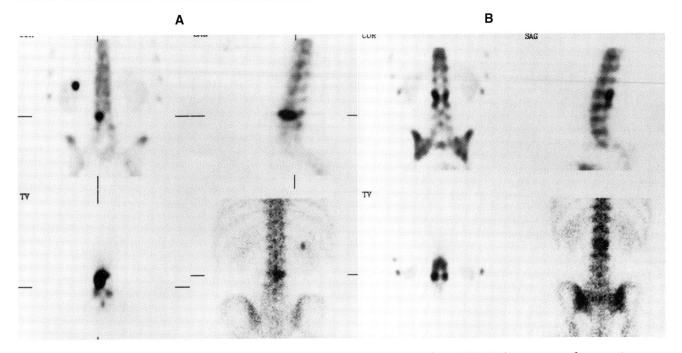

Three-view format of selected coronal, sagittal slices, and transaxial images from SPECT bone scans of two patients with cancer and low back pain. The bottom right images are the posterior projection preprocessed raw images.

1. Describe the scintigraphic SPECT findings in studies *A* and *B*.

2. Give the likely diagnosis in both patients.

3. Why is accuracy of lumbar spine SPECT higher than for planar imaging?

4. How can bone SPECT be clinically helpful in diagnosing disease in a patient with recurrent pain 1 year after spinal surgery?

Skeletal System: Improved Specificity with Bone Scan Lumbar SPECT

1. *A,* Uptake in the region of the L4 right pedicle, extending to the vertebral body. *B,* Uptake in the region of the L2 facet joints bilaterally, right greater than left.

2. *A,* Metastatic tumor. *B,* Articular facet osteoarthritis.

3. SPECT improves the target-to-background ratio by removing overlying activity from adjacent slices and allows for three-dimensional display.

4. One year after surgery a healed fusion has no more than minimally increased activity, whereas a pseudoarthrosis shows active bony repair with increased activity.

References

Sarkaya I, Sarikaya A, Holder LE: The role of single photon emission computed tomography in bone imaging, *Semin Nucl Med* 31:3-16, 2001.

Gates GF: SPECT bone scanning of the spine, *Semin Nucl Med* 28:78-94, 1998.

Cross-Reference

Nuclear Medicine: THE REQUISITES, ed 2, pp 128-129.

Comment

Bone scans are very sensitive for the detection of osseous disease. Although increased uptake is the rule, cold lesions caused by lytic or destructive lesions are not rare with malignant disease and may not always be obvious on two-dimensional planar images because of overlying activity. Thus SPECT can increase the sensitivity and localization of spine abnormalities.

The specificity of bone scanning is its major problem. Benign and malignant causes can appear similar. Specificity often can be improved by determining the distribution of the abnormal uptake. Spine disease can be particularly problematic because of overlapping activity of the anterior and posterior elements. Ascertaining whether the increased focal spine uptake is in the pedicle, body, or posterior elements can improve the specificity and aid in the differential diagnosis. Malignant lesions involve the pedicle and may extend into the vertebral body. Articular facet osteoarthritis, a common cause of bone scan abnormalities, involves the posterior elements of the vertebral body. Posterior oblique views sometimes can be helpful in making this distinction but often do not answer the question. SPECT, with its three-dimensional display, permits differentiation between vertebral body, pedicle, and posterior element uptake. Thus SPECT often can confirm or exclude malignant disease.

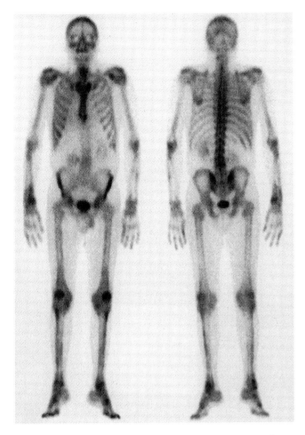

A patient was referred for bone scan because of joint pain.

1. Describe the scintigraphic bone findings.

2. Describe any soft tissue findings. What is the likely cause?

3. What other imaging study should be ordered?

4. What is the diagnosis and most likely common cause for this scan pattern?

Skeletal System: Pulmonary Hypertrophic Osteoarthropathy

1. Diffuse increased uptake in the upper and lower extremities and periarticular regions of the elbow, wrist, and ankle joint. Uptake in the seventh right rib anteriorly.

2. Diffuse uptake in the right thorax. The most common cause is malignant pleural effusion.

3. Chest x-ray.

4. Hypertrophic pulmonary osteoarthropathy. Bronchogenic cancer of the lung.

Reference

Silberstein EB, Elgazzar AH, Fernandez-Ulloa M, et al: Skeletal scintigraphy in non-neoplastic osseous disorders. In Henkin RE, editor: *Nuclear medicine,* St Louis, 1996, Mosby, pp 1185-1186.

Cross-Reference

Nuclear Medicine: THE REQUISITES, ed 2, p 123.

Comment

Hypertrophic osteoarthropathy is characterized clinically by the presence of periostitis causing bone pain and arthralgia, and clubbing of the fingers and toes. The characteristic radiographic and scintigraphic changes usually precede the development of clinical symptoms and signs. The hypertrophic changes regress after successful therapy of the underlying disease.

The bone scan changes of hypertrophic pulmonary osteoarthropathy are evident before radiographic changes. The pattern consists of generally increased activity in long bones and increased activity in the periarticular regions of the long bones, phalanges, scapula, and clavicle. Pericortical striping along the medial and lateral aspects of the lower extremities (railroad tracking) is characteristic.

The pathophysiological process of hypertrophic pulmonary osteoarthropathy is poorly understood. It is seen in a large number of benign and malignant conditions of the chest and abdomen. Thoracic benign and malignant tumors are the most common; the majority are bronchogenic carcinoma. Other less common causes of hypertrophic osteoarthropathy include mesothelioma, pulmonary metastases, bronchiectasis, and lung abscess. In children, it has been reported with asthma, cystic fibrosis, bronchiectasis, mediastinal disease (Hodgkin's disease), cardiovascular disease (cyanotic heart disease, bacterial endocarditis), and gastrointestinal disease (regional enteritis, ulcerative colitis, congenital biliary atresia).

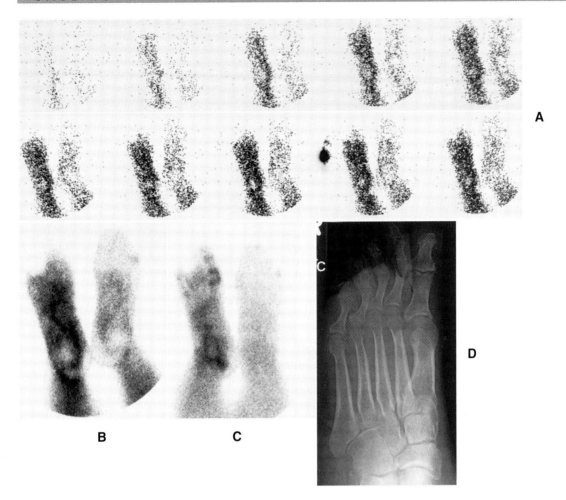

A

B   C

D

A patient with diabetes was referred with cellulitis of the right lower leg to rule out osteomyelitis.

1. Discuss the advantage of a three-phase bone scan compared with the delayed phase only.

2. Describe the scintigraphic bone scan findings. Flow *(A)*, blood pool *(B)*, delayed *(C)*, *D*, Radiograph.

3. Provide the differential diagnosis.

4. What is the most likely diagnosis?

Skeletal System: Gangrene of Toes

1. The flow and blood pool phases increase the specificity of the diagnosis and narrow the differential diagnosis.

2. Diffuse increased blood flow and blood pool to the foot and ankle of the right lower extremity. No blood flow, pool, or uptake of the right third and fourth toes, mild increase in all bones on the delayed image, slightly worse at the first metatarsophalangeal (MTP) joint.

3. Vascular insufficiency, prior surgery, acute osteomyelitis, frostbite, replacement by tumor, artifact.

4. Arterial insufficiency and gangrene of the third and fourth toes; cellulitis; mild arthritis of first MTP joint.

References

Tomas MB, Patel M, Marwin SE, et al: The diabetic foot, *Br J Radiol* 73:443-450, 2000.

Rehm PK, Delahay J: Epiphyseal photopenia associated with metaphyseal osteomyelitis and subperiosteal abscess, *J Nucl Med* 39:1084-1086, 1998.

Cross-Reference

Nuclear Medicine: THE REQUISITES, ed 2, pp 134-136.

Comment

Artifacts such as a lead shield or metal object causing attenuation should be excluded as a cause of nonvisualization. With nonvisualization of bony structures, the radiologist should consider prior surgery, which can be confirmed easily by history, physical inspection, or radiography. In this case, amputation is excluded by the radiograph that shows all digits. An adequate vascular supply is required for delivery of the radiopharmaceutical for deposition to occur. Nonvisualization of the third and fourth toes indicates absent flow, which could result from acute or chronic arterial insufficiency or venous occlusion. In a patient with diabetes, chronic arterial insufficiency is the most likely cause. Acute photopenic osteomyelitis occurs more commonly in children.

A three-phase bone scan can provide additional important diagnostic information on vascular status of the limb or digit and on the degree of active bone remodeling. Osteomyelitis is classically three-phase positive with increased flow, blood pool, and delayed uptake at the site of osteomyelitis. The sensitivity of this finding is high, however, the specificity is less so. Fractures, tumors, and Charcot's joint may produce a similar three-phase positive pattern. A radiolabeled leukocyte study often is needed to confirm the diagnosis in nonvirgin bone. Rarely, acute osteomyelitis in children may show abnormalities on the early phases of the bone scan with a normal delayed phase if imaging is performed early after onset.

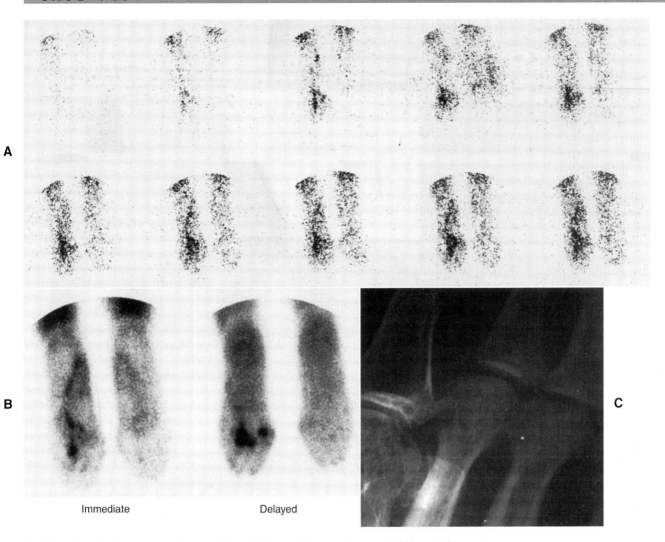

A, Flow. B, Immediate and delayed plantar images.

Immediate   Delayed   C

1. Describe the bone scan abnormality. *A,* Flow. *B,* Immediate and delayed plantar images.

2. Provide the differential diagnosis.

3. Given the radiograph *(C),* name the entity. List at least three other sites that are subject to the same process.

4. List at least three conditions associated with this entity.

Skeletal System: Avascular Necrosis of Metatarsal Head (Freiberg's Disease)

1. The three-phase bone scan demonstrates abnormal increased blood flow and blood pool activity in the region of the second and third metatarsal heads. The delayed bone phase demonstrates increased activity in the bones in the same distribution.

2. Fracture, osteotomy, osteomyelitis, primary or secondary neoplasm, avascular necrosis.

3. Avascular necrosis. Tarsal navicular, carpal lunate, femoral head, humeral head, ring apophyses of the spine, tibial tubercle.

4. Trauma, hypercortisolism, collagen vascular disease, chronic renal disease, aspirin, sickle cell disease, alcoholism, dysbaric conditions.

References

Sartoris DJ: *Musculoskeletal imaging: the requisites,* St Louis, Mosby, 1996, pp 183-193, 375.

Groshar D, Gorenberg M, Ben-Haim S, et al: Lower extremity scintigraphy: the foot and ankle, *Semin Nucl Med* 28:62-67, 1998.

Cross-Reference

Nuclear Medicine: THE REQUISITES, ed 2, pp 132-134.

Comment

This patient's bone scan is an example of Freiberg's disease, one of the osteochondroses, a heterogeneous group of disorders that radiographically display the features of increased density and fragmentation, with or without flattening of the epiphysis or apophysis, as seen on the radiograph involving the third and, to a lesser extent, the second metatarsal head. The causes include osteonecrosis, trauma, and normal variation.

Avascular necrosis, osteonecrosis, and ischemic necrosis are terms applied to the results of inadequate blood flow to bone. Compared with other portions of the bone, the epiphyseal ends of long bones are predisposed because they have relatively limited arterial and venous pathways, which are even more pronounced while growth plates are present. Typically the epiphysis is supplied by a single artery, which increases risk. When the dominant blood supply is compromised, severe ischemia, and, if prolonged, necrosis, occur. Mechanisms of vascular compromise include obstruction, compression, or disruption. Causes or associated conditions include trauma, hypercortisolism, chronic renal disease, aspirin, collagen vascular disease, sickle cell disease, alcoholism, dysbaric conditions (caisson disease). Although it can occur at any joint surface, the sites listed are the most frequently involved.

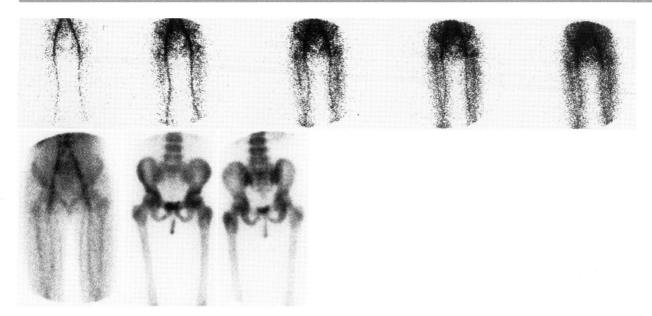

A bone scan was requested for evaluation of hip pain and low-grade fever in an 11-year-old. The hip radiograph was normal.

1. What imaging instructions should be given to the technologist?

2. Describe the scintigraphic findings (*above,* blood flow; *below left,* blood pool; *below middle and right,* delayed images).

3. Provide the differential diagnosis.

4. Bone biopsy: neuroblastoma. Name another radiopharmaceutical used in this disease.

Skeletal System: Neuroblastoma Mimicking Osteomyelitis

1. Three-phase bone scan with attention to the hips because of the acute nature of the symptoms and infection is a clinical consideration.

2. Moderately increased flow, blood pool, and delayed uptake in the proximal right femur metaphysis.

3. Osteomyelitis, fracture, primary or secondary malignant tumor (monostotic), fibrous dysplasia.

4. ^{131}I metabenzylguanidine (MIBG) and ^{111}In pentetreotide, a somatostatin receptor radiotracer.

Reference

Treves ST, Connolly LP, Kirkpatrick, et al: Bone. In Treves ST, editor: *Pediatric nuclear medicine,* ed 2, New York, 1995, Springer-Verlag, pp 287-292.

Cross-Reference

Nuclear Medicine: THE REQUISITES, ed 2, pp 124, 126.

Comment

Neuroblastoma occurs most frequently in early childhood. Fifty percent of patients with neuroblastomas are younger than 2 years, and 75% are younger than 4; the disease is rare after the age of 14. The site of the primary tumor varies; 70% originate in the retroperitoneum, 30% in the adrenal gland, and 10% in the abdominal sympathetic chain. Others occur in the cervical, thoracic, and pelvic sympathetic side chains. The distribution contrasts with pheochromocytoma, which occurs in the adrenal gland in 90% of adults and 25% of children. The most common clinical presentations of neuroblastoma are palpation of a large abdominal mass or manifestations of metastatic disease.

Skeletal scintigraphy is a sensitive detector of metastatic spread to bone and is abnormal weeks before radiographic changes. Uptake on ^{99m}Tc MDP bone scans in the primary tumor is most intense in younger patients. Even when the primary tumor shows no radiographic evidence of calcification, the bone scan often shows primary tumor uptake. A bone metastasis mimicking osteomyelitis, as seen in this case, is not common. The metastatic pattern may be increased symmetric uptake in the proximal humeri, distal femurs, and proximal tibias. This uptake may be subtle and is most prominent in the metaphyseal areas. Chemotherapy may reduce abnormal uptake toward normal; however, this does not indicate tumor eradication. The combination of bone scan with ^{131}I MIBG has the best sensitivity for tumor detection and evaluation of response to therapy.

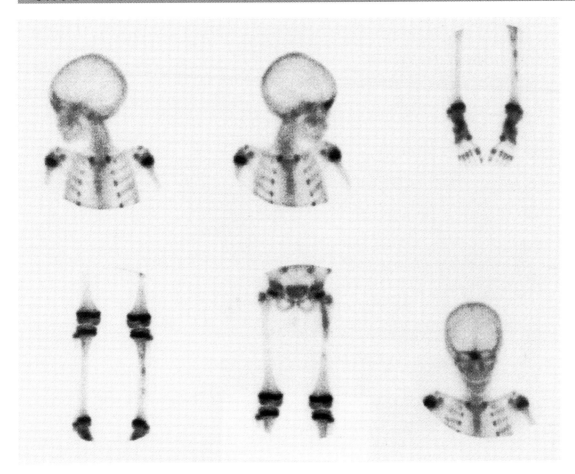

A 5-year-old with precocious puberty.

1. Name two findings that might be seen when examining this patient.

2. Describe the scan findings.

3. What bone lesion is most likely?

4. Name the syndrome that this patient has.

Skeletal System: Fibrous Dysplasia, McCune-Albright Syndrome

1. Pigmented "café-au-lait" skin lesions, gynecomastia.

2. Abnormal uptake is seen in the frontal bone, left femur, left tibia, with a nonuniform pattern of uptake in the long bones.

3. Polyostotic fibrous dysplasia.

4. McCune-Albright syndrome.

References

Greenfield GB: *Radiology of bone diseases,* ed 4, Philadelphia, 1986, Lippincott, pp 127-129.

Machida K, Makita K, Nishikawa J, et al: Scintigraphic manifestation of fibrous dysplasia, *Clin Nucl Med* 11:427-429, 1986.

Cross-Reference

Nuclear Medicine: THE REQUISITES, ed 2, p 127.

Comment

Fibrous dysplasia is a developmental abnormality that results in localized proliferation of fibroblasts that replace normal cancellous bone. The abnormal fibrous tissue results in a trabecular pattern of immature woven bone, the radiographic density of which varies depending on the amount of bone present. The condition may be monostotic, monomelic, or polyostotic. The disease begins in childhood and may be seen in infants. Pathological fracture of the abnormally weak bone is the most frequent complication.

Scintigraphy is helpful in determining the activity and distinguishing monostotic from polyostotic disease. The majority of lesions in fibrous dysplasia are tracer avid on ^{99m}Tc MDP bone scans. Seven percent to 14% of lesions have uptake equivalent to normal bone; however, the remainder show supranormal uptake.

Localized abnormal pigmentation, café-au-lait spots, are present in approximately one third of patients with polyostotic disease. These skin lesions have an irregular outline ("coast of Maine") in contrast to the smoothly marginated ("coast of California) pigmented lesions seen in neurofibromatosis. Several endocrine manifestations can be seen in these patients. Hyperthyroidism may occur in up to 5% of patients. Sexual precocity occurs in up to 30% of females with polyostotic disease, is rare in males, and is referred to as McCune-Albright syndrome.

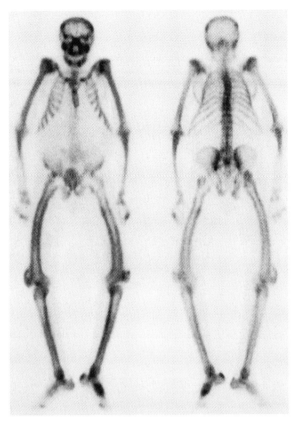

1. Describe the bone scan skeletal abnormalities.

2. Provide the differential diagnoses for the bone abnormalities.

3. Describe the ancillary nonbone abnormalities.

4. Given the presence of nonbone and bone abnormalities, provide the most likely diagnosis.

Bone: Renal Osteodystrophy

1. Increased cortical radiotracer activity in the long bones of the upper and lower extremities. "Railroad tracking" and bowing of the femurs. Bilateral hip prostheses.

2. Hypertrophic osteoarthropathy, vitamin A intoxication, fluorosis, renal osteodystrophy, thyroid acropachy, melorheostosis.

3. High bone-to-soft tissue uptake ratio. Renal nonvisualization. Minimal bladder activity. Additional history: patient is undergoing dialysis following a failed kidney transplant.

4. The scan is characteristic of renal osteodystrophy. Prior hip replacements for avascular necrosis caused by steroid therapy related to the kidney transplant.

References

Greenspan A: *Orthopedic radiology: a practical approach,* Philadelphia, 2000, Williams & Wilkins, pp 655-662.

Sartoris DJ: *Musculoskeletal imaging: the requisites,* St Louis, 1996, Mosby, pp 297-298.

Cross-Reference

Nuclear Medicine: THE REQUISITES, ed 2, pp 121, 138.

Comment

Renal osteodystrophy occurs in patients with chronic renal failure resulting from abnormal vitamin D metabolism and secondary hyperparathyroidism. The former occurs because the kidney is the site of conversion of inactive 25-hydroxyvitamin D to the active form 1,25-dihydroxyvitamin D. Secondary hyperparathyroidism occurs because phosphate retention depresses serum calcium levels, prompting an increase rise in parathyroid hormone levels. Often the radiographic features show evidence of rickets, osteomalacia, or secondary hyperparathyroidism. Osteosclerosis is seen more often in secondary than primary hyperparathyroidism, predominantly in the axial skeleton.

The term *superscan* signifies a bone scan that appears to be of excellent quality because of the high target-to-soft tissue ratio with minimal or no evidence of urinary activity. Patient factors unrelated to the skeleton can result in a "beautiful" bone scan, e.g., enhanced renal clearance because of imaging delay greater than usual, good hydration and renal function, and little soft tissue. The differential for superscan includes renal osteodystrophy, diffuse skeletal metastases, myelofibrosis, fluorosis, mastocytosis, and pyknodysostosis and overlaps the gamut for diffuse osteosclerosis with that of some normal well-conditioned athletes. However, this patient's bone scan is clearly not normal and very characteristic of renal osteodystrophy. Characteristic increased uptake in renal osteodystrophy commonly is seen throughout the calvaria and mandible, costochondral junctions (beading), axial skeletal, and sternum (tie sign).

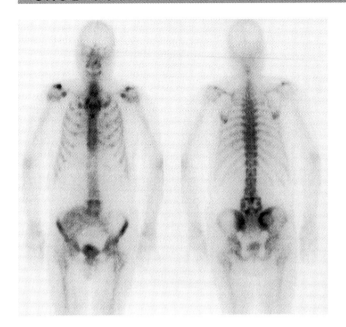

Newly diagnosed prostate cancer.

1. List the abnormalities demonstrated in the bones.

2. Provide the most likely diagnosis.

3. List any other abnormalities.

4. What is most likely diagnosis?

Skeletal System: Lumbar Spinal Fusion, Renal Transplant

1. Abnormal contour at the L4 and L5 level, with relative increase in the diameter of the apparent vertebrae, central photopenia in a well-defined geometrical pattern surrounded by increased activity. Abnormal increased uptake in a crescent pattern in the right sacral ala.

2. Posterior fusion with bone graft material seen lateral to the expected contour of the vertebra. The photopenia is caused by orthopedic hardware (pedicle screws and plates). The right iliac crest is the bone graft donor site.

3. Nonvisualization of kidneys in the expected location; tracer excretion is present in the bladder. Faint soft tissue uptake overlying and extending superior to the right ilium.

4. Lumbar spinal fusion. Renal transplant in the right iliac fossa.

Reference
Palestro CJ: Radionuclide imaging after skeletal interventional procedures, *Semin Nucl Med* 25:3-14, 1995.

Cross-Reference
Nuclear Medicine: THE REQUISITES, ed 2, p 128.

Comment
Spinal fusion is not an uncommon procedure and frequently may be seen as an incidental finding on a bone scan. Further questioning of the patient or comparison with radiographs if they exist can be useful to confirm the nature of the findings. The clue is the abnormality of contour, which in some patients can be even more pronounced than in this case. The intensity of the uptake may vary depending on the duration since surgery and whether continuing abnormal stress or mobility exist at the fusion site. If bone graft material only and no hardware is present, no photopenic defects will be present. The bone graft donor site in this case is obvious, but depending on its location and the duration since surgery, it may not be evident.

The nature of the soft tissue uptake seen in the right lower abdomen is more easily explained if the absence of native kidneys is noted. This can be distinguished as soft tissue uptake rather than abnormal uptake in the ileum, in that the superior medial contour does not conform to the shape of the ileum, and abnormal uptake is not present in the right ileum on the posterior view in that distribution. If the location is uncertain, anterior oblique views or SPECT would provide further information as to its location and separation from the right ilium.

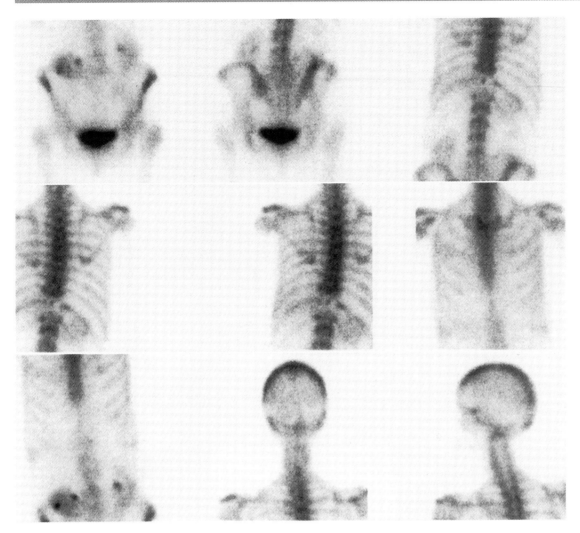

1. The patient was referred for back pain. Describe the bone findings.
2. Describe any other nonosseous findings.
3. Provide the differential diagnosis for the bone abnormality.
4. List three possible primary neoplasms.

Skeletal System: Metastases to Bone (Cold) and Adrenal Gland

1. Photopenia of a low thoracic vertebra, probably T11.

2. Ptotic kidneys, abnormal soft tissue uptake seen between the posterior right eleventh and twelfth ribs.

3. Primary or metastatic neoplasm, attenuation from external or internal source, e.g., buckle on back of clothing, metallic orthopedic hardware, or prior vertebroplasty.

4. Breast, colon, lung; neuroblastoma in a child, but clearly this patient is an adult.

Reference

Silberstein EB, McAfee JG, Spasoff AP: *Diagnostic patterns in nuclear medicine,* Reston, Va, 1998, Society of Nuclear Medicine, p 207.

Cross-Reference

Nuclear Medicine: THE REQUISITES, ed 2, pp 117-125.

Comment

The differential diagnosis for a solitary cold lesion on bone scan is long, but can be shortened by considering the pattern of the abnormality, its location, and the patient's age. On careful inspection, the spinous process is visible, while the remainder of the vertebra appears photopenic. Benign or malignant primary neoplasms such as hemangioma, brown tumor of hyperparathyroidism, or myeloma/plasmacytoma could have this appearance. Metastases that result in primarily lytic lesions, e.g., thyroid and renal, should be considered. However, more often photopenic lesions in adults are caused by common malignancies, such as breast or lung. The majority of metastases from breast or lung scintigraphically show increased activity or occasionally photopenic centers with "hot" margins, but some appear photopenic, as this case. The lung cancer metastasis to the right adrenal gland shows abnormal soft tissue uptake.

Both kidneys are noted to be ptotic and located near the iliac crests on the anterior and posterior views of the abdomen. If one failed to note this, the finding in the right posterior flank could easily be overlooked. The bone scan was obtained with the patient standing. Ptosis rather than ectopia can be confirmed by imaging the patient in the supine position.

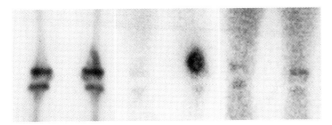

Limited bone scan *(left)* in patient with left distal femur osteosarcoma. A different type of nuclear study was done before *(middle)* and after chemotherapy *(right)*.

1. Describe the bone scan findings.
2. Is a whole-body bone scan warranted?
3. What is the second radiopharmaceutical used?
4. Describe the findings of the second study. What is the clinical significance of the scan findings before and after chemotherapy?

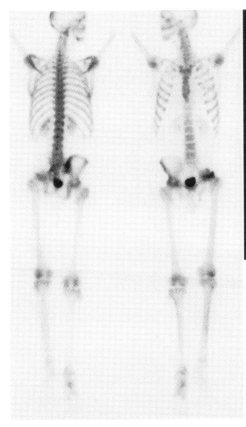
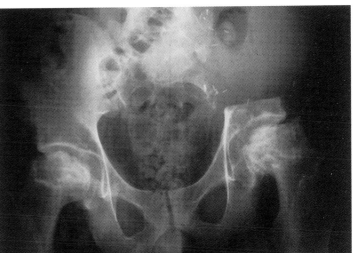

Previously resected chondrosarcoma. Evaluate for metastases.

1. Describe the bone scan findings.
2. Provide the differential diagnoses.
3. List at least three conditions that predispose patients to this condition.
4. List two other sites that are subject to the same process.

CASE 146

Bone: Osteosarcoma and ^{201}Tl

1. Increased uptake in the lateral margin of the distal metaphysis compatible with the known osteosarcoma. Relative photopenia medial to this uptake.

2. Yes, for staging to detect other sites of tumor.

3. ^{201}Tl. ^{99m}Tc sestamibi can be used for the same purpose.

4. Prechemotherapy: very increased uptake in the osteosarcoma. Postchemotherapy: resolution of the uptake. The degree of decrease in ^{201}Tl uptake after therapy correlates with tumor response to chemotherapy and tumor necrosis.

Reference

Imbriaco M, Yet SD, Yeung H, et al: Thallium-201 scintigraphy for the evaluation of tumor response to preoperative chemotherapy in patients with osteosarcoma, *Cancer* 80:1507-1512, 1997.

Cross-Reference

Nuclear Medicine: THE REQUISITES, ed 2, pp 125-127, 136.

Comment

Imaging of osteosarcoma with ^{201}Tl or ^{99m}Tc sestamibi can provide clinical information for evaluation of tumor response to chemotherapy. The degree of decrease in the amount of ^{201}Tl or ^{99m}Tc sestamibi uptake are directly proportional to the degree of tumor necrosis found on histopathology. This is important in preoperative management before limb-sparing surgery, now possible for many patients who previously would have undergone amputation. These agents also are useful for differentiating residual or recurrent tumor from posttherapy changes, as significant residual uptake is suggestive of residual or recurrent tumor. A quantitative assessment of uptake can be made using tumor-to-background ratios by comparing a contralateral or adjacent normal region, adding an objective component to visual assessment.

^{201}Tl and ^{99m}Tc sestamibi are both nonspecific tumor imaging radiopharmaceuticals. ^{201}Tl is a less than ideal agent because of its low energy (69 to 83 keV) and low administered dose, 3 mCi versus 20 to 25 mCi for ^{99m}Tc sestamibi. Although ^{99m}Tc sestamibi has theoretical advantages, less data are available to confirm its usefulness for this purpose. Evaluation of skeletal lesions in the trunk may be compromised because of sestamibi physiological activity in the heart, gastrointestinal tract, or bladder.

Notes

CASE 147

Skeletal System: Avascular Necrosis of Femoral Heads

1. Nonvisualization of the left ilium; leg length discrepancy as a result of high-riding left hip; and increased uptake both femoral heads, left worse than right.

2. The ilium has been surgically resected. Femoral heads: avascular necrosis, fractures, osteotomies; slipped capital femoral epiphyses in the appropriate age group.

3. Trauma, steroid administration, sickle cell disease, collagen vascular disease, chronic renal disease, aspirin, alcoholism, dysbaric conditions.

4. Humeral head, tarsal navicular.

Reference

Sartoris DJ: *Musculoskeletal imaging: the requisites,* St Louis, 1996, Mosby, pp 183-193, 375.

Cross-Reference

Nuclear Medicine: THE REQUISITES, ed 2, pp 132-134.

Comment

When confronted with an imaging study with a gross abnormality, the radiologist easily can become distracted from the less-glaring abnormality. This patient demonstrates scintigraphic and radiographic findings of advanced avascular necrosis of both femoral heads. Likely causes would be steroid administration in the course of chemotherapy or trauma related to severely altered stresses as a result of altered weight bearing.

Avascular necrosis, osteonecrosis, and *ischemic necrosis* are terms applied to the results of inadequate blood flow to bone. Compared with other portions of the bone, the epiphyseal ends of long bones are predisposed because they have relatively limited arterial and venous supply. Mechanisms of vascular compromise include obstruction, compression, or disruption. Although vascular compromise can occur at any joint surface, the femoral and humeral heads are more commonly involved. Scintigraphically the earliest stage may demonstrate photopenia, which often is missed because of the delay in obtaining the scan compared with the onset of symptoms. Later, increased activity is seen as a result of active bone remodeling caused by reparative bone formation. Frequently late in the course, scintigraphic and radiographic changes appear on both sides of the joint as a result of secondary osteoarthritis; the severity of these changes depends on the degree of distortion of the articular surface.

Notes

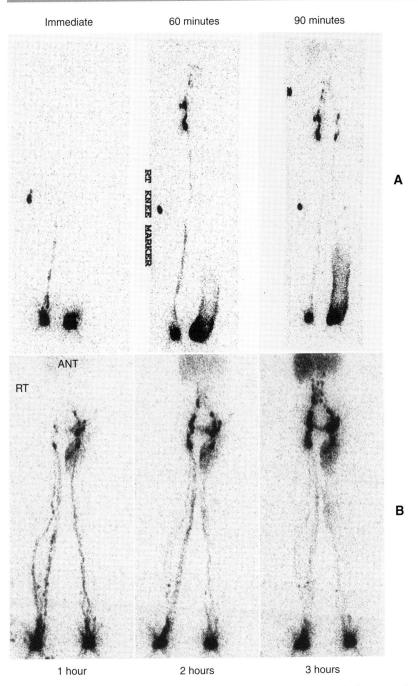

Immediate   60 minutes   90 minutes

RT KNEE MARKER

A

ANT

RT

B

1 hour   2 hours   3 hours

Patient *A* is a 50-year-old woman with recurrent cellulitis and chronic edema of the left lower extremity. Patient *B* is a 60-year-old man with swelling in the left upper thigh for several months after femoral artery surgery. Radionuclide lymphoscintigraphy was performed for both patients.

1. What radiopharmaceutical is most commonly used in the United States for lymphoscintigraphy?

2. What is the differential diagnosis of chronic lower extremity edema if systemic disease, e.g., cardiac, hepatic, renal, have been excluded?

3. Describe the lymphoscintigraphic pattern in these two patients.

4. What are the diagnoses?

Musculoskeletal System: Lymphoscintigraphy of the Lower Extremities

1. Filtered ^{99m}Tc sulfur colloid.

2. Chronic venous insufficiency and lymphedema, primary or secondary.

3. *A,* Normal deep lymphatic flow to femoral and inguinal nodes on the right. Dermal backflow pattern on the distal left lower extremity. *B,* Abnormal focal accumulation in the medial left thigh. One superficial collateral lymphatic vessel on the right.

4. *A,* Lymphatic obstruction *(left)*. *B,* Extravasation into a lymphocele *(left)*. *Right,* Asymptomatic; normal.

References

Gloviczki P, Calcagno D, Shirger A, et al: Noninvasive evaluation of the swollen extremity: experiences with 190 lymphoscintigraphic examinations, *J Vasc Surg* 9:145-152, 1989.

Weissleder H, Weissleder R: Lymphedema: evaluation of qualitative and quantitative lymphoscintigraphy in 238 patients, *Radiology* 167:729-735, 1988.

Cross-Reference

Nuclear Medicine: THE REQUISITES, ed 2, pp 226-227.

Comment

Lymphedema usually is progressive. Early in the disease, edema predominates; later, chronic soft tissue inflammation and ultimately irreversible fibrosis result. Lymphedema can be a primary condition (aplasia, hypoplasia, lymphangiectasia), but most commonly is secondary (infection, inflammation, trauma, malignancy, surgical or radiation therapy). Venous and lymphatic causes may coexist. Lymphedema usually is diagnosed on a clinical basis; imaging studies can confirm or exclude lymphatic obstruction. Contrast lymphangiography is technically difficult to perform; especially in this patient group, it does not allow functional assessment of lymph flow and may produce lymphadenitis.

Radionuclide lymphoscintigraphy demonstrates the physiology of lymphatic flow. Radiolabeled colloid particles are injected subcutaneously between web spaces of the second and third toes. In patients without lymphatic disease, lymphoscintigraphy shows lymph flowing along the medial aspect of the leg to lymph nodes in the groin, pelvis, and paraaortic region. Abnormal patterns of obstruction include no or delayed flow, collateral vessel flow, dermal backflow because of obstructed or nonfunctioning lymph channels with interstitial dermal lymph transport (case *A*), extravasation into lymphoceles or fistula (case *B*), and lymphangiectasia.

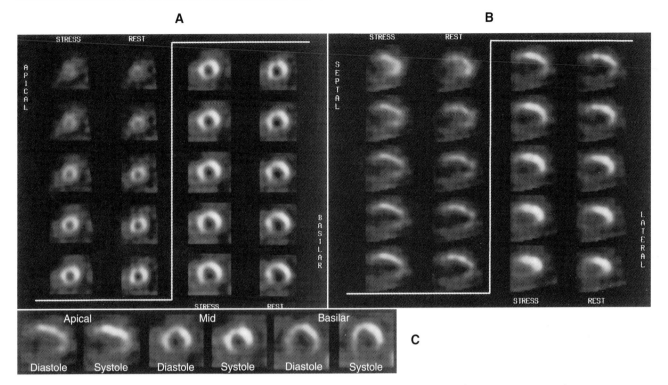

A 48-year-old patient with COPD and claudication. She has asthma. SPECT perfusion images (*A*, short-axis; *B*, vertical long-axis; and *C*, select gated poststress SPECT images). The left ventricular ejection fraction (LVEF) is 20%.

1. What is the appropriate stress technique for this patient? In what other patients is this the stress method of choice?

2. Why is this considered a second-line pharmacological stress agent?

3. Describe the SPECT image findings in this case.

4. What is the mechanism of cardiac uptake for ^{99m}Tc sestamibi and ^{99m}Tc tetrofosmin?

Cardiovascular System: Dobutamine Stress

1. Dobutamine stress. Patients who are not candidates for either exercise, e.g., claudication, or vasodilator stress, e.g., patients with asthma.

2. The common occurrence of side effects including angina and the inability of a significant number of patients to tolerate the required dose.

3. Mild fixed anteroseptal perfusion defect with decreased wall thickening. Severe fixed inferior defect with absent wall thickening. Dilated left ventricular cavity. No reversibility. Myocardial thickening and wall motion signify functioning viable myocardium.

4. ^{99m}Tc sestamibi, an isonitrile monovalent cation, diffuses passively from the blood into myocardial cells because of its lipophilicity, then localizes in the mitochondria. ^{99m}Tc tetrofosmin, a diphosphene, has a similar uptake mechanism.

Reference
Travain MI, Wexler JP: Pharmacological stress testing, *Semin Nucl Med* 29:298-318, 1999.

Cross-Reference
Nuclear Medicine: THE REQUISITES, ed 2, pp 85-86.

Comment
Dobutamine is a synthetic catecholamine that acts on α- and β-adrenergic receptors (inotropic and chronotropic properties). It increases coronary blood flow by increasing myocardial oxygen demand (increased heart rate, systolic blood pressure, contractility). The protocol for intravenous dobutamine infusion is infusion of increasingly higher dose rates up to a maximum of 40 μg/kg/min under constant ECG monitoring. Because of its short half-life, side effects can be managed by discontinuing the infusion.

Typical candidates for dobutamine are those who cannot exercise because of arthritis, peripheral vascular disease, or lower extremity weakness or patients with bronchospastic pulmonary disease, e.g., COPD or patients with asthma who cannot be given adenosine. Dobutamine also can be used in patients in whom xanthine-containing medications or foods were not discontinued before the appointment for adenosine or dipyridamole stress. Patients with low systolic blood pressure also may be candidates because blood pressure tends to increase with dobutamine but tends to decrease with adenosine and dipyridamole. Relative contraindications to dobutamine are recent myocardial infarction or unstable angina, significant left ventricular outflow obstruction, atrial tachyarrhythmias, ventricular tachycardia, uncontrolled severe hypertension, aortic dissections, or aneurysms.

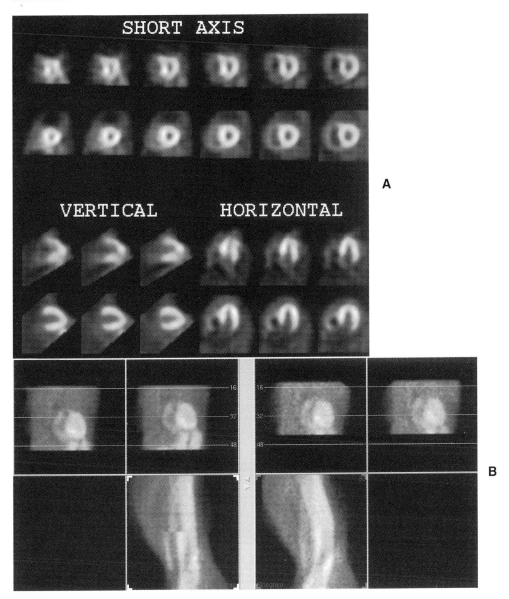

A, Exercise myocardial SPECT perfusion studies. The patient's initial stress study acquisition *(above)* and repeat acquisition *(below). B,* Sinograms for the first *(left)* and second *(right)* scans.

1. Describe the findings based on the SPECT images and sinograms.

2. Describe the purpose of the sinogram.

3. List other techniques in addition to the sinogram that can be used similarly.

4. Provide the diagnosis.

Cardiovascular System: Patient Movement Artifact

1. *A,* The first study *(above)* shows an abnormal configuration of the anterior wall; the repeat study *(below)* is normal. *B,* The initial sinogram shows a discontinuity or break; the second is normal.

2. To visually present the raw unprocessed projection images to evaluate for patient motion.

3. Review SPECT projection data, image by image, or in cinematic display.

4. Artifact caused by patient motion.

Reference

DePuey EG: Artifacts in SPECT myocardial perfusion imaging. In DePuey EG, Garcia EV, Berman DS, editors: *Cardiac SPECT imaging,* ed 2, Philadelphia, 2001, Lippincott Williams & Wilkins, pp 232-262.

Cross-Reference

Nuclear Medicine: THE REQUISITES, ed 2, pp 42-43, 75-79.

Comment

Artifact should be considered when the myocardium appears irregular in shape and contour. Linear rays of activity (comet tails) are present in the initial study, strongly suggestive of motion, but are not seen on the repeat study. The radiologist also should consider center of rotation error as a mechanism for the artifact. Sinograms are constructed by stacking all raw projection images of a single cross-sectional slice. The histogram plane is indicated by the horizontal line crossing the cardiac projection images in *B (above).* The first sinogram shows an abnormal sharp step-off or discontinuity; the second shows a normal, smooth-curving appearance.

The unprocessed projection images from the SPECT acquisition should be inspected before image reconstruction. As seen in this study, motion can severely degrade the quality of the SPECT scan. Greater than two pixels of movement often produces artifacts. Some gamma camera–computer systems offer motion correction software that can be used to adjust for horizontal or vertical motion of the patient. However, it cannot correct for off-plane motion. When practical, imaging should be repeated if significant patient motion has occurred. This is feasible with ^{99m}Tc myocardial perfusion agents that fix in myocardial cells, but much less possible for ^{201}Tl stress imaging with ongoing dynamic wash-in and washout of the radiopharmaceutical.

Regular gamma camera quality control procedures are even more critical for SPECT than for planar imaging. Factors determining image quality include center of rotation, pixel size, uniformity, spatial resolution and linearity, and detector head alignment, and head matching if a multiheaded camera is used.

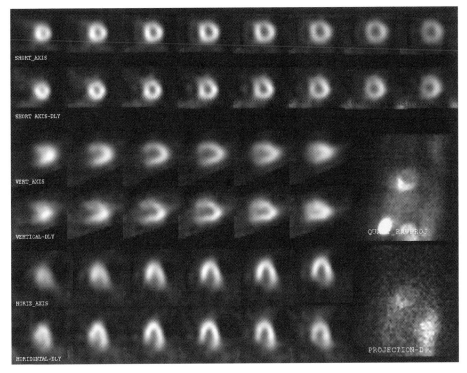

Stress and rest SPECT myocardial perfusion images and a single projection of unprocessed acquisition data from a cine loop *(right)* are provided.

1. What radiopharmaceuticals can be used for this stress study?

2. Describe the SPECT findings and any additional information available from the cine loop stress and rest projection images.

3. List the differential diagnosis.

4. List the advantages of adding ECG-synchronization (gating) to SPECT myocardial perfusion imaging.

Cardiovascular System: Breast Attenuation

1. ^{99m}Tc sestamibi (Cardiolite), tetrofosmin (Myoview), and not ^{201}Tl because the gall bladder is seen.

2. Mild fixed defect in the anterior wall. Projection images: decreased uptake in the upper half of the heart at stress and rest in a curvilinear configuration.

3. Breast attenuation, anterior wall myocardial scar (infarction).

4. Assessment of regional wall motion, wall thickening, and ejection fraction.

Reference

DePuey EG: Artifacts in SPECT myocardial perfusion imaging. In DePuey EG, Garcia EV, Berman DS, editors: *Cardiac SPECT imaging*, ed 2, Philadelphia, 2001, Lippincott Williams & Wilkins, pp 232-262.

Cross-Reference

Nuclear Medicine: THE REQUISITES, ed 2, pp 67-68, 73-79.

Comment

Breast tissue often causes attenuation of photons arising from the heart, reducing the number of counts available for image reconstruction in that region. This can lead to spurious defects varying in location depending on the breast position at the time of imaging. Breast attenuation defects most commonly occur in the anterior and anterolateral walls but also are seen in the anteroseptal and lateral walls, depending on the location, density, and mobility of breast tissue. Breast attenuation would be expected to appear as a "fixed" defect; however, with a change in breast position between the stress and rest images, a stress-rest pattern can be seen that may mimic ischemia. Unprocessed acquisition projection image data should be reviewed to confirm the presence of attenuation and determine whether the breast has changed position between stress and rest.

Various interventions have been used to minimize attenuation, including the use of a breast binder to flatten and hold the breasts in the same position for both scans, or imaging the patient with the bra on to ensure similar positioning on both studies. Others image with the bra off, contending that gravity will flatten the breast (decreasing its thickness and attenuation). Gated SPECT can help to differentiate attenuation effects from myocardial infarction in patients with fixed defects. Infarcts show abnormal motion and thickening; attenuation defects have normal function. Note the focal hot spot seen in the right lower corner on the stress projection image caused by gallbladder filling. ^{99m}Tc sestamibi and tetrofosmin both have hepatobiliary clearance.

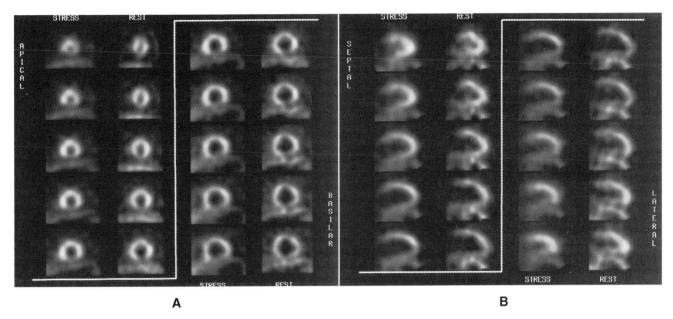

A   B

Dipyridamole (Persantine) sestamibi SPECT myocardial perfusion study. Short-axis *(A)* and vertical long-axis images *(B)* are shown.

1. List the mechanism of action of dipyridamole. List foods and medications that counteract its pharmacological effect.
2. Describe the timing of radiotracer injection with respect to dipyridamole administration and the management of dipyridamole side effects.
3. Describe the SPECT image findings.
4. List maneuvers to deal with the problem of abdominal (liver and intestinal) activity.

Cardiovascular System: Dipyridamole, Inferior Ischemia, Overlying Bowel Activity

1. Dipyridamole inhibits the action of adenosine deaminase, thus increasing endogenous adenosine, a potent coronary artery vasodilator. Coffee, tea, caffeine-containing soft drinks or foods such as chocolate, theophylline, and aminophylline.

2. Dipyridamole is infused for 4 minutes. Radiotracer is given 3 minutes after completion of the dipyridamole infusion. Side effects can be reversed with intravenous aminophylline.

3. Mild to moderate fixed defect of the anterior wall. Severe, mostly fixed defect involving the entire inferior wall, but a small area of reversibility in the inferoapical-apical region. Dilated left ventricle.

4. Obtain delayed SPECT to allow additional hepatic clearance or movement of bowel activity, have the patient drink water, or both.

Reference

Rehm PK, Atkins FB, Ziessman HA, et al: Frequency of extracardiac activity and its effect on Tc-99m sestamibi cardiac SPECT interpretation, *Nucl Med Commun* 17:851-856, 1996.

Cross-Reference

Nuclear Medicine: THE REQUISITES, ed 2, pp 66-72, 85, 390, 392-393.

Comment

The radiopharmaceutical is injected at peak dipyridamole effect, which occurs 2 to 3 minutes after complete infusion. Relative contraindications to dipyridamole and adenosine include asthma or bronchospastic pulmonary disease, hypotension, severe bradycardia, or heart block greater than first-degree. Adverse effects can be treated with a slow intravenous injection of 125 to 250 mg of aminophylline and can be repeated 2 to 5 minutes later if necessary. Because dipyridamole's duration of action is longer than that of aminophylline, a subsequent injection of aminophylline may be necessary if side effects recur.

Extracardiac subdiaphragmatic activity can cause interpretation problems, whether related to liver or hepatobiliary clearance of ^{99m}Tc perfusion agents into the intestines. Abdominal activity is common on rest or vasodilator stress studies because of increased splanchnic distribution compared with exercise stress studies. With exercise, splanchnic flow is diverted to the muscles. In this study case, curvilinear activity is noted adjacent to the inferior wall, but the ischemia can be seen separate from bowel activity. However, at times extracardiac activity may overlie the inferior wall or cause significant scatter, making it difficult or impossible to evaluate that portion of the myocardium.

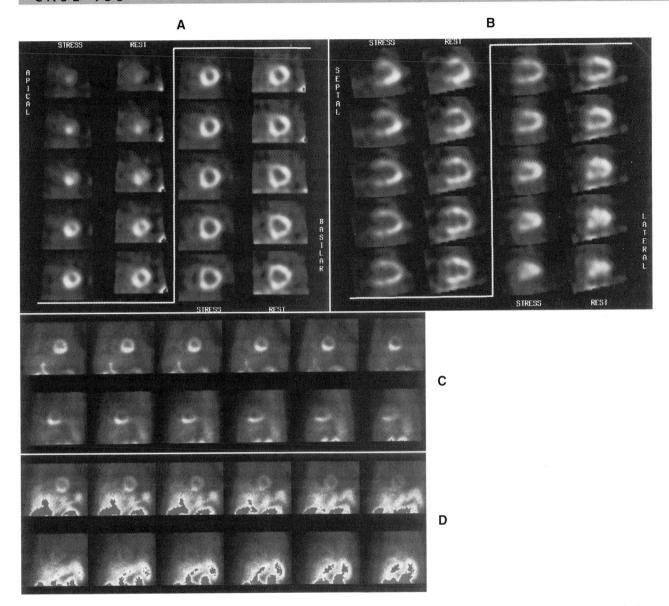

A 45-year-old woman with hypercholesterolemia. *A,* Short-axis and *B,* vertical long-axis SPECT stress myocardial perfusion images, and raw data sequential projection images from the stress *(C)* and rest *(D)* scans.

1. Describe the SPECT perfusion image findings.

2. List three reasons to review the raw data projection images.

3. Provide any information available from the acquisition projection images.

4. What is the most likely diagnosis?

Cardiovascular System: Attenuation Caused by Change of Breast Position

1. Partially reversible perfusion defect in the apical-antero-septal wall. Mild fixed defect in the inferolateral wall. Dilated left ventricle.

2. To detect patient motion, camera malfunction, or attenuation.

3. Decreased radiotracer in the upper portions of the myocardium that appears somewhat different in location on the stress and rest projection images.

4. Position-dependent breast artifact. Concomitant ischemia may or may not be present.

Reference

DePuey EG: Artifacts in SPECT myocardial perfusion imaging. In DePuey EG, Garcia EV, Berman DS, editors: *Cardiac SPECT imaging,* ed 2, Philadelphia, 2001, Lippincott Williams & Wilkins, pp 232-262.

Cross-Reference

Nuclear Medicine: THE REQUISITES, ed 2, pp 67-68, 73-79.

Comment

Attenuation artifacts most commonly occur in the anterior and lateral walls, and less often in the anteroseptal wall, depending on location, size, density, and mobility of breast tissue. The apparent reduced uptake in the superior portion of the heart on the stress projection images is different in the two studies, extending more inferiorly at rest. Breast attenuation would be expected to be a "fixed" defect; however, a change in breast position between stress and rest can mimic ischemia. Thus this stress-rest perfusion pattern could be caused by changing attenuation alone or may be caused by ischemia and breast movement. A standardized protocol improves the likelihood that the breasts are in the same position for both studies, e.g., both with or both without bra or binding.

An increased incidence of false-positive stress SPECT myocardial perfusion studies occurs in young women. This case illustrates one reason. Another is predicted by Bayes' theorem. Patient groups with a low pretest probability of disease have an increased false-positive rate, whereas those with a high pretest likelihood have increased false-negative results. Thus the best use of this study for CAD diagnosis is to select patients at intermediate risk. Young women with few risk factors have a low likelihood of disease. A similar problem occurs with other screening tests, e.g., human immunodeficiency virus (HIV). Screening patients at risk results in relatively few false-positive results; however, mass screening results in more false-positive than true-positive results. Myocardial perfusion studies are performed not only for diagnosis, but importantly, also for risk stratification and prognosis in patients with known disease.

A

B

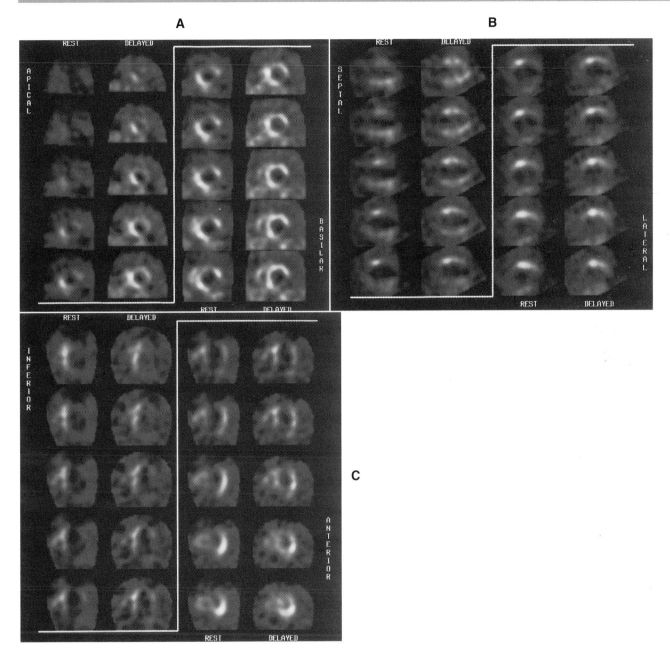

C

A 62-year-old man with known CAD had fixed defects with no reversibility on a ^{99m}Tc perfusion SPECT study at another hospital. This is a rest-rest ^{201}Tl SPECT study. *A,* Short-axis, *B,* vertical long-axis; *C,* horizontal long-axis.

1. Describe the SPECT findings on the initial rest and the 4-hour delayed rest study.

2. What is the clinical significance of these findings?

3. Based on the available evidence, should revascularization be considered?

4. What is hibernating myocardium?

CASE 154

Cardiovascular System: ^{201}Tl Viability Study

1. Initial rest images show extensive defects: (1) the anterior wall extending to the apex, septum, and anterolateral wall; and (2) the inferolateral wall extending to the inferior and lateral regions. Delayed rest images show some improvement in perfusion in the anterior wall extending to the apex and septum and anterolateral region.

2. There is viable myocardium in the left anterior descending (LAD) artery distribution.

3. Yes.

4. Chronic myocardial ischemia where both blood flow and function (contractility) are reduced. Although the myocardium is viable, the lack of wall motion mimics infarction.

References

Canty JM Jr, Fallavollita JA: Chronic hibernation and chronic stunning: a continuum, *J Nucl Cardiol* 7:509-527, 2000.

Schelbert HR: Merits and limitations of radionuclide approaches to viability and future developments, *J Nucl Cardiol* 1(2 Pt 2):S86-96, 1994.

Cross-Reference
Nuclear Medicine: THE REQUISITES, ed 2, p 92.

Comment

Distinguishing chronic ischemic ("hibernating myocardium") from scarred myocardium is critical for appropriate clinical management. Depending on the extent of hibernation, revascularization improves cardiac function manifested by improvement in wall motion, LVEF, and long-term patient outcome. Patients with "viable" myocardium have better survival from revascularization than from medical management. Those with infarction do not benefit from revascularization. They may be candidates for cardiac transplantation like patients with nonischemic cardiomyopathies. Identifying candidates who require cardiac transplantation is critical given the high cost, risk, and morbidity of cardiac transplantation compared with the relatively low cost and widespread availability of coronary revascularization procedures.

Rest-rest ^{201}Tl imaging is a proven alternative to ^{18}F FDG-PET imaging. Improved ^{201}Tl uptake on delayed images is indicative of myocardial viability and the likelihood of improvement after revascularization. "Stunned" myocardium refers to myocardium that is reperfused after occlusion, either through spontaneously recanalization or commonly after angioplasty. Blood flow is normal or even increased with stunning, but wall motion is decreased because of the severe ischemic event. This stunned myocardium usually regains function with time, usually a few weeks.

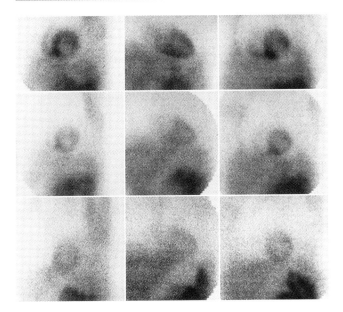

Stress *(top row)*, 4-hour delay *(middle row)*, and 24-hour *(bottom row)* planar ^{201}Tl planar images obtained in a patient too heavy for the SPECT table.

1. What is the mechanism for ^{201}Tl uptake at stress and rest?

2. What is redistribution?

3. Name the three views and describe the scintigraphic findings.

4. List other circumstances in which planar imaging may be preferable to SPECT.

CASE 155

Cardiovascular System: Planar ²⁰¹Tl with Ischemia

1. ²⁰¹Tl behaves like a potassium analogue using the ATPase sodium-potassium pump. Almost 90% of thallium is extracted on first pass through the coronary circulation at normal flow. Uptake is proportional to blood flow. At high flow rates, extraction is less. Five percent of the administered dose localizes in the myocardium.

2. After initial cellular uptake, ²⁰¹Tl undergoes redistribution throughout the body. As ²⁰¹Tl clears from the myocardium, it is replaced by circulating ²⁰¹Tl. This is the basis for the stress redistribution imaging strategy. Cold defects seen on early images are the result of decreased flow and therefore decreased ²⁰¹Tl delivery. Ischemic myocardium will "fill in" on 2- to 4-hour delayed imaging. No fill-in is seen with infarct. With severe ischemia, e.g., hibernating myocardium, fill-in may require a longer time, up to 24 hours.

3. *Left:* left lateral; *middle:* anterior; *right:* left anterior oblique. Reduced radiotracer in the inferolateral-inferior region, which partially normalizes on the delayed 4-hour redistribution images and completely redistributes by 24 hours.

4. Claustrophobia. Some patients do not tolerate the SPECT camera, particularly a multiheaded camera.

Reference
Gerson MC: *Cardiac nuclear medicine,* ed 3, New York, 1997, McGraw-Hill.

Cross-Reference
Nuclear Medicine: THE REQUISITES, ed 2, pp 66-68, 76-79, 82.

Comment
²⁰¹Tl has a physical half-life of 73 hours and decays by electron capture to ²⁰¹Hg. The photons available for imaging are mercury k-alpha and k-beta characteristic x-rays in the range of 69 to 83 keV (95% abundant) and thallium gamma rays of 167 keV (10% abundant) and 135 keV (3% abundant).

Many studies have addressed the issues of sensitivity and specificity of thallium myocardial scintigraphy for diagnosis of coronary artery disease (CAD). Reported sensitivity of ²⁰¹Tl ranges from 60% to 95%, with specificity ranging from 50% to 90%. These wide variations in results relate in part to differences in the populations studied. Specificity results are affected by breast attenuation and by selection bias. A reasonable estimate of sensitivity for CAD is 85% to 90%, and specificity is 80% to 85%. Planar imaging was used successfully for many years to diagnose CAD. However, SPECT is now the standard methodology. Today, ²⁰¹Tl studies are more commonly performed to evaluate for risk assessment and prognosis.

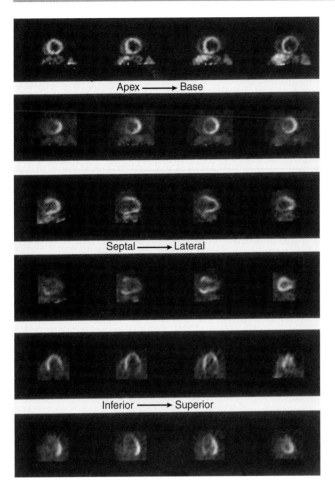

Apex ⟶ Base

Septal ⟶ Lateral

Inferior ⟶ Superior

PET cardiac study using two different radiopharmaceuticals. Short, vertical, and horizontal long-axis images are shown. Top row of each set is ^{13}N ammonia. The bottom images are ^{18}F FDG.

1. What physiological parameter does the ^{13}N ammonia distribution reflect?

2. Similar information could be obtained using what other clinically used positron radiopharmaceutical?

3. What is the rationale for the use of ^{18}F FDG?

4. Describe the image findings and interpret the results.

Cardiovascular System: ^{13}N Ammonia/FDG Cardiac Viability Study

1. Myocardial perfusion.

2. ^{82}Rb.

3. FDG is taken up by ischemic myocardium.

4. The ^{13}N ammonia study shows decreased perfusion in the proximal two thirds of the lateral wall extending to the anterolateral and inferolateral regions. The FDG uptake is mismatched. Increased FDG uptake indicating ischemia is seen where the ^{13}N ammonia images show hypoperfusion. Diagnostic of myocardial viability (hibernating myocardium).

Reference

Schelbert HR: ^{18}F deoxyglucose and the assessment of myocardial viability, *Semin Nucl Med* 32:60-69, 2002.

Cross-Reference

Nuclear Medicine: THE REQUISITES, ed 2, pp 89-93.

Comment

^{13}N ammonia has a physical half-life of 10 minutes; therefore an on-site cyclotron is required for its use in patient studies. It is rapidly taken up by the myocardium where it fixes through incorporation into ^{13}N glutamine. ^{82}Rb has a half-life of 75 seconds and is obtained from a ^{82}Sr/^{82}Ru generator on-site. It is administered with an infusion pump directly routed from the generator. This generator should be replaced on a monthly basis. However, it is expensive and a large cardiac patient volume is needed for cost-effectiveness. In the usual clinical setting where FDG (t½ of 110 minutes) is the only positron radiopharmaceutical available, the FDG-PET images must be compared with a ^{201}Tl or ^{99m}Tc sestamibi/tetrofosmin image. This is a clinical setting where gamma camera PET (SPECT-PET), using a two-headed gamma camera modified with coincidence circuitry and collimator removed, offers an advantage. A dual-isotope study can be obtained sequentially with the patient in the identical position.

An important myocardial application of ^{18}F FDG is to identify viable hibernating myocardium. Areas of hibernating myocardium demonstrate decreased stress and rest perfusion but increased FDG uptake, and thus perfusion and metabolism appear mismatched. This occurs because hibernating myocardium has increased FDG uptake because of the metabolic shift in ischemic myocardium to glycolysis from the normal utilization of free fatty acids in the nonischemic state.

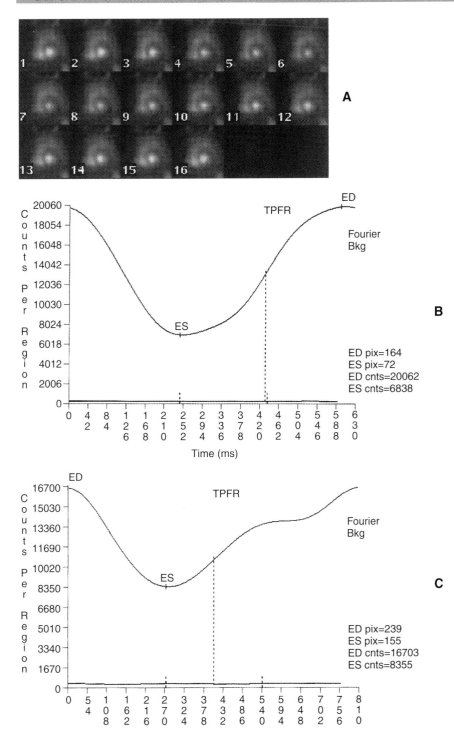

A

B

ED pix=164
ES pix=72
ED cnts=20062
ES cnts=6838

C

ED pix=239
ES pix=155
ED cnts=16703
ES cnts=8355

A 40-year-old patient with malignant lymphoma was treated with doxorubicin (Adriamycin). A radionuclide ventriculogram (RVG) performed at the time of initial diagnosis reported a 60% LVEF. *A,* Follow-up RVG with all 16 image frames and left ventricular time-activity curves (TACs) before *(B)* and after *(C)* chemotherapy.

1. Discuss sequential images and the TACs.

2. What is the likely diagnosis?

3. List features that should be included in reporting RVG or MUGA studies.

4. List three reasons why radionuclide ventriculography is preferred to echocardiography for monitoring left ventricular function.

Cardiovascular System: Doxorubicin Toxicity

1. Sequential images *(A)* show a LVEF within normal range. The ventricle appears mildly dilated. End-systole is image number 7. TACs show counts for each of 16 frames of the gated acquisition. *B* is normal. *C* shows deterioration from baseline with a slower, broad diastolic upslope and decreased stroke volume (ESV-EDV). The pattern is compatible with ventricular dysfunction, predominantly diastolic, and deterioration compared with the baseline study. LVEF was calculated to be 50%.

2. Doxorubicin toxicity.

3. Qualitative assessment of cardiac chambers and great vessels in terms of size and relationships, regional wall motion based on review of cinematic display, and quantitative analysis (LVEF).

4. Echocardiography is operator dependent, relies on visual estimates of LVEF, and may not be technically feasible in up to 30% of patients because of poor acoustic window. RVG is relatively free of operator-dependent factors, is generally reproducible within an institution and across institutions, and is not limited by acoustic windows.

Reference
Borges-Neto S, Coleman RE: Radionuclide ventricular function analysis, *Radiol Clin North Am* 31:817-830, 1993.

Cross-Reference
Nuclear Medicine: THE REQUISITES, ed 2, p 101.

Comment
Doxorubicin chemotherapy is associated with a risk of cardiotoxicity and cardiomyopathy. Doxorubicin cardiotoxicity rarely occurs with cumulative doses less than 400 mg/m². Doses in excess of 550 mg/m² result in cardiotoxicity in approximately one third of patients. However, some patients can tolerate considerably higher doses. The latter patients should have LVEF measured both before and during each treatment. A decrease in LVEF suggests drug-related cardiotoxicity. Doxorubicin usually is withheld from patients with baseline LVEFs below 30%. The drug usually is discontinued if the LVEF decreases by more than 10% below a pretreatment level of 50%. Functional recovery of cardiotoxicity after cessation of doxorubicin therapy is poor. This is now the most common indication for radionuclide ventriculography. Cardiac biopsy is an invasive alternative to radionuclide ventriculography to determine cardiotoxicity.

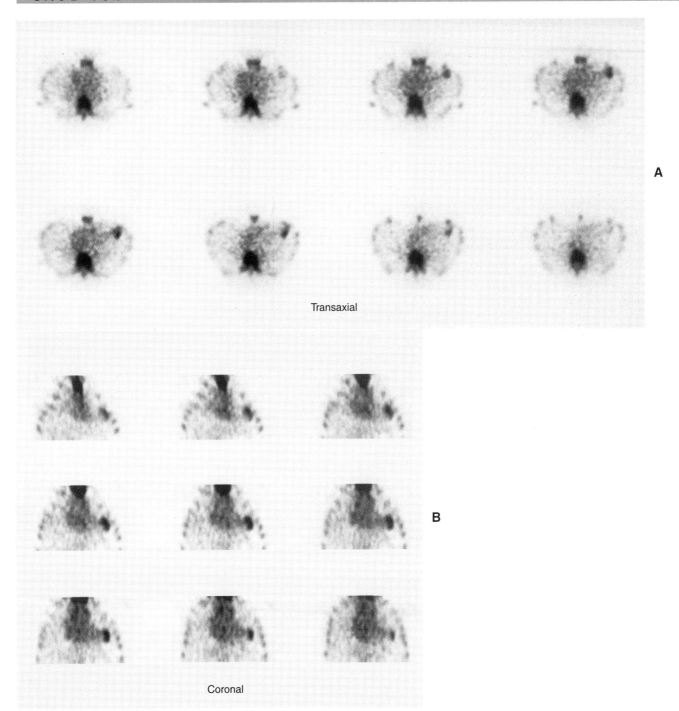

Transaxial

B

Coronal

A ^{99m}Tc pyrophosphate study is obtained to evaluate for myocardial infarct in a patient with equivocal ECG and borderline enzyme levels.

1. What information should be obtained before the injection?

2. Describe the scintigraphic SPECT (*A*, transverse; *B*, coronal) findings in this patient.

3. Give a differential diagnosis of the scan finding.

4. Name another infarct-avid radiopharmaceutical.

Cardiac: Pyrophosphate SPECT Infarct

1. The time of the suspected event. Depending on the time of the event and whether chest pain is ongoing, a perfusion SPECT study may be more appropriate.

2. Focal abnormal uptake is seen at the left apex.

3. Focal apical myocardial infarct, severe ischemia, aneurysm, focal myocarditis, focal pericardial calcification.

4. [111]In antimyosin.

Reference

Gerson MC, Lenihan DJ: Selection of noninvasive test in the emergency room and in the coronary care unit. In Gerson MY, editor: *Cardiac nuclear medicine,* ed 3, New York, 1997, McGraw-Hill, pp 466-470.

Cross-Reference

Nuclear Medicine: THE REQUISITES, ed 2, pp 88-89, 105-108.

Comment

[99m]Tc pyrophosphate accumulates in a myocardial infarction within a few hours after the acute event if the coronary artery is patent, or later if it remains occluded. Maximum uptake is present 24 to 72 hours after infarction. Uptake remains detectable, but decreasingly, for 6 to 10 days after the event. Usually no uptake is seen at a site of old infarction, but occasionally infarcts nearly a year old have uptake. [99m]Tc pyrophosphate uptake parallels calcium deposition.

[99m]Tc pyrophosphate is indicated for patients with a nondiagnostic ECG and enzyme studies. Not only can it confirm infarct, but it also shows its location. Uptake also may occur with chronic ongoing ischemia, aneurysm, myocarditis, pericarditis, or amyloidosis. Similar to diphosphonate bone tracers, ^{99m}Tc pyrophosphate scans have skeletal uptake. Therefore if a focal hot area is present because of a bone abnormality superimposed on the heart, it may be mistaken on planar scans as myocardial uptake. SPECT can be helpful in this situation and can aid localization of the abnormal uptake. The uptake at the fracture site also provides the cause for pain.

Myosin, one of the myofibrillar proteins, is not exposed to circulating antibodies unless the sarcolemma has been disrupted, as in cases of infarction. The ^{111}In antimyosin uptake is highly specific for myocyte necrosis. Positive images may be seen 12 hours after injection, but optimal images require 24 to 48 hours. In addition to myocardial infarction, myocyte necrosis can occur in myocarditis and cardiac allograft rejection, both of which can demonstrate uptake of ^{99m}Tc pyrophosphate or ^{111}In antimyosin.

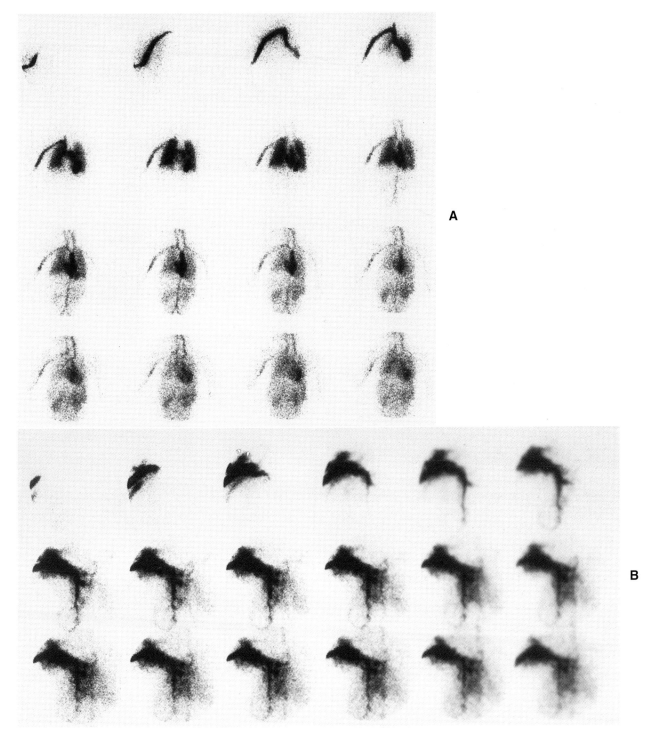

A

B

Two patients have radionuclide blood flow imaging after right upper extremity injection.

1. Describe the route of the radiotracer in patient *A*. Give an interpretation.

2. What are the image findings and interpretation of patient *B?*

3. What radiopharmaceuticals could be used for this study?

4. What is the framing rate (seconds/frame) and minimum injected dose required to obtain a good flow study?

Cardiovascular System: Superior Vena Cava Obstruction

1. Subclavian vein, superior vena cava, right ventricle, lungs, left ventricle, carotids, aorta. Normal flow pattern.

2. Venous occlusion at the superior vena cava with collateral flow over the anterior chest. (This patient had lung cancer.)

3. Any ^{99m}Tc radiopharmaceutical. All that is needed is enough activity for a good flow study. ^{99m}Tc DTPA often is used because it is cleared rapidly by the kidneys and can be repeated if necessary.

4. 1 to 3 seconds/frame; 5 mCi or greater.

Reference

Mishkin FS, Freeman LM: Miscellaneous applications of radionuclide imaging. In Freeman LM, editor: *Freeman and Johnson's clinical radionuclide imaging,* ed 3, Philadelphia, 1984, WB Saunders, pp 1400-1419.

Cross-Reference

Nuclear Medicine: THE REQUISITES, ed 2, pp 48-62.

Comment

Radionuclide flow studies can be a rapid, easily performed method for evaluation of the patency of venous access lines. Rapid acquisition images provide a sensitive means for detecting obstruction of axillary, subclavian, or innominate veins. This is particularly important in modern medicine when patients frequently have central venous access lines for infusion of various therapeutic drugs that increase the risk of thrombosis. A good bolus is required to maximize the diagnostic information of the flow sequence. Although resolution is poor compared with a contrast study, this "poor man's" noninvasive dynamic vascular study can provide valuable diagnostic information.

Radionuclide blood flow studies commonly are used to study a variety of arterial and venous abnormalities. A vascular sequence is performed routinely for three-phase bone scans to diagnose osteomyelitis or to estimate the age of a stress fracture. Flow studies are performed in association with renography to assess renal arterial blood flow, e.g., to diagnose renal artery stenosis, acute transplant rejection, or kidney viability. With a gastrointestinal bleeding study, occasionally the site of increased vascularity can be detected from the flow study when there is no evidence of active bleeding, e.g., angiodysplasia. With HIDA imaging, increased blood flow sometimes can be seen in the region of the gallbladder fossa with acute cholecystitis.

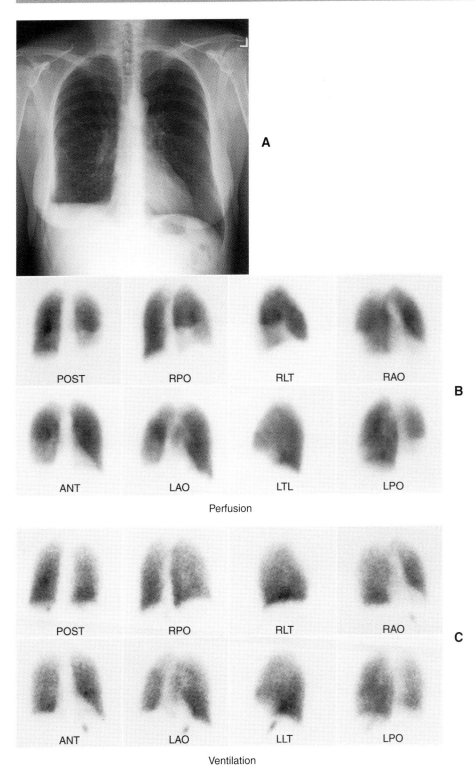

A 62-year-old patient with right-sided chest discomfort and shortness of breath. *A,* Posteroanterior chest radiograph; *B,* perfusion; *C,* ventilation.

1. Describe the ventilation perfusion image findings.

2. Interpret the study. Give your reasoning.

3. What is the likelihood of pulmonary embolus in this patient?

4. What are the most common chest x-ray findings in patients with pulmonary emboli?

Pulmonary System: High Probability of Pulmonary Embolus

1. Perfusion: decreased right lower lobe except for the superior segment. Ventilation: normal except for mildly truncated right lower lobe consistent with subpulmonic effusion.

2. High probability of pulmonary embolus. Mismatch between perfusion and ventilation in the basal segments. The perfusion defect is considerably larger than the pleural effusion on the radiograph.

3. Greater than 80%.

4. Most common: normal. Next most common: atelectasis. These are also the most common x-ray findings in patients determined by angiography not to have emboli.

References

Freitas JE, Sarosi MG, Nagle CC, et al: Modified PIOPED criteria used in clinical practice, *J Nucl Med* 36:1573-1578, 1995.

Juni J, Alavi A: Lung scanning in the diagnosis of pulmonary embolism: the emperor redressed, *Semin Nucl Med* 21:281-296, 1991.

Cross-Reference

Nuclear Medicine: THE REQUISITES, ed 2, pp 150-161.

Comment

The criterion that a perfusion defect larger than the radiographic abnormality is high probability by PIOPED definition should be used cautiously. The chest radiograph is obtained with maximal inspiration. The lung scan image is acquired during tidal breathing. Thus the heart is more horizontal on the lung scan than the radiograph, and the lung fields appear smaller on the lung scan than the radiograph. However, in this case the perfusion defect is definitely larger than the radiographic finding. No ventilatory defects are apparent; only the lower lung field is truncated.

A patient with a high-probability scan has a greater than 80% probability of pulmonary embolus. However, fewer than half of patients determined to have pulmonary embolus by angiography have a high-probability scan. Thus a high-probability scan is not sensitive for the diagnosis of pulmonary embolus, but it is fairly specific. Conversely, this also means that 20% of patients have another diagnosis. The most common cause is lung cancer. A mediastinal tumor often preferentially occludes the pulmonary vessels, which are easily compressible in contrast to the more rigid bronchi. Old emboli are another common cause of a false-positive study for pulmonary embolus. Vasculitis or sickle cell disease are other less common causes.

A

B

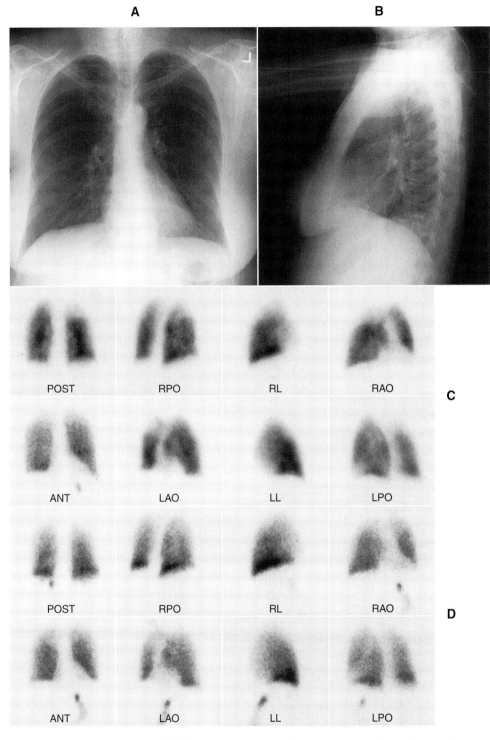

C

D

A 59-year-old patient with COPD complains of right-sided chest discomfort and shortness of breath.
A, Posteroanterior chest radiograph; B, lateral chest; C, perfusion; D, ventilation.

1. Describe the ventilation-perfusion image findings.

2. Interpret the study.

3. What is a stripe sign and what is its significance?

4. What is the physiological basis of a stripe sign?

Pulmonary System: Stripe Sign

1. Decreased perfusion in the right upper lobe (apical and anterior segments). Stripe sign of the posterior segment of the right upper lobe. Normal ventilation.

2. Two segmental mismatches. High probability of pulmonary embolus.

3. Its presence signifies perfused lung tissue between a perfusion defect and the adjacent pleural surface. Its presence can be used to classify a segment as not related to pulmonary embolus, and in some cases, lower the probability of a scan from intermediate to low.

4. Usually a manifestation of airway obstruction. The sign has been correlated with CT and PET showing spared perfusion of the cortex of the lung in asthma and emphysema.

References

Freitas JE, Sarosi MG, Nagle CC, et al: Modified PIOPED criteria used in clinical practice, *J Nucl Med* 36:1573-1578, 1995.

Sostman HD, Gottschalk A: Prospective validation of the stripe sign in ventilation-perfusion scintigraphy, *Radiology* 184:455-459, 1992.

Cross-Reference

Nuclear Medicine: THE REQUISITES, ed 2, p 160.

Comment

The stripe sign is seen in only 5% of ventilation-perfusion studies. To be defined as a stripe sign, the finding needs only to be seen in one projection. It is an ancillary sign that in some cases helps lower the probability from intermediate to low probability. The stripe sign only is useful for evaluating the segment in question. The sign is not totally specific for nonembolic causation. It also can be seen in areas of reperfused lung previously obstructed by emboli.

The natural history of pulmonary embolism is clot fragmentation in the right side of the heart, which induces multivessel segmental embolization of the pulmonary vasculature with preservation of segmental ventilation. Most emboli occur in the lower lobes and have a random distribution. Evidence against pulmonary embolus in this case is the fact that the abnormal perfusion is limited to adjacent upper lobe segments is unusual. Thus even though this finding might indicate a high-probability scan by established criteria, this pattern is atypical. Published data also have suggested that the specificity for pulmonary embolus is maximized in patients with cardiopulmonary disease if three segmental mismatches are present. Thus it would not be incorrect to classify this study as indeterminate or intermediate probability.

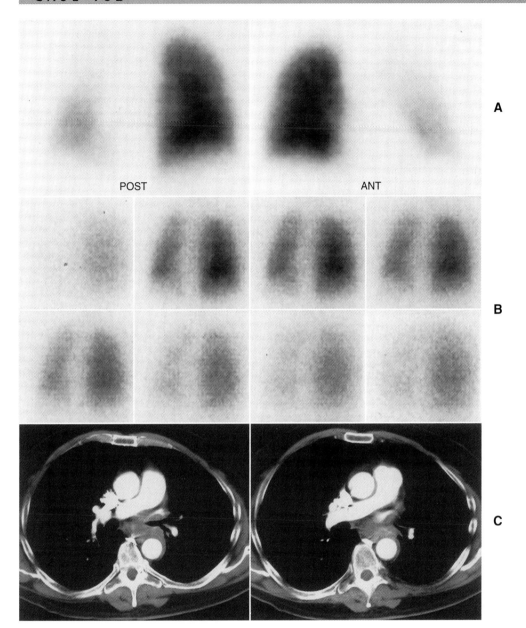

POST   ANT

A

B

C

A ventilation-perfusion lung scan is ordered for increasing shortness of breath. Chest radiograph (not shown) findings were negative.

1. Describe the scintigraphic findings (*A*, perfusion, anterior and posterior only; *B*, ^{133}Xe washin-washout ventilation image sequence; *C*, CT).

2. What pulmonary embolus probability category would you assign?

3. Provide the differential diagnosis.

4. A chest CT was performed to further evaluate for the symptoms. What is the most likely diagnosis?

Pulmonary System: Unilateral Matched Ventilation-Perfusion Abnormality

1. Perfusion images: global decreased perfusion to the entire left lung, more striking than the ventilation. ^{133}Xe ventilation images: decreased and delayed ventilation of the entire left lung. Washout images show no significant air trapping.

2. Low probability.

3. Hilar mass (lung cancer or adenopathy), severe unilateral parenchymal lung disease, Swyer-James syndrome, hypoplastic pulmonary artery, prior shunt for congenital heart disease.

4. Lung cancer.

Reference

Datz FL: *Gamuts in nuclear medicine,* ed 3, St Louis, 1995, Mosby, pp 188-189.

Cross-Reference

Nuclear Medicine: THE REQUISITES, ed 2, pp 147-148, 154-157.

Comment

Lung cancer and hilar adenopathy can result in perfusion defects disproportionate to ventilation. This is the most common cause for a false-positive high probability ventilation-perfusion study. A high-probability ventilation-perfusion scan has an 80% positive predictive value for pulmonary embolus. The other 20% must have another cause. The majority are related to hilar masses. A proximal pulmonary embolus may manifest as a unilateral, whole lung mismatch; however, the latter should always raise the question of tumor. An easy memory device is to think of the mass as abutting the hilar structures. The thin-walled vessels (veins and arteries) are relatively compressible compared with the thick-walled bronchi; thus ventilation is relatively preserved compared with perfusion. A good posteroanterior and lateral chest radiograph usually narrows the differential, and if not, the question can be resolved by CT. Pathological study is needed to ensure the correct diagnosis.

Swyer-James syndrome, a variant of postinfectious obliterative bronchiolitis, shares some common radiographic features with congenital unilateral absence of the pulmonary artery, including a small lung manifested by cardiac and mediastinal shift, absence of pulmonary arterial shadow, elevation of the hemidiaphragm, and a decrease in pulmonary vessels on the affected lung with oligemia. Swyer-James syndrome, caused by bronchiolitis, is associated with air trapping which can be documented by an expiration radiograph or a ^{133}Xe ventilation scan.

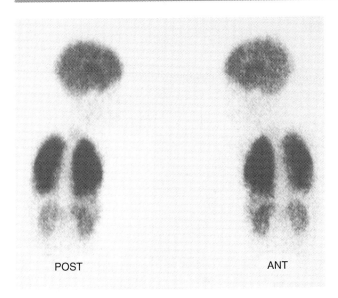

POST   ANT

A 3-year-old child was referred for a ^{99m}Tc macroaggregated albumin (MAA) study.

1. Describe the scintigraphic findings.
2. What is the diagnosis?
3. Describe the radiopharmaceutical's mechanism of uptake.
4. What are contraindications to this study?

Pulmonary System: Right-to-Left Shunt Demonstrated by ^{99m}Tc MAA

1. Uptake of the radiotracer in the brain, lungs, kidneys, and liver.

2. Right-to-left shunt.

3. ^{99m}Tc MAA particles are larger than capillary size. When given intravenously, the particles occlude the first arteriolar-capillary bed they reach normally, the lungs. With a right-to-left shunt, some will bypass the lungs and be delivered systemically in proportion to the size of the shunt.

4. Relative contraindications include pregnancy, severe pulmonary hypertension, and right-to-left shunt. There are no absolute contraindications.

Reference

Treves ST, Packard AB: Lungs. In Traves ST, editor: *Pediatric nuclear medicine,* ed 2, New York, 1995, Springer-Verlag, pp 168-190.

Cross-Reference

Nuclear Medicine: THE REQUISITES, ed 2, pp 145-161.

Comment

This case study was requested for a child known to have a right-to-left shunt to quantify the size of the shunt. Quantification of a right-to-left shunt can be estimated by drawing regions of interest on computerized data to determine the percent of the total activity outside the lung field. In this case, the shunt was calculated to be 20%.

Particle size range of ^{99m}Tc MAA is 10 is 90 μm (mean 30 to 40 μm). Capillary size is 7 μm. The particles occlude only 1/1000 to 1/10,000 of the arteriolar capillary bed. Pulmonary infarction does not occur because of the dual circulation of the lung, and the nature of the particles. The particles are malleable, cause partial occlusions, and break down rapidly into smaller particles that pass through the lungs. The direct injection of ^{99m}Tc MAA particles into the carotid artery has been done experimentally in humans to map cerebral perfusion without serious adverse affect. In a patient with known severe pulmonary hypertension, or a right-to-left shunt, the usual approach would be to reduce the number of ^{99m}Tc MAA particles. A minimum of 60,000 particles is required to provide adequate uniformity, and 100,000 or more are usually recommended. A perfusion study generally has 300,000 to 400,000 particles. To maximize the count rate with a reduced number of particles, a high-specific activity ^{99m}Tc pertechnetate is required.

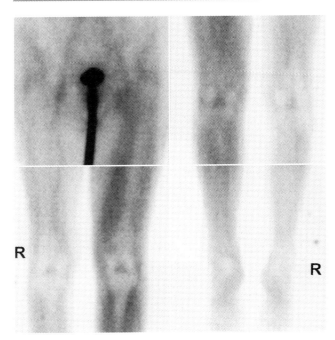

A 55-year-old patient with a remote history of thrombophlebitis in the left thigh has recurrent similar pain. A Foley catheter is in place.

1. What is the radiopharmaceutical and scintigraphic study?
2. What is its mechanism of uptake?
3. What are the scintigraphic findings?
4. What are its clinical indications?

Thrombophlebitis: AcuTect (^{99m}Tc apcitide)

1. Radionuclide venogram with AcuTect (^{99m}Tc apcitide).

2. AcuTect is a synthetic peptide that binds to the glycoprotein GPIIB/IIIa receptors on the surface of activated platelets.

3. Increased uptake in the left deep venous system extending from the proximal to distal thigh consistent with acute deep venous thrombophlebitis. Diffuse increased uptake is seen throughout the soft tissue of the left lower extremity.

4. To differentiate acute thrombophlebitis from old inactive thrombophlebitis. It also can be used to diagnose acute thrombophlebitis when Doppler ultrasonography is nondiagnostic.

Reference

Taillefer R, Edell S, Innes G, et al: Acute thromboscintigraphy with (99mTc)-apcitide: results of the phase 3 multicenter clinical trial comparing 99mTc-apcitide scintigraphy with contrast venography for imaging acute DVT. Multicenter trial investigators, *J Nucl Med* 41:1214-1223, 2000.

Cross-Reference

Nuclear Medicine: THE REQUISITES, ed 2, pp 163-165.

Comment

Acute deep venous thrombophlebitis is a common problem and the source of most pulmonary emboli. Approximately 50% of patients with acute thrombophlebitis develop long term sequelae, such as the postphlebitic syndrome. Clinical history and examination are notoriously unreliable for diagnosing thrombophlebitis.

Although contrast venography arguably is considered the "gold standard" for diagnosis of deep venous thrombophlebitis, this invasive procedure is no longer commonly performed for numerous reasons. Duplex ultrasonography with Doppler is the standard diagnostic modality. However, in many patients, the method is nondiagnostic, e.g., in the setting of postoperative trauma, casts, and obesity. Partial obstructions to flow may be missed. Importantly, it often cannot differentiate new from old thrombophlebitis.

With thrombus formation, platelets receive humoral signals that cause activation and aggregation. The latter is dependent on the GPIIb/IIIa receptors expressed on activated platelets. AcuTect binds to these receptors. Because AcuTect binds to activated platelets only, the study detects acute but not chronic thrombophlebitis. Aspirin and heparin therapy do not seem to adversely affect its accuracy.

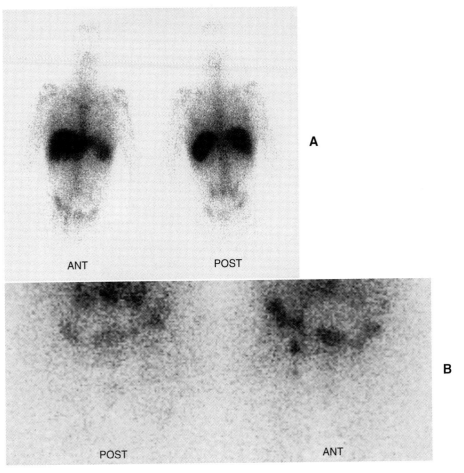

A 56-year-old paraplegic patient has fever of uncertain origin. No localizing signs or symptoms are present.

1. Which radiopharmaceutical was used? What others could be used for this purpose?
2. Which organ receives the highest radiation absorbed dose? Estimate the dose.
3. What is your interpretation of this whole-body scan (A) and pelvic spot (B)?
4. What is the photopeak(s) of the radionuclide used? What is its half-life?

Infection and Inflammation: [111]In Oxine WBCs—Right Ileum Osteomyelitis

1. [111]In oxine or ^{99m}Tc HM-PAO leukocytes. [67]Ga could also be used. The intense spleen uptake is consistent with a radiolabeled leukocyte study; ^{111}In oxine leukocytes were used. The image resolution is poor compared with ^{99m}Tc leukocytes.

2. Spleen, approximately 15 to 20 rads.

3. Abnormal focal uptake in right groin (there has been a femoral line) and in the right ileum, indicating osteomyelitis.

4. 173, 247 keV. Physical half-life is 77 hours.

References

Kipper SL: Radiolabeled leukocyte imaging of the abdomen. In Freeman M, editor: *Nuclear medicine annual 1995,* New York, 1995, Raven Press, pp 81-128.

Coleman RE, Datz FL: Detection of inflammatory disease using radiolabeled cells. In Sandler M, Coleman RE, editor: *Diagnostic nuclear medicine,* Baltimore, Md, 1996, Williams & Wilkins.

Cross-Reference

Nuclear Medicine: THE REQUISITES, ed 2, pp 177-190.

Comment

Choosing the appropriate infection-seeking radiopharmaceutical in a particular clinical setting requires weighing of the advantages and disadvantages of each. [67]Ga detects tumor and infection; therefore it can be useful for patients with fever of unknown origin. Radiolabeled leukocytes are preferable if infection localization is the clinical question. Both require cell labeling, at least a 2-hour procedure and with the potential problem of blood-borne disease. [99m]Tc HM-PAO leukocytes provide better image quality because of the ^{99m}Tc radiolabel and larger administered dose, but have the disadvantage of clearance through the kidneys and biliary system, interfering with intraabdominal visualization. Abdominal imaging by 1 to 2 hours, before intraabdominal clearance, obviates this problem. [111]In oxine is not cleared intraabdominally and thus is preferable for intraabdominal infection. Otherwise the distribution is similar to spleen, liver, and bone marrow. Image quality is lower with ^{111}In oxine because of the lower administered dose (500 μCi versus 10 mCi for ^{99m}Tc HM-PAO), higher energy photopeaks (173, 247 keV), and the need for a medium-energy collimator. Images are usually obtained at 24 hours.

[111]In oxine diffuses through the neutrophil cell membrane. Intracellularly it dissociates and the ^{111}In binds to intracellular proteins, whereas oxine diffuses back out of the cell. In addition to labeling leukocytes (granulocytes, lymphocytes, monocytes), erythrocytes and platelets are labeled. Red blood cells and platelets are removed with sedimentation and settling agents early in the labeling procedure.

A

B

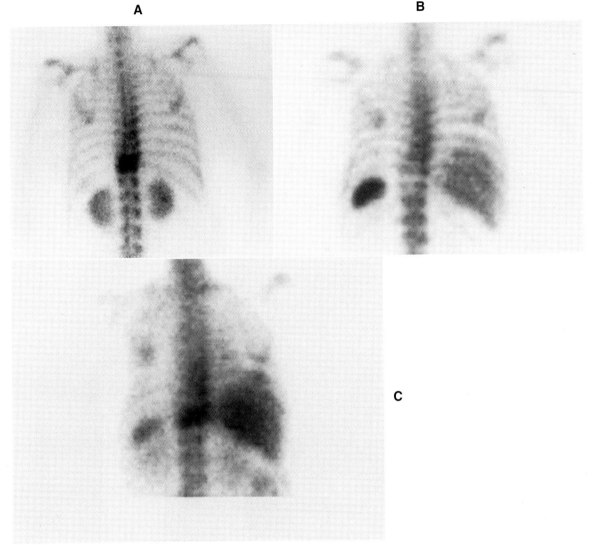

C

A 67-year-old patient has low-grade fever, back pain, and suspected osteomyelitis of the lumbar spine. *A,* ^{99m}Tc MDP bone scan; *B,* ^{111}In oxine leukocyte study; and *C,* Ga-67 study. Negative radiograph.

1. Describe the scintigraphic findings of these three studies.
2. What is the differential diagnosis of the ^{111}In study alone?
3. What is your interpretation of the three studies?
4. What is the false-negative rate for ^{111}In oxine leukocyte studies for vertebral osteomyelitis?

Infection and Inflammation: Osteomyelitis of the Spine

1. Bone scan shows increased uptake of the T11 vertebrae. [111]In oxine leukocyte study shows decreased uptake in the same region. [67]Ga shows increased uptake that matches the bone scan in relative intensity.

2. Osteomyelitis, fracture, infarction, metastasis, orthopedic hardware, surgical defect, localized radiation therapy, myelofibrosis, Paget's disease.

3. Osteomyelitis in this clinical setting. Many of the diseases listed can be excluded by history and radiographs.

4. As high as 40%.

Reference

Palestro CJ, Kim CK, Swyer AJ, et al: Radionuclide diagnosis of vertebral osteomyelitis: indium-111-leukocyte and Tc-99m MDP scintigraphy, *J Nucl Med* 32:1861-1865, 1991.

Cross-Reference

Nuclear Medicine: THE REQUISITES, ed 2, p 189.

Comment

Vertebral osteomyelitis usually occurs in adults and is most commonly in the lumbar spine, followed by thoracic and cervical locations. *Staphylococcus aureus* is the most common causative organism. Predisposing conditions include urinary tract infection and instrumentation, intravenous drug abuse, cancer, and diabetes mellitus. Plain radiographs are not sensitive and may be nonspecific for the diagnosis in nonvirgin bone. Osteomyelitis originates as a septic embolus that lodges in an end arteriole of the vertebral body. The embolus propagates retrograde and circumferentially around the vertebral body, occluding other arteries and causing septic infarction and osteomyelitis.

Radiolabeled leukocyte studies have a high accuracy for diagnosis of osteomyelitis except in the spine. The reason for decreased rather than increased uptake of leukocytes with vertebral osteomyelitis has not been well explained, but is a common finding (photopenia compared with adjacent vertebras). The cause may be concomitant infarction. [67]Ga is sensitive for osteomyelitis but is not specific because uptake can be seen whenever bone remodeling occurs for any reason, e.g., prior trauma or infection, orthopedic hardware. The ^{67}Ga study result is interpreted as positive if the uptake is greater than the bone scan or in a different distribution. In this case the ^{67}Ga uptake is equal to bone; however, in the presence of a normal x-ray, the bone scan alone is highly suspicious for osteomyelitis, which is further indicated by the ^{67}Ga scan.

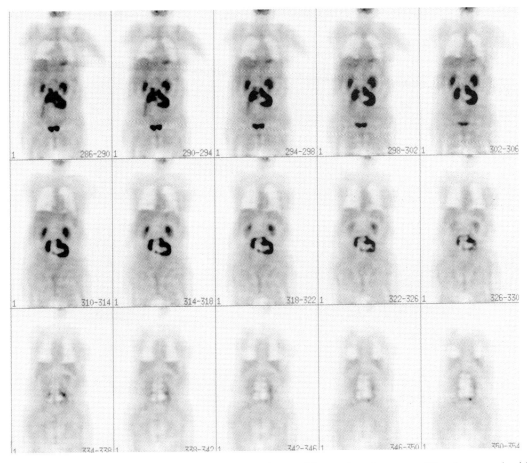

A 64-year-old woman has non-Hodgkin's lymphoma. Tumor involvement of lumbar vertebral bodies required resection and fusion. Pain and low-grade fever were noted 12 weeks after surgery.

1. Describe the FDG-PET findings.

2. Give your interpretation.

3. Can infection have increased FDG uptake? Why?

4. What is the energy photopeak of ^{18}F? What is the photopeak of ^{11}C, ^{13}N, ^{15}O?

Inflammation and Infection:
FDG—PET-Paraspinal Infection

1. Intense uptake involving the retroperitoneum anterior to the recent lumbar fusion surgery. Note the spinal fusion site on the lower right hand posterior coronal images.

2. Consistent with postoperative infection. Although this could be tumor, CT showed bilateral heterogenous and enlarged psoas muscles thought likely to be due to abscess or hematoma. (Subsequently proved by biopsy to be infection, not tumor.)

3. Yes. Leukocytes and macrophages utilize glucose.

4. All positron emitters have a 511-keV photopeak, i.e., ^{18}F, ^{11}C, ^{13}N, ^{15}O.

References

Bakheet SM, Powe J: Benign causes of 18-FDG uptake on whole body imaging, *Semin Nucl Med* 28:352-358, 1998.

Sugawara Y, Zasadny KR, Kison PV, et al: Splenic FDG uptake by granulocyte colony-stimulating factor therapy: PET imaging results, *J Nucl Med* 40:1456-1462, 1999.

Cross-Reference
Nuclear Medicine: THE REQUISITES, ed 2, pp 205-214.

Comment

Increased FDG uptake occurs not only with tumors, but also with inflammation and infection. Generally uptake with tumors is higher than with infection, but overlap exists. Subacute, chronic, and indolent infections tend to have low-grade uptake; however, at times, uptake is high and indistinguishable from tumor. Acute infections, as in this case, may have intense uptake. FDG uptake has been reported with arthritis, thyroiditis, sinusitis, herpes encephalitis, radiation pneumonitis, mastitis, empyema, gingivitis, alveolitis, pneumonia, sarcoidosis, tuberculosis, aspergillosis, blastomycosis, histoplasmosis, and histocytosis. Sensitivity for detection of these infections is unknown.

Positron decay occurs in nuclides that are neutron poor. When a positron (positive electron) is ejected from the nucleus, it loses its kinetic energy and interacts with an electron. Annihilation of both particles occurs and they are converted to energy, two 511-keV photons emitted 180 degrees apart. These simultaneously emitted photons are detected by the coincidence circuitry of PET cameras.

Granulocyte-stimulating factor is a hormone that regulates proliferation and differentiation of granulocyte precursors. Human colony-stimulating factor, produced by recombinant DNA technology, is a drug used to reduce the chemotherapy-induced neutropenia often seen in cancer patients. Increased bone marrow FDG uptake often is seen in patients receiving this drug.

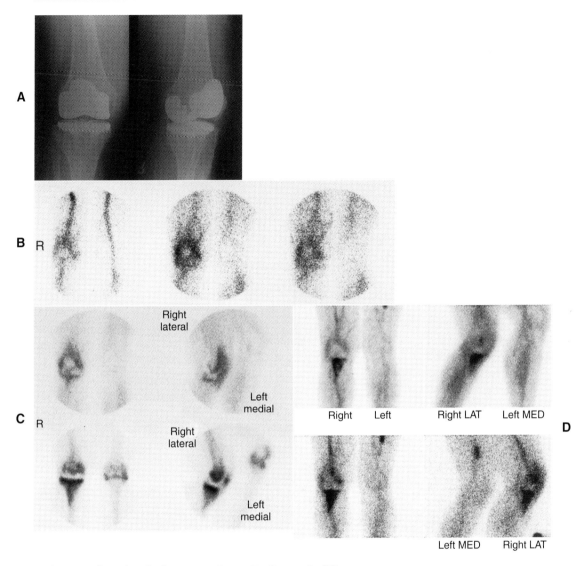

Rule out infected right knee prosthesis. Radiograph *(A)*.

1. Describe the three-phase bone scan findings. *B*, Flow; *C*, immediate *(above)* blood pool and delayed *(below)* images.

2. Describe the ^{99m}Tc HM-PAO leukocyte study *(D, above)* and ^{99m}Tc sulfur colloid study *(D, below)*.

3. What is the purpose of the ^{99m}Tc sulfur colloid study?

4. Interpret the study.

315

Infection and Inflammation: Knee Arthroplasty—Rule Out Infection

1. Increased blood flow to the right knee.

2. Increased uptake in the proximal tibia on both.

3. Serves as a template for normal marrow distribution.

4. Negative for infected prosthesis.

References

Palestro CJ, Swyer AJ, Kim CK, et al: Infected knee prosthesis: diagnosis with In-111 leukocyte, Tc-99m SC and Tc-99m MDP imaging, *Radiology* 179:645-648, 1991.

Elgazzar AH, Abdel-Dayem M: Imaging skeletal infections: evolving considerations. In Freeman M, editor: *Nuclear medicine annual 1999,* Philadelphia, 1999, Lippincott Williams & Wilkins.

Cross-Reference

Nuclear Medicine: THE REQUISITES, ed 2, pp 177-190.

Comment

The role of ^{99m}Tc MDP bone scanning in the diagnosis of total knee arthoplasty infection is limited because of persistent periprosthetic uptake of radiotracer for many years after prosthetic implantation. The intensity of periprosthetic uptake cannot be used to differentiate infected from uninfected prosthesis.

Radiolabeled leukocyte studies, whether ^{111}In oxine or ^{99m}Tc HM-PAO, are sensitive for the diagnosis of infected prostheses. However, specificity is a problem because implantation of an orthopedic prosthesis produces alterations in the distribution of bone marrow. The distribution of radiolabeled leukocytes in a noninfected knee is similar to that seen with ^{99m}Tc SC. Thus regions of increased marrow may exist that could be interpreted as infection with a leukocyte-only study, but when compared with a bone marrow study, the pattern is that of altered distribution, not infection. Although marrow is often not present in the normal bones of the knee, one study of patients with knee prostheses found normal marrow in 50% of noninfected knees. When infection is severe, the marrow scan may show decreased uptake at the site of infection. The radiolabeled leukocyte study should be performed first. If no increased periprosthetic activity is visible, a marrow study is not needed. The combined leukocyte-marrow study has proved particularly valuable for hip prostheses.

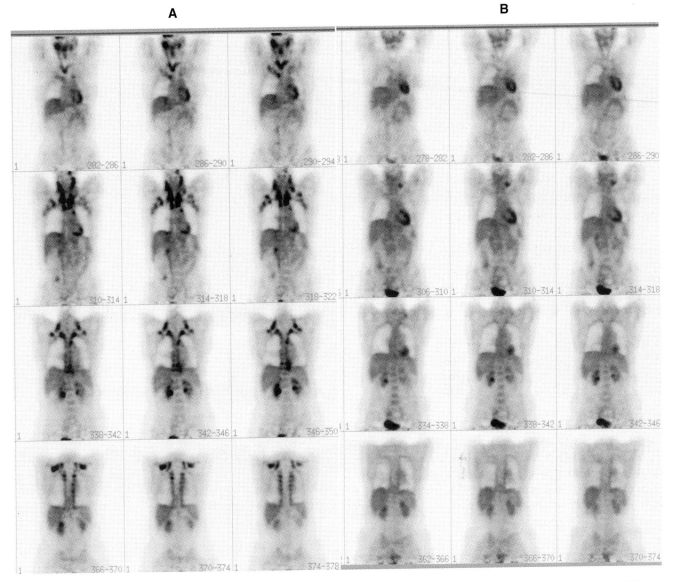

A   B

A 34-year-old woman with recently diagnosed Hodgkin's disease presenting as a left neck mass. Two ^{18}F FDG-PET scans were performed 3 days apart.

1. What is the mechanism of uptake of this radiopharmaceutical?

2. Describe the findings of the first study *(A)* and the second study *(B)* and explain how the study could have changed so dramatically in only 3 days.

3. What is the half-life of [18]F? [15]O, ^{13}N, [11]C?

4. What is the radiation dose to the target organ? What other organs have high uptake?

Oncology: FDG—Hodgkin's Disease and Muscle Tension Artifact

1. FDG is a glucose analogue. Increased FDG uptake occurs with increased glucose metabolism. It is taken up intracellularly and phosphorylated similar to glucose; however, unlike glucose, it cannot be metabolized further and is intracellularly trapped.

2. *A,* Intense multifocal uptake bilaterally in the neck, upper chest, and paraspinal regions. *B,* Uptake limited to left neck. Study *A* abnormalities are caused by muscle tension. Diazepam, 5 mg, was taken just before study *B.*

3. Approximately 110 minutes. 2, 10, and 20 minutes. It is important to remember that the half-lives of many positrons are very short.

4. 3.2 rads/5 mCi to the urinary bladder. Brain and heart.

Reference

Shreve PD, Anzai Y, Wahl RL: Pitfalls in oncological diagnosis with FDG PET imaging: physiologic and benign variants, *Radiographics* 19:61-77, 1999.

Cross-Reference

Nuclear Medicine: THE REQUISITES, ed 2, pp 207-209.

Comment

Because FDG whole-body uptake is a physiological map of relative glucose metabolism, strenuous exercise or muscle tension can result in uptake. Normal physiological uptake can be seen in laryngeal muscles in patient who talk after injection. Relative distribution in the brain varies depending on whether the patient's eyes are open or closed or whether the patient is listening to music or the room is quiet.

FDG distribution is not related only to glucose metabolism. Unlike glucose, FDG is normally excreted by the kidneys into the bladder. However, glucosuria is not normal, occurring only in patients with diabetes. Some laboratories routinely insert a bladder catheter in oncology patients to allow for better pelvic evaluation. Others insert a catheter only when disease is likely to reside in the pelvis, e.g., ovarian or rectal cancer. Many clinics routinely hydrate patients. Only a few routinely use diuretics to clear the bladder. Physiological FDG uptake may be seen at sites of arthritis, ostomy sites, healing fractures, and postoperative wounds because leukocytes use glucose.

The use of radiopharmaceuticals with very short half-lives, e.g., ^{11}C, ^{13}N, ^{15}O (2 to 20 minutes), requires an on-site cyclotron. The 110-minute half-life of ^{18}F allows for production and delivery from a more distant site. FDG is now available on a unit-dose basis from many regional radiopharmacies.

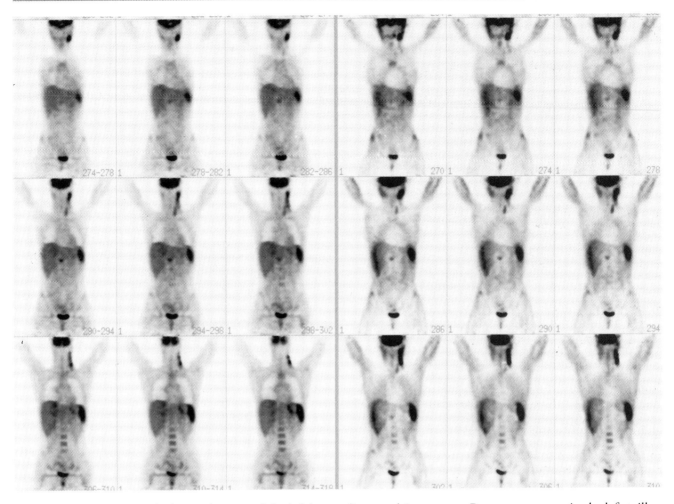

A 34-year-old woman with skin melanoma of the left breast diagnosed 3 years ago. Recent recurrence in the left axilla. Treated with resection and interferon therapy.

1. Both coronal image sets *(left, right)* of FDG-PET are acquired in the same patient on the same day. What is the reason for the difference in appearance?

2. Why do tumors have increased FDG uptake?

3. Is there a patient preparation for FDG-PET studies? If so, what is it, and why?

4. How much myocardial uptake is expected?

Oncology: ¹⁸F FDG—Melanoma

1. The images on the left are corrected for attenuation; the ones on the right are not. Both show increased uptake in the left neck consistent with tumor adenopathy.

2. Tumors have increased glucose metabolism compared to most normal tissues. A partial explanation is increased glucose transporter protein activity, higher levels of hexokinase, and lower levels of glucose-6-phosphatase.

3. Yes. 4- to 12-hour fast. Nonlabeled glucose due to hyperglycemia (fasting or postprandial) competes for FDG uptake.

4. In the fasting state the heart preferentially metabolizes free fatty acids. However, despite fasting the heart uptake is highly variable.

Reference
Holder WD, White RL, Zuger JH, et al: Effectiveness of positron emission tomography for the detection of melanoma metastases, *Ann Surg* 227:764-769, 1998.

Cross-Reference
Nuclear Medicine: THE REQUISITES, ed 2, pp 213, 226-227.

Comment
Note the difference between attenuation-corrected *(left)* and nonattenuation-corrected images *(right)*. In the noncorrected images, organs at depth have apparent decreased activity. Note the liver. The lateral surface of the liver is well seen in nonattenuated images; centrally there is much less activity. With attenuation correction the liver uptake appears more uniform; however, there is now an attenuation-correction artifact along the medial border of the liver. Without attenuation correction the lungs appear to have mildly increased uptake compared with adjacent soft tissue, heart, and mediastinum. This is reversed with attenuation correction. Surface soft tissue uptake is exaggerated with nonattenuation-corrected images. Anatomical definition is better with attenuation correction. With an obese patient, attenuation correction assumes increased importance.

Malignant melanoma is rapidly increasing in incidence around the world and accounts for 3% of cancers. The prognosis for melanoma is directly related to the depth of invasion of the primary lesion (Clark's level). The tumor initially grows vertically in the skin, then spreads to regional lymph nodes. For high-risk patients (lesion >4 mm in depth), FDG-PET is used to detect metastases. In this case the patient has new metastases in the left neck and upper abdominal periaortic region.

Coronal

Transverse

A 56-year-old man with newly diagnosed esophageal carcinoma. FDG-PET was performed on a two-headed SPECT camera adapted for coincidence imaging.

1. Describe the findings on the transverse and coronal sequential SPECT slices.

2. Give your interpretation of the study.

3. What are the advantages of this gamma camera–based PET technology?

4. What are the disadvantages of this camera–based PET technology?

Oncology: Gamma Camera FDG-PET

1. Large focus of uptake in the right lobe of the liver with a hypermetabolic rim and central photopenic region and a second small hypermetabolic focus in the region of the distal esophagus.

2. Primary esophageal cancer in the distal esophagus with metastatic tumor to the right lobe of the liver; the photopenic center indicates central necrosis.

3. Most nuclear medicine laboratories have two-headed SPECT cameras, obviating the need for a relatively expensive, dedicated PET camera in a small hospital or clinic.

4. Poorer image quality and sensitivity than a dedicated PET camera for detection of smaller tumors. Longer acquisition time for whole-body imaging.

References

Abdel-Dayem HM, Luo J-Q, Sadek S, et al: Multifunctional gamma camera coincidence imaging. In Freeman LM, editor: *Nuclear medicine annual,* Philadelphia, 2000, Lippincott Williams & Wilkins, pp 1-52.

Fahey FH: Positron emission tomography instrumentation, *Radiol Clin North Am* 39:919-930, 2001.

Cross-Reference

Nuclear Medicine: THE REQUISITES, ed 2, pp 33-47, 214.

Comment

PET imaging no longer requires an on-site cyclotron because regional radiopharmacies can deliver FDG on a daily basis in most metropolitan areas. PET imaging merely requires a camera with coincidence detectors. Dedicated PET cameras are expensive compared with traditional gamma cameras, although the price difference between multiheaded gamma cameras and low-end PET systems is decreasing. Smaller clinics cannot fully use a dedicated PET camera. Thus gamma camera PET, with collimators removed and coincidence detectors in place, offers the flexibility of using the two-headed camera for PET when required and routine nuclear medicine studies at other times.

The system resolution of the SPECT/PET cameras is quite similar to that of many dedicated PET cameras (± 5 mm). An important difference, however, is the count rate capability, which is considerably lower with the gamma camera–based systems. This translates into poorer image quality and lower detectability for smaller lesions. Gamma camera PET can detect approximately 75% of the lesions seen with dedicated PET systems. This should be considered in selecting suitable patients for PET imaging. For example, detection of a 1-cm CT lesion may not be indicated, but gamma camera PET may be very useful for larger tumors.

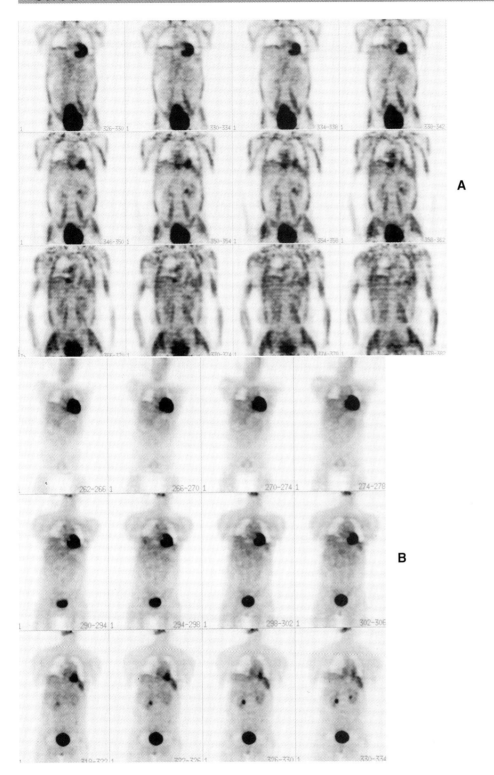

A

B

A 56-year-old patient with insulin-dependent diabetes was referred for an ^{18}F FDG-PET scan. These two studies (*A* and *B*) were performed 1 week apart on the same patient.

1. What patient preparation is required for patients without diabetes and those with diabetes? Why?

2. What serum glucose concentration is acceptable before FDG-PET imaging?

3. What is the effect of insulin on image quality?

4. What could explain the difference in quality between study *A* and *B*?

Oncology: [18]F FDG—Patient with Diabetes

1. For patients without diabetes: fast for 4 to 12 hours before FDG injection. Serum glucose competes with FDG for uptake. For patients with diabetes: good glucose control required. The optimal method for preparing patients with insulin-dependent diabetes is uncertain. Some recommend fasting, and others recommend a light meal and reduced insulin injection at least 2 hours before FDG injection. A blood glucose level determination is required before FDG injection.

2. Blood glucose concentration should be less than 140 mg/dl, although some accept values <180 mg/dL.

3. Insulin drives glucose and FDG into muscle and liver cells.

4. *A,* Poor diabetic control and insulin administration just before ^{18}F FDG administration. *B,* Good diabetic control. Insulin given more than 2 hours before ^{18}F FDG administration.

References

Engel H, Buck A, Berthold T, et al: Whole-body PET: physiological and artifactual fluorodeoxyglucose accumulations, *J Nucl Med* 37:441-446, 1996.

Shreve PD, Anzai Y, Wahl RL: Pitfalls in oncologic diagnosis with FDG PET imaging: physiologic and benign variants, *Radiographics* 19:61-78, 1999.

Cross-Reference

Nuclear Medicine: THE REQUISITES, ed 2, pp 207-209.

Comment

Fasting before a FDG study maximizes tumor uptake and minimizes heart uptake, allowing for better tumor visualization in the chest. High serum glucose levels interfere with FDG tumor uptake because of competitive inhibition. Unfortunately, fasting does not always ensure low cardiac uptake, suggesting that other mechanisms besides glucose competition are at work.

In patients with hyperglycemia, image quality is poor, heart uptake high, and tumor uptake low. Insulin can reduce the serum glucose level, but it also drives glucose and FDG into liver and muscle cells, thus degrading image quality and hindering tumor detection, as seen in this case.

A fasting blood glucose level should be determined before FDG infusion in all patients with diabetes. In this patient the serum glucose concentration was 276 mg/dL. Insulin was administered, and the serum glucose level decreased to 120 mg/dL. [18]F FDG was administered and imaging was performed an hour later; study *A* resulted. The patient was instructed to return another day under better diabetic control. Study *B* is the repeat study with the patient in good diabetic control (blood glucose concentration 120 mg/dL).

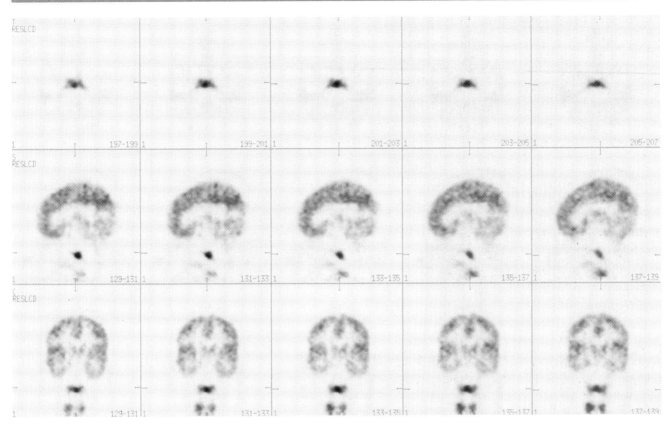

A 51-year-old man with AIDS. MRI scan (not shown) showed a cystic mass in the medulla oblongata.

1. What is the differential diagnosis in this clinical setting?

2. What are the FDG-PET imaging findings? Transverse *(above)*, sagittal *(middle)*, coronal *(below)*.

3. What is your interpretation?

4. Can this differentiation of tumor versus infection be made using single photon radiopharmaceuticals?

Oncology: Brain Lymphoma Versus Infection in AIDS

1. Tumor, especially lymphoma, versus infection, e.g., toxoplasmosis.

2. Increased FDG uptake in the medulla oblongata.

3. Consistent with malignancy.

4. Yes, with ^{201}Tl or ^{99m}Tc sestamibi.

References

O'Malley JP, Ziessman HA, Kumar PN, et al: Diagnosis of intracranial lymphoma in patients with AIDS: value of 201 Tl-single photon computed tomography, *Am J Radiol* 163:417-421, 1994.

Hoffman JM, Washkin HA, Schifter T, et al: FDG-PET in differentiating lymphoma from non-malignant central nervous system lesions in patients with AIDS, *J Nucl Med* 34:567-575, 1993.

Cross-Reference

Nuclear Medicine: THE REQUISITES, ed 2, pp 314-316.

Comment

Intracerebral masses in patients with AIDS are caused by a variety of infectious and neoplastic processes. Conventional imaging with CT or MRI is not reliable for distinguishing tumor and infectious causes. The most common causes are toxoplasmosis and malignant lymphoma, although other opportunistic infections and multifocal leukoencephalopathy must be considered. Radiographic features suggestive of lymphoma include a central location, lack of multifocality, size greater than 2 cm, and a lesion crossing midline. However, diagnosis frequently is uncertain and biopsy is required. Malignant lymphomas in patients with AIDS are aggressive and survival is poor. Early treatment is optimal; however, these patients often are treated empirically for toxoplasmosis because it is common and treatable. Using this approach a biopsy is performed only when therapy fails. However, response to antitoxoplasmosis therapy can take weeks.

FDG-PET and ^{201}Tl SPECT also have been used to make this differentiation, both with good success. Increased uptake of ^{201}Tl is consistent with malignant tumor, whereas no or very low uptake is most consistent with an infectious process, with a 90% accuracy. A positive test result would allow for early biopsy and definitive treatment. ^{99m}Tc sestamibi could be used in a similar manner. It offers the advantage of the ^{99m}Tc radiolabel and higher administered dose, resulting in superior image quality. A potential disadvantage of sestamibi is normal uptake in the choroid plexus.

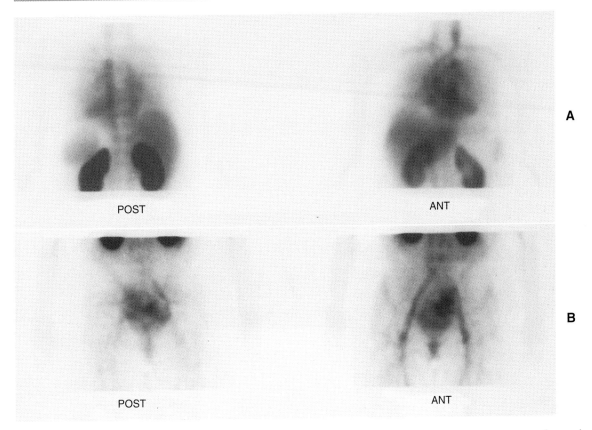

A 56-year-old woman, with a history of colorectal carcinoma, underwent resection 1 year ago and now has a rising serum carcinoembryonic antigen (CEA) level. A ^{99m}Tc CEA planar study is shown.

1. Describe the scintigraphic findings and give your interpretation.

2. What is the relative accuracy of this study compared with CT?

3. List clinical indications for a ^{99m}Tc CEA study.

4. What other radiopharmaceuticals have been used to localize colorectal carcinoma?

Oncology: ^{99m}Tc CEA Colorectal Carcinoma Recurrence

1. Large abnormal region of increased uptake in the pelvis consistent with recurrent tumor. A large tumor is present in the left pelvis adjacent to the bladder in addition to multiple small sites of tumor uptake.

2. ^{99m}Tc CEA is superior to CT in the extrahepatic abdomen and pelvis but equal to CT in detecting tumor in the liver.

3. Rising serum CEA level with negative CT findings. Potentially resectable recurrent disease, usually in the liver, done to exclude other metastases that would preclude surgery.

4. ^{111}In OncoScint and ^{18}F FDG-PET.

References

Willkomm P, Bender H, Bangard M: FDG PET and immunoscintigraphy with 99mTc-labeled antibody fragments for detection of the recurrence of colorectal carcinoma, *J Nucl Med* 41:1657-1663, 2000.

Hughes K, Pinsky CM, Petrelli NJ, et al: Use of carcinoembryonic antigen radioimmunodetection and computed tomography for predicting the resectability of recurrent colorectal cancer, *Ann Surg* 226:621-631, 1997.

Cross-Reference

Nuclear Medicine: THE REQUISITES, ed 2, pp 214-219.

Comment

^{99m}Tc is radiolabeled to a Fab′ fragment of the CEA antibody IMMU-4. The removal of the Fab′ fragment from the Fc portion of the IgG eliminates much of the immunogenicity seen with mouse-derived whole antibodies. Another advantage of the antibody fragment is its rapid clearance from the kidneys allowing for an early high tumor-to background ratio and imaging on the day of injection. More than 95% of colorectal carcinomas express CEA on the cell surface. It is shed into the blood stream and is detectable in approximately 65% of patients. The serum CEA level does not have to be elevated for the scan result to be positive. Of patients with recurrent tumor, one third do not have elevated serum CEA levels. ^{99m}Tc CEA has better image quality and higher tumor detectability than ^{111}In OncoScint, particularly in the liver. The ^{99m}Tc radiolabel is a distinct advantage. Uptake of the radiopharmaceutical in a patient with increasing CEA levels can localize the previously undetected tumor, in a patient with an indeterminate liver lesion can confirm or exclude tumor, and in patients with a potentially resectable liver tumor can exclude other metastases that prohibit surgery. FDG-PET is used increasingly to provide similar information. The incidence of elevated human anti-mouse antibody (HAMA) levels with CEA-SCAN is less than 1%.

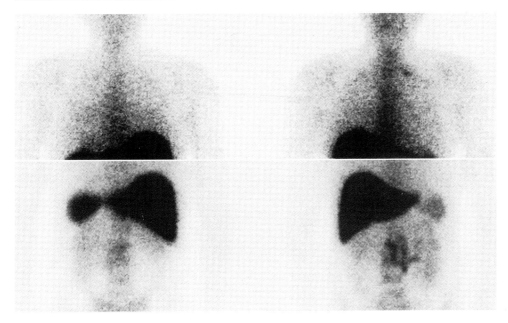

A 64-year-old man had prostatectomy for prostate cancer 3 years ago. Now the serum prostate-specific antigen (PSA) level is increasing. Bone scan and CT findings are negative. ^{111}In ProstaScint scan is shown.

1. What is the mechanism of uptake?

2. Compare the accuracy of CT and MRI with ^{111}In ProstaScint for detecting prostate cancer metastases after prostatectomy.

3. What are the abnormal imaging findings on this study? Give your interpretation.

4. How does the ProstaScint study affect the patient's therapy plan?

Oncology: [111]In ProstaScint—Prostate Cancer

1. ^{111}In-labeled monoclonal antibody directed against the prostate-specific membrane antigen, a glycoprotein expressed by normal and prostate cancer cells.

2. CT and MRI sensitivity ranges from 5% to 20%. Overall reported accuracy of [111]In ProstaScint is 70%.

3. Paraaortic upper abdominal uptake consistent with tumor adenopathy. Focal uptake in the left upper chest consistent with tumor.

4. Recurrent tumor limited to the prostate bed or metastatic pelvic lymph nodes require different radiation ports. Extrapelvic metastases require systemic therapy.

References

Manyak MJ, Hinkle GH, Olsen JO, et al: Immunoscintigraphy with In-111-capromab pendetide: evaluation before definitive therapy in patients with prostate cancer, *Urology* 54:1058-1063, 1999.

Blend MJ, Sodee DB: Prostascint: an update. In Freeman LM, editor: *Nuclear medicine annual 2001,* Philadelphia, 2001, Lippincott Raven, pp 109-138.

Cross-Reference

Nuclear Medicine: THE REQUISITES, ed 2, pp 220-223.

Comment

Examination, histopathological Gleason's score, and serum PSA level are used to stage prostate cancer. After primary therapy for prostate cancer the patient is monitored with the serum PSA level as a marker of tumor activity. An increasing PSA level suggests recurrence of tumor. Because bone metastases are common in metastatic prostate cancer, the ^{99m}Tc bone scan is obtained first. If bone scan results are negative, CT or MRI may be performed; however, their sensitivity for detection of recurrent prostate cancer is very low. [111]In ProstaScint (capromab pendetide) is a monoclonal antibody directed against intact prostate cells. It is a murine immunoglobulin reactive with prostate-specific membrane antigen (PMSA), a glycoprotein expressed by more than 95% of prostate cancers. It is clinically indicated for detection of soft tissue metastases. Extrapelvic metastases in the abdomen sometimes can be diagnosed with planar imaging, as seen in this patient. However, SPECT is mandatory to detect prostate bed and pelvic tumor adenopathy. ProstaScint is less sensitive for bone metastases than the ^{99m}Tc bone scan. Images are interpreted in conjunction with blood pool imaging to aid in anatomical localization, either by imaging on the day of injection when blood pool activity is high or using ^{99m}Tc RBCs as a dual-isotope study on imaging day 4 to 6.

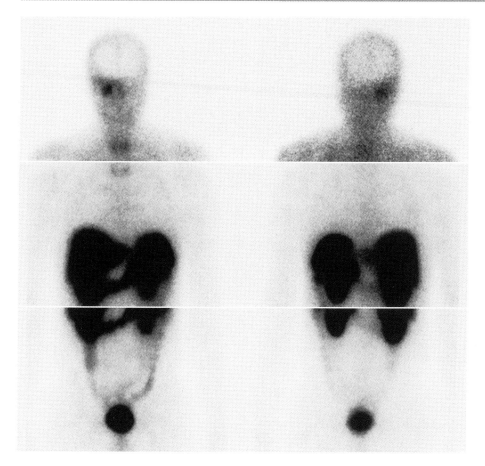

A patient with a neuroendocrine disorder and pulsatile tinnitus in the right ear. CT study shows a mass in the right temporal bone.

1. What radiopharmaceuticals are applicable?

2. Based on the biodistribution, what agent was used?

3. Describe the findings in the head and neck.

4. Provide the most likely diagnosis and a differential diagnosis.

Oncology: OctreoScan—Glomus Tympanicum

1. [111]In OctreoScan (octreotide), ^{131}I MIBG.

2. Prominent liver, spleen, and kidney uptake is seen with [111]In OctreoScan.

3. Focal abnormal uptake in the right temporal bone that correlates with CT report.

4. Paraganglioma (glomus tympanicum) considering the patient's history; also meningioma or neuroendocrine tumor metastasis.

References

Grossman RI, Yousem DM: *Neuroradiology: the requisites,* St Louis, 1994, Mosby, p 345.

Telischi FF, Bustillo A, Whiteman ML, et al: Octreotide scintigraphy for the detection of paragangliomas, *Otolaryngol Head Neck Surg* 122:358-362, 2000.

Cross-Reference

Nuclear Medicine: THE REQUISITES, ed 2, pp 223-225, 383-384.

Comment

Glomus tympanicum and glomus jugulare arise from paraganglioma tissue in the middle ear. Glomus tympanicum, associated with the ninth cranial nerve, usually manifests as pulsatile tinnitus, although other entities can present similarly, e.g., high jugular bulb, aberrant carotid artery, dural arteriovenous malformation, cavernous carotid fistula, meningioma. Glomus tympanicum usually produces symptoms early in the clinical course as a small soft tissue mass behind the tympanic membrane that markedly enhances. It is critical in preoperative assessment to distinguish among the various vascular tympanic masses to avoid a patient with a vascular abnormality being inadvertently sent to the operating room without the surgeon's foreknowledge.

[111]In pentetreotide (OctreoScan) is a somatostatin analogue that binds to somatostatin receptors on neuroendocrine tumors and numerous other malignancies, e.g., breast cancer, small cell lung cancer, and lymphoma. The radiopharmaceutical's sensitivity for detection of tumors varies by malignancy. It has a very high accuracy for carcinoid, gastrinoma, small cell lung cancer (80% to 95%), but the accuracy is lower for insulinoma and medullary carcinoma of the thyroid (30% to 50%). The sensitivity for paragangliomas has been reported to be 86%.

The ^{111}In radiolabel allows for delayed imaging at 24 to 48 hours when the target-to-background ratio is optimal. This is an advantage because of the high uptake in the liver and kidneys (see images). A ^{99m}Tc-labeled somatostatin analogue (Neotect) has been approved for small cell and non-small cell lung cancer. Similar analogues labeled with therapeutic radionuclides are being investigated.

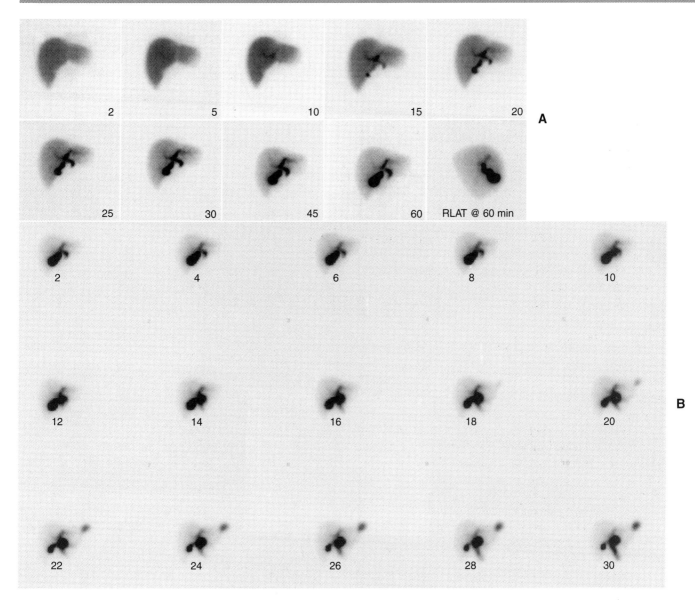

A 10-year-old girl has acute abdominal pain. A cholescintigraphy scan taken at 60 minutes *(A)* was followed by 30-minute cholecystokinin (CCK; sincalide) infusion *(B)*.

1. Describe the cholescintigraphic findings.

2. What is the likely diagnosis?

3. What other clinical presentations are common in patients with this problem?

4. What is the cause, pathological condition, and appropriate therapy for this entity?

Hepatobiliary System: Choledochal Cyst

1. *A,* Good hepatic uptake and clearance into the gallbladder, common hepatic, and proximal common bile duct at 60 minutes. No biliary-to-bowel transit. *B,* The gallbladder contracts with sincalide infusion; however, focal increasing accumulation of radiotracer occurs just medial to the proximal portion of the common bile. The proximal common duct activity empties into the duodenum. Note enterogastric reflux.

2. Likely choledochal cyst. Partial biliary obstruction also would result in radiotracer retention within the more proximal biliary ducts.

3. Cholangitis, sepsis, pancreatitis, or obstruction.

4. Congenital anomaly. Localized dilation of the biliary tract, either fusiform or diverticular outpouching. Surgery is the appropriate therapy.

References

Camponovo E, Buck JL, Drane WE: Scintigraphic features of choledochal cyst, *J Nucl Med* 30:622-628, 1989.

Kim OH, Chung HJ, Choi BG: Imaging of the choledochal cyst, *Radiographics* 15:69-87, 1995.

Cross-Reference

Nuclear Medicine: THE REQUISITES, ed 2, p 243.

Comment

A choledochal cyst is a congenital anomaly characterized by saccular dilation of the extrahepatic biliary tract. It is not a true cyst. The most common form is characterized by a fusiform dilation of the common bile duct. A second type is a diverticular outpouching of the common bile duct, and the third is a small saccular dilation of the distal common bile duct. Less common intrahepatic ductal dilation is referred to as Caroli's disease.

Recognition and appropriate early treatment of a choledochal cyst are critical because of the risk of severe cholangitis, obstruction, and adenocarcinoma (10% occurrence rate) if the cyst is left unattended. The diagnosis is made preoperatively in only 27% to 80% of patients in different published reports. A lower surgical morbidity is associated with a preoperative diagnosis. Ultrasonography is the best screening method for small children; CT has been advocated for older children and adults. Cholescintigraphy is used to noninvasively confirm the diagnosis, i.e., to ensure that the cystic structure connects with the biliary tract and sometimes to help identify the type. Definitive diagnosis is made by ECRP or intraoperative cholangiography.

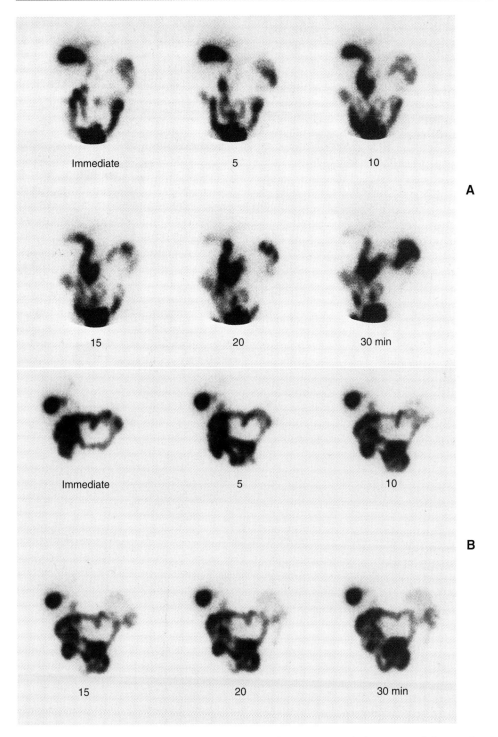

Two patients (*A* and *B*) have a similar history of recurrent, colicky upper abdominal pain and negative test results. They were referred for CCK cholescintigraphy to confirm the clinical diagnosis of chronic acalculous cholecystitis (CAC). Images were acquired during sincalide infusion.

1. What is CAC, and how does it differ from chronic calculous cholecystitis?

2. Why is sincalide cholescintigraphy required to make the diagnosis of CAC?

3. The calculated gallbladder ejection fraction (GBEF) was greater than 80% for patient *A* and 10% for patient *B*. What are their diagnoses?

4. What is the accuracy of CCK cholescintigraphy for confirming the diagnosis of CAC?

Hepatobiliary System: Chronic Acalculous Cholecystitis

1. CAC is clinically and pathologically identical to chronic calculous cholecystitis, except for the absence of gallstones.

2. Anatomical imaging diagnosis depends heavily on visualization of gallstones. CCK cholescintigraphy allows quantification of gallbladder contraction. Diseased gallbladders do not contract.

3. Findings consistent with chronic acalculous cholecystitis in patient *B* but not *A*.

4. A low GBEF has a positive predictive value of more than 90% that cholecystectomy will cure the patient's symptoms and that the diagnosis will be confirmed by pathological gallbladder examination.

Reference

Ziessman HA: Cholecystokinin cholescintigraphy: clinical indications and proper methodology, *Radiol Clin North Am* 39:997-1006, 2001.

Cross-Reference

Nuclear Medicine: THE REQUISITES, ed 2, pp 240-241.

Comment

The symptoms of chronic cholecystitis overlap with many causes of abdominal pain. Before the availability of CCK cholescintigraphy, clinicians had no objective method to diagnose CAC before surgery. CCK cholescintigraphy should be performed only in the proper clinical setting, i.e., in outpatients with recurrent symptoms suggestive of the disease who have been evaluated to exclude other diseases and with follow-up of many months' duration to allow time for other diseases to manifest. The test should not be performed in acutely ill patients, and patients should not be taking drugs that inhibit gallbladder contraction, e.g., progesterone, nifedipine, atropine, phentolamine, and morphine.

Proper methodology is important. CCK administered as a bolus results in spasm of the gallbladder neck and ineffective contraction. One- to 3-minute infusions using 0.01 or 0.02 μg/kg also often result in ineffective contraction in one third of normal subjects. However, infusions of 30 to 60 minutes using the same total dose result in good contraction in these same subjects. With 1- to 3-minute infusions, up to half of patients have abdominal cramps and nausea as a result of the rapid rate of infusion and not because of a gallbladder pathological condition. With 30- to 60-minute infusions, no adverse symptoms occur. Reproduction of the patient's pain with CCK is not diagnostic of the disease. With a 30-minute infusion an abnormal GBEF is less than 30% and with a 60-minute infusion is less than 40%.

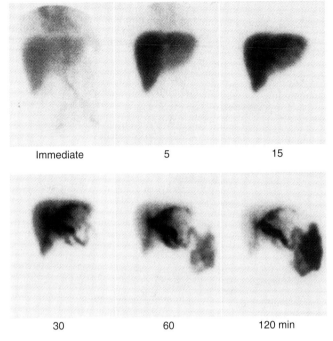

Immediate   5   15

30   60   120 min

A 46-year-old woman 8 months after cholecystectomy and removal of common bile duct stone has recurrent upper abdominal pain.

1. Describe the cholescintigraphic findings.

2. Provide a differential diagnosis at 60 minutes. What is the likely diagnosis at 2 hours?

3. Give the differential diagnosis for the postcholecystectomy syndrome.

4. What is sphincter of Oddi dysfunction?

Hepatobiliary System: Postcholecystectomy Syndrome

1. Prompt hepatic uptake (blood pool clearance by 5 minutes), clearance into biliary ducts by 15 to 30 minutes, retention of activity in ducts, apparently dilated proximal hepatic and common ducts, biliary-to-bowel clearance by 60 minutes. At 120 minutes, further small bowel clearance but prominent retention in common duct with apparent cutoff distally.

2. 60 minutes: partial common duct obstruction versus post-biliary duct obstruction surgery with nonobstructed persistent bile duct dilation. 120 minutes: suspected partial obstruction.

3. Common duct stone, inflammatory stricture of the common duct, sphincter of Oddi dysfunction, inflamed cystic duct remnant.

4. Sphincter of Oddi dysfunction is a partial biliary obstruction at the level of the sphincter of Oddi not caused by stones or stricture.

Reference

Ziessman HA, Zeman RK, Akin EA: Cholescintigraphy: correlation with other hepatobiliary imaging modalities. In Sandler MP, Coleman RE, et al, editors: *Diagnostic nuclear medicine,* ed 4, Baltimore, 2002, Williams & Wilkins.

Cross-Reference

Nuclear Medicine: THE REQUISITES, ed 2, pp 245-246.

Comment

Severe recurrent abdominal pain symptoms occur in up to 10% of patients after cholecystectomy. The most common causes are common duct stones and inflammatory fibrosis causing biliary obstruction. Typical cholescintigraphic findings are a partial biliary duct obstruction and nonclearing of the common duct. Biliary-to-bowel transit may or may not be delayed. As many as 50% of patients with partial common duct obstruction have biliary-to-bowel transit by 60 minutes. In this case, nonclearance of the common hepatic and common bile duct at 2 hours is consistent with partial obstruction; clearance would have excluded obstruction. An alternative to obtaining delayed imaging would be administration of sincalide. With no obstruction the sphincter of Oddi relaxes and the common duct drains. An obstructed duct has continued retention. The diagnosis of sphincter of Oddi dysfunction usually is considered when a stricture or stone is excluded and delayed contrast drainage is seen on endoscopic retrograde cholangiopancreatography (ERCP). Sphincter of Oddi manometry demonstrating elevated pressure is more specific for making the diagnosis. However, manometry generally is not available and is technically demanding. Cholescintigraphy has been used to make this diagnosis, and the findings are those of a partial biliary obstruction. Cholecystokinin has been used during cholescintigraphy to increase bile flow "stress" a partial obstruction, thus improving the sensitivity for cholescintigraphic detection. Treatment is sphincterotomy.

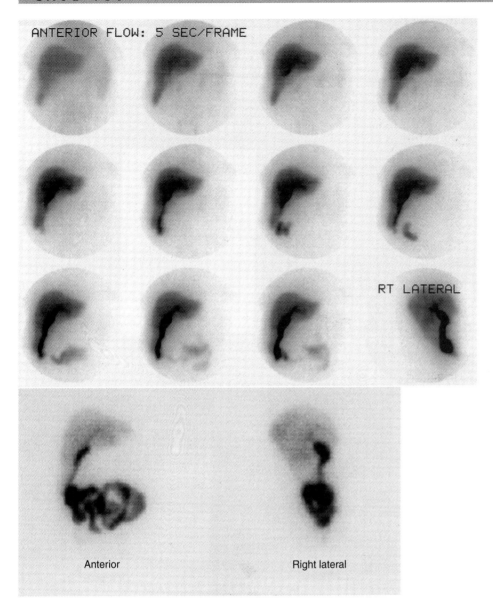

ANTERIOR FLOW: 5 SEC/FRAME

RT LATERAL

Anterior   Right lateral

A patient has a history of biliary diversion of unknown type and now has abdominal pain.

1. Describe the scintigraphic findings.

2. What is the biliary diversion?

3. Are the study results normal or abnormal?

4. Could ultrasonography have provided the same information?

Hepatobiliary System: Cholecystojejunostomy

1. Prompt hepatic uptake and rapid biliary-to-bowel clearance through the gallbladder.

2. Cholecystoduodenostomy or cholecystojejunostomy.

3. Normal postoperative study results.

4. Nondiagnostic examinations are frequent with ultrasonography, occurring in up to 67% of patients, usually as a result of gas in the anastomotic bowel segment. Persistent biliary dilation is often present without obstruction.

Reference

Ziessman HA, Zeman RK, Akin EA: Cholescintigraphy: correlation with other hepatobiliary imaging modalities. In Sandler MP, Coleman RE, et al: Diagnostic nuclear medicine, ed 4, Baltimore, 2002, Lippincott Williams & Wilkins.

Cross-Reference

Nuclear Medicine: THE REQUISITES, ed 2, pp 243-244.

Comment

Cholescintigraphy is used to evaluate the postoperative biliary tract after creation of a biliary-enteric anastomosis. Evaluation of acute and early complications of surgery and long-term follow-up for biliary patency is possible. Knowledge of the postoperative anatomy of the patient is important when imaging the postoperative biliary tract. Biliary scintigraphy commonly is used to evaluate a choledochojejunostomy, which is a direct anastomosis of the extrahepatic portion of the common bile duct or the common hepatic duct to a Roux-en-Y of jejunum. It also is used to evaluate intrahepatic cholangiojejunostomies. The latter is more complex, requiring direct anastomosis between small bowel and intrahepatic ducts that must be dissected out deep with the liver. Choledochoduodenostomy, cholecystoduodenostomy, and cholecystojejunostomy also can be studied. The latter two procedures frequently are used in benign disease states.

Many complications can occur postoperatively after creation of biliary diversion. Biliary leakage is among the most common. Recurrent biliary obstruction is a major problem and is well suited for cholescintigraphic evaluation. Cholescintigraphy is the only noninvasive technique that can distinguish obstructed dilated ducts from those that are persistently dilated.

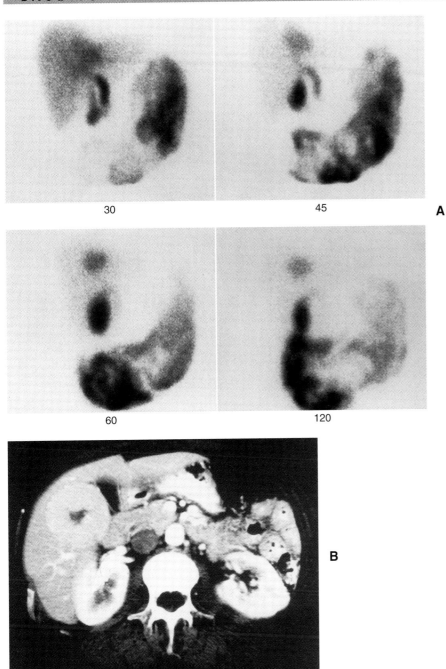

A 35-year-old woman has abdominal pain. Cholescintigraphy *(A)* images at 30 to 120 minutes. The CT scan *(B)* shows a large, circumscribed lesion at the juncture of the right and left lobes.

1. Describe the cholescintigraphic findings.

2. What is the differential diagnosis? What is the diagnosis in this case?

3. What is the appropriate therapy for each of these diagnoses?

4. What other radiopharmaceutical could confirm the diagnosis in this case?

Hepatobiliary System: Focal Nodular Hyperplasia (FNH)

1. Increased radiopharmaceutical uptake that corresponds to the lesion seen on CT. The uptake is retained after liver washout.

2. Benign and malignant tumors that have hepatocytes, e.g., hepatic adenoma, hepatoma, focal nodular hyperplasia. The latter is the correct diagnosis.

3. FNH usually requires no specific therapy. Hepatic adenoma requires discontinuation of oral contraceptives and surgical removal, and hepatoma requires resection.

4. ^{99m}Tc sulfur colloid.

Reference

Boulahdour H, Cherqui D, Charlotte F, et al: The hot spot hepatobiliary scan in focal nodular hyperplasia, *J Nucl Med* 34:2105-2110, 1993.

Cross-Reference

Nuclear Medicine: THE REQUISITES, ed 2, pp 246-247.

Comment

FNH and hepatic adenoma are benign liver tumors that occur as solid intrahepatic lesions in young and middle-aged women. The natural history of the two is quite different. Although hepatic adenomas may manifest as a mass, often the initial presentation is an abdominal crisis because of intraperitoneal hemorrhage. Hepatic adenoma has a strong association with contraceptive use. Pathologically adenomas consist of sheets of hepatocytes without structure, bile ducts, or Kupffer cells. FNH has only a weak association with contraceptive use, usually produces no symptoms, and usually is discovered incidentally. Pathologically FNH tumors have a stellate fibrous core (see CT) and contain all three liver cell types.

^{99m}Tc SC is taken up by liver Kupffer cells. Two thirds of FNH tumors take up ^{99m}Tc SC to varying degrees. Hepatic adenoma and hepatoma do not have uptake because they do not usually have Kupffer cells. On cholescintigraphy, FNH has a characteristic appearance: increased flow, normal or increased uptake, and delayed clearance compared with adjacent uninvolved liver, probably as a result of immature biliary canaliculi. Hepatic adenomas have no uptake; the reason is uncertain. With hepatocellular carcinoma, images during the first hour demonstrate a cold defect; however, delayed imaging at 2 to 4 hours shows uptake within the tumor as the normal liver washes out. This pattern occurs because hepatocellular carcinoma cells are hypofunctional compared with normal liver, with delayed uptake and clearance. The low-level uptake also is easier to visualize when the normal liver has washed out. Sensitivity for detection of FNH with cholescintigraphy is greater than 90%.

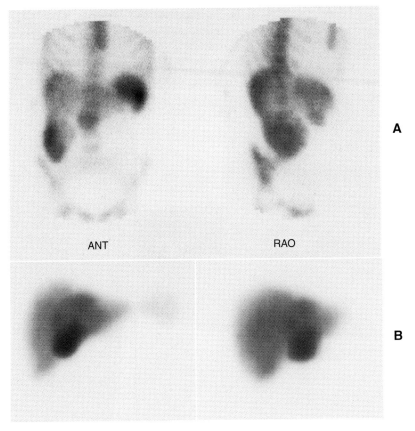

ANT   RAO

A

B

^{99m}Tc sulfur colloid liver-spleen scans in two patients. *A*, A 50-year old with abnormal liver function and hepatosplenomegaly. *B*, A 59-year-old with a liver mass on CT in the quadrate lobe. Anterior *(left)* and right anterior oblique views *(right)* in both studies.

1. What is the mechanism of ^{99m}Tc sulfur colloid uptake?

2. What is the normal distribution of this radiopharmaceutical?

3. What are the image findings and diagnoses in these two patients?

4. List three other causes for hot spots ^{99m}Tc sulfur colloid spleen scans.

Hepatobiliary System: Hot Spot ^{99m}Tc Sulfur Colloid Imaging

1. Uptake by the reticuloendothelial system.

2. More than 85% of ^{99m}Tc sulfur colloid is taken up by the Kupffer cells of the liver, 10% by the spleen, and 5% by the bone marrow.

3. *A,* The central, large cold region may be caused by an intrahepatic mass, but the pattern has been stable and CT shows cirrhosis. There is colloid shift to the spleen and bone marrow. The relatively increased uptake in the inferior aspect of the right lobe and dome of the liver is the best functioning portion of the liver, related to preferential damage more centrally, or alternatively, possibly areas of regeneration. *B,* Increased uptake in the region of the quadrate lobe, consistent with FNH.

4. Superior vena cava syndrome (arm injection), inferior vena cava obstruction (leg injection), Budd-Chiari syndrome.

Reference

Welch TJ, Sheedy HF, Johnson M, et al: Focal nodular hyperplasia and hepatic adenoma: comparison of angiography, CT, US, and scintigraphy, *Radiology* 156:593-595, 1985.

Cross-Reference

Nuclear Medicine: THE REQUISITES, ed 2, pp 256-258.

Comment

^{99m}Tc sulfur colloid liver imaging is uncommon since the advent of CT scanning; however, it occasionally is ordered to evaluate the degree of hepatic insufficiency in patients with cirrhosis, e.g., colloid shift indicates portal hypertension. A liver tumor must have Kupffer cells to take up ^{99m}Tc sulfur colloid. With cirrhosis the liver is fibrotic and poorly functional, seen as decreased uptake in a shrunken liver and increased uptake in the spleen and bone marrow. FNH, with all three liver cell types (hepatocytes, biliary ducts, and Kupffer cells) often takes up ^{99m}Tc sulfur colloid. Approximately one third of patients with FNH have increased, one third decreased, and one third uptake equivalent to adjacent liver. Thus in two thirds of patients with FNH the diagnosis can be made. Hepatic adenomas have few or no Kupffer cells; nor do other primary or secondary liver tumors. With the Budd-Chiari (hepatic vein thrombosis) syndrome, poor liver function is caused by impaired venous drainage from the liver, except for the caudate lobe, which connects separately to the inferior vena cava. In superior vena cava syndrome, collateral thoracic and abdominal vessels communicate with the recanalized umbilical vein, delivering increased blood flow and radiotracer to the region of the quadrate lobe through the left portal vein when the radiopharmaceutical is injected in the arm. With a lower extremity injection the distribution is normal.

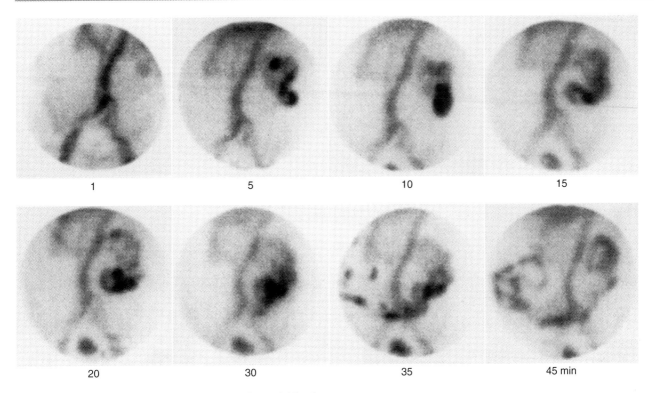

1   5   10   15

20   30   35   45 min

A 46-year-old man has a second episode of rectal bleeding.

1. What is the radiopharmaceutical, and what method of labeling was likely used?

2. Describe the scintigraphic bleeding study findings.

3. Provide a diagnosis.

4. List common causes for bleeding from this portion of the gastrointestinal tract.

Gastrointestinal System: ^{99m}Tc-labeled RBCs—Small Bowel Bleeding

1. ^{99m}Tc-labeled RBCs. The in vitro method of labeling was used. The modified in vivo method would be an acceptable alternative.

2. Evidence for active bleeding, first seen at 5 minutes, starting in the left upper abdomen and moving in a serpiginous pattern across the mid to lower abdomen to the right lower and then right mid abdomen.

3. Small bowel bleeding originating from the region of the jejunum.

4. Arteriovenous malformations and tumors.

References

Lewis BS: Small intestinal bleeding, *Gastroenterol Clin North Am* 29:67-95, 2000.

Ziessman HA: The gastrointestinal tract. In Harbert JC, Eckelman WC, Neuman RD, editors: *Nuclear medicine, diagnosis and therapy,* New York, 1996, Thieme Medical Publishers, pp 617-627.

Cross-Reference
Nuclear Medicine: THE REQUISITES, ed 2, pp 280-287.

Comment

Major bleeding from the small intestine is uncommon and often difficult to localize because of the organ's length, its free intraperitoneal location, and the nature of the lesions that bleed in the small bowel. Causes include arteriovenous malformations (e.g., angiodysplasia), tumors (e.g., leiomyoma, leiomyosarcoma, and adenocarcinoma), Meckel's diverticulum, and Crohn's disease. In approximately 5% of all patients with gastrointestinal bleeding, no cause for the bleeding is evident after an extensive evaluation and is referred to as gastrointestinal bleeding of obscure origin. Almost 30% of these patients have lesions in the small bowel.

The pattern of movement of radiolabeled RBCs in this case is characteristic of small bowel bleeding. It is important to distinguish this pattern from colonic bleeding. Frequent image acquisition is important to determine the site of bleeding. Although the case images are taken every 5 to 10 minutes, the study was acquired on the computer at a framing rate of 1 minute per frame. Thus reviewing the cinematic display on the computer can be very helpful in confirming the origin of the bleeding.

The in vitro method of radiolabeling erythrocytes is optimal. Labeling efficiency is greater than 98%. The modified in vivo method, performed by drawing the patient's blood back into a syringe containing ^{99m}Tc pertechnetate after intravenous injection of stannous chloride or pyrophosphate, is an alternative method with labeling efficiency of approximately 85% to 90%.

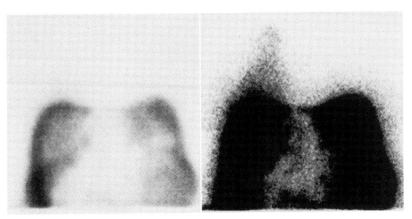

A 54-year-old man with a history of cirrhosis and ascites has shortness of breath and a right pleural effusion. The clinical service requests a radionuclide study.

1. What question can nuclear medicine address regarding the effusion?

2. Describe the procedure.

3. What radiotracer is preferred?

4. What other radiopharmaceutical can be used to demonstrate the peritoneal fluid flow?

Gastrointestinal System:
Peritoneal-Pleural Scan

1. Is there a connection between the pleural effusion and the ascites?

2. Inject radiotracer into the peritoneum in an area where ascites is present. Ultrasound guidance may be helpful. Immediate and delayed images are obtained to evaluate transit from the peritoneum to the pleural space, confirming transdiaphragmatic flow.

3. ^{99m}Tc sulfur colloid.

4. ^{99m}Tc MAA is the tracer of choice to establish the patency of a peritoneal-venous shunt catheter, such as a Le Veen or Denver shunt. Uptake in the lungs of the ^{99m}Tc MAA confirms patency of the shunt.

References

Armstrong P, Wilson AG, Dee P, et al, editors: *Images of diseases of the chest,* ed 3, St Louis, 2000, Mosby, p 749.

Sing A: Peritoneovenous shunts: patency studies. In Henkin RE, Boles MA, Dillehay GL, et al, editors: *Nuclear medicine,* St Louis, 1996, Mosby, pp 1041-1052.

Cross-Reference

Nuclear Medicine: THE REQUISITES, ed 2, pp 253, 261.

Comment

Pleural effusion in a patient with cirrhosis is not uncommon. When other causes for pleural effusion have been excluded, e.g., cardiac, pulmonary, or pleural, the term *hepatic hydrothorax* is used for the transudative effusion in patients with cirrhosis. The effusion varies in size, is more common on the right, but can occur on the left side alone or bilaterally. Transdiaphragmatic passage of fluid is the most important mechanism explaining a hepatic hydrothorax. The development of pleural effusion by this mechanism depends on the presence of ascites. Postmortem examinations have shown that defects exist in the diaphragm, usually in the tendinous part of the diaphragm, and probably are tears resulting from stretching caused by abdominal distention by ascites. The right-sided prevalence of hepatic hydrothorax may be because the tendinous diaphragm is more exposed on the right side while it is covered by the heart on the left.

^{99m}Tc sulfur colloid can be used for this investigation because these particles diffuse poorly through peritoneal or visceral surfaces (slow systemic absorption may occur), and its appearance above the diaphragm confirms a pleural-peritoneal connection. ^{99m}Tc MAA particles cannot be absorbed systemically because they are considerably larger particles (10 to 90 μm versus 0.1 to 1.0 μm). These are advantageous for peritoneal venous shunts because uptake in the lungs confirms venous access and patency.

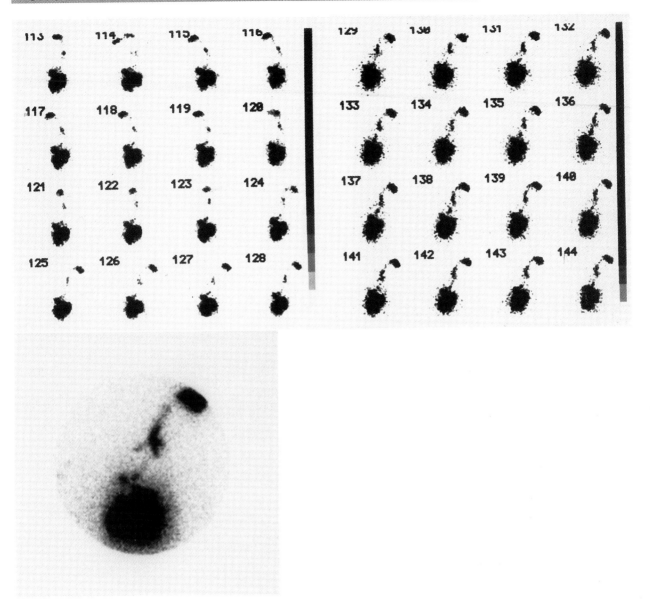

A 2-year-old was referred for "salivagram" (esophageal transit study) to diagnose suspected aspiration (anterior imaging). The result of a gastroesophageal reflux ("milk") study was positive for reflux but negative for aspiration.

1. What are the clinical symptoms of pulmonary aspiration?

2. What radiopharmaceutical is used for the salivagram, and what is the method of administration?

3. What are the scintigraphic findings in this case?

4. What is the advantage of the salivagram over the milk study?

Gastrointestinal System: Pulmonary Aspiration

1. Recurrent pneumonia, cough, asthma, failure to thrive, apnea, sudden infant death.

2. ^{99m}Tc sulfur colloid in a small volume of fluid placed on the tongue and allowed to mix with oral secretions and swallowed.

3. Poor bolus progression noted in the dynamic esophageal swallow study with entrance into the main bronchi bilaterally and then into the right lower lobe.

4. The milk study is very sensitive for reflux; however, it is insensitive for aspiration. The salivagram is sensitive for small amounts of pulmonary aspiration.

References

Heyman S, Respondek M: Detection of pulmonary aspiration in children by radionuclide "salivagram," *J Nucl Med* 30:667-679, 1989.

Bar-Sever Z, Connolly LP, Treves ST: The radionuclide salivagram in children with pulmonary disease and a high risk of aspiration, *Pediatr Radiol* 24(Suppl 1):S180-S183, 1995.

Cross-Reference

Nuclear Medicine: THE REQUISITES, ed 2, pp 272-273.

Comment

The aspiration of gastric contents can result in bronchospasm and severe bronchopneumonia that can be life-threatening. Aspiration often is associated with patients who have neurological dysfunction or gastroesophageal reflux or after surgery to the upper airway or digestive tract.

Radionuclide milk studies are considerably more sensitive for diagnosing reflux than the barium swallow study. However, the sensitivity for diagnosis of aspiration is significantly lower, and the diagnosis is rarely made on the basis of a "milk" scan even in patients with significant reflux. Many patients with aspiration have associated esophageal motor abnormalities and gastroesophageal reflux. The esophageal swallow portion of the salivagram study is acquired in a rapid dynamic mode (15- to 30-second frames) that allows visualization of esophageal swallowing physiology. To perform the test, 250 μCi ^{99m}Tc sulfur colloid in 10 mL of water is placed on the tongue or posterior pharynx. Once the transit study is completed, the remaining meal volume is fed and further imaging can be obtained. Esophageal swallow studies also have been used to diagnose or follow the effectiveness of therapy in patients with achalasia, esophageal spasm, or scleroderma.

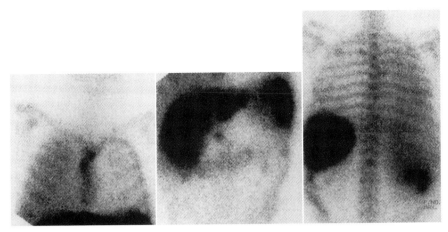

A patient who had peritoneal-venous shunt for intractable ascites years ago is now experiencing increasing ascites. Images obtained 30 minutes after injection are submitted.

1. What is the clinical question to be addressed?

2. What tracer(s) could be used, and what was used?

3. Describe the injection procedure.

4. Describe the findings and provide a conclusion.

Gastrointestinal System: Peritoneal Scan—Patent Denver Shunt

1. Is the peritoneal-venous shunt patent, or occluded and causing the increased ascites?

2. ^{99m}Tc MAA or sulfur colloid; ^{99m}Tc sulfur colloid.

3. The radiotracer is injected into the peritoneal cavity.

4. Uptake of the radiotracer is seen in the liver and spleen (which appears enlarged), indicating shunt patency. There is transdiaphragmatic transit into the right hemithorax.

Reference

Stewart CA, Sakimura IT, Applebaum DM, et al: Evaluation of peritoneovenous shunt patency seen by intraperitoneal Tc-99m macroaggregated albumin: clinical experience, *Am J Roentgenol* 147:177-180, 1986.

Cross-Reference

Nuclear Medicine: THE REQUISITES, ed 2, pp 253-254.

Comment

Le Veen or Denver-type peritoneovenous shunts are used to decompress the peritoneal cavity in patients with significant ascites refractory to medical management. The shunt drains into a large vein in the neck or thorax. The caudal end is located within the peritoneal cavity and contains a one-way valve that opens when increasing ascites results in increased intraperitoneal pressure. Fibrinous deposits at the valve in the peritoneal space may cause shunt obstruction, which is manifest as increasing ascites in a patient with a shunt. Patency can be demonstrated by intraperitoneal injection of ^{99m}Tc sulfur colloid or MAA, subsequent identification of organ extraction of the radiotracer (liver for sulfur colloid, lungs for MAA). Flow through the shunt requires sufficient pressure to open the valve. Therefore patients who have limited ascites are inappropriate for the test. In patients who have had therapeutic paracentesis, shunt patency evaluation should be postponed until reaccumulation of adequate fluid. A normally functioning shunt results in lung uptake within 10 minutes. The shunt tubing usually is visible. In cases in which organ extraction does not occur within the first 30 minutes, delayed images may be useful to distinguish partial from complete shunt obstruction. ^{99m}Tc MAA offers an advantage in that the site of uptake (lungs) is further removed from the site of injection (peritoneum) than sulfur colloid, which demonstrates uptake in the liver and spleen. However, if bilateral effusions are present, ^{99m}Tc MAA may enter the thorax by transdiaphragmatic flow, which can complicate interpretation.

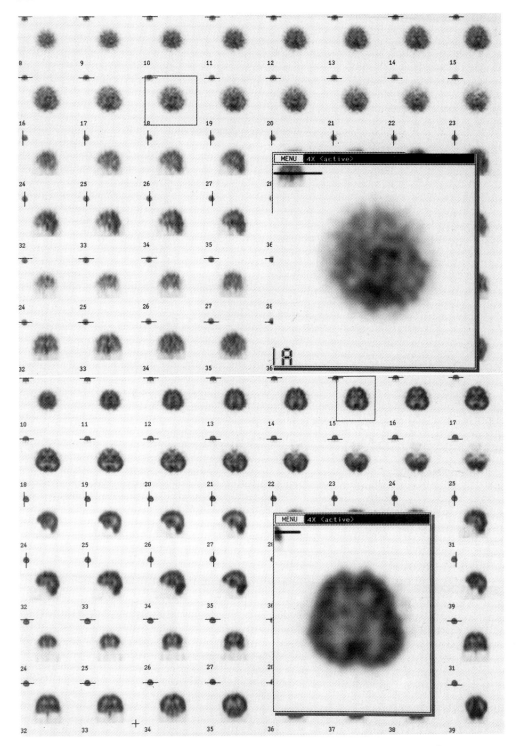

A SPECT ^{99m}Tc HM-PAO cerebral perfusion study. Single transverse slices from two separate SPECT acquisitions of the same patient are shown. *A,* Initial study. *B,* Repeat study.

1. Image quality is very poor. What are questions that should be asked?

2. What camera quality control should be performed daily for all gamma cameras?

3. What special quality control is required for SPECT?

4. What is the difference between an intrinsic and extrinsic flood?

Central Nervous System: Gamma Camera Quality Control

1. Was the camera set at the correct photopeak? Did the patient move? What did the flood and spatial resolution tests look like in the morning? How do they look now?

2. Field uniformity. A flood source of radioactivity is used to test gamma camera uniformity of response across its field of view. Spatial resolution and linearity, using a four-quadrant bar phantom, is acquired weekly.

3. Uniformity flood acquired for 30 million counts for SPECT (1 million to 5 million counts for planar), center of rotation.

4. An extrinsic flood is acquired with the collimator on; an intrinsic flood is done with the collimator off.

Reference

Siegel BA, editor: *Nuclear radiology* (third series), Chicago, 1993, American College of Radiology, pp 22-31.

Cross-Reference

Nuclear Medicine: THE REQUISITES, ed 2, pp 27-30, 42-43.

Comment

Routine gamma camera quality control is mandatory to ensure proper function and high-quality diagnostic images. In this case the technologist forgot to change the gamma camera photopeak to 140 keV from 122 keV used for the cobalt flood source acquisition before this first study of the morning; this is a common error. Floods are performed in the early morning before the start of clinical studies. A commonly used flood source is one with ^{57}Co embedded in a solid plastic encasement. It is placed directly on the collimator. ^{57}Co is commonly used because of its long half-life (122 days) and energy photopeak (122 keV) is close, although not identical to ^{99m}Tc (140 keV). The alternative method used in some laboratories is insertion of ^{99m}Tc pertechnetate mixed with water in a plastic refillable disk. Its disadvantage is the need for daily refilling because of ^{99m}Tc's short (6-hour) physical half-life. Both methods are referred to as extrinsic floods, i.e., extrinsic to the collimator. An intrinsic flood is performed by placing a hot source at a distance from the gamma camera with the collimator off. A well-tuned camera with proper photomultiplier tube and correction circuitry performance should appear uniform. Photomultiplier tube drift or failure can be seen as an area of decreased activity. Cracked crystals and collimator damage can be detected. Floods should be performed on a daily basis.

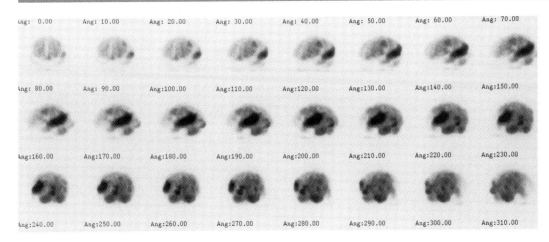

A 29-year-old man with recent onset of fever and headache has no prior medical problems.

1. Describe the ^{99m}Tc HM-PAO SPECT reconstructed volume display in this patient. Angle 0 is the anterior projection, angle 90, the left lateral view, and so forth.

2. What is the physiological correlate of this imaging pattern?

3. What is the differential diagnosis of this scintigraphic pattern in this patient?

4. What is the likely diagnosis considering the patient's history?

Central Nervous System: Herpes Encephalitis

1. Increased uptake in the left temporal lobe.

2. Increased blood flow to this region.

3. Seizure focus (ictal injection), infection, tumor.

4. Herpes encephalitis.

References

Meyer MA, Hubner KF, Raja S, et al: Sequential positron emission tomography evaluations of brain metabolism in acute herpes encephalitis, *Neuroimaging* 4:104-105, 1994.

Ackerman ES, Tumeh SS, Charon M, et al: Viral encephalitis: imaging with SPECT, *Clin Nucl Med* 13:640-643, 1988.

Cross-Reference

Nuclear Medicine: THE REQUISITES, ed 2, pp 300-301.

Comment

Because of its poor prognosis and rapid progression, early diagnosis and treatment of herpes encephalitis is critical. The disease is life-threatening and may result in permanent memory and cognitive brain dysfunction for those who survive. The clinical diagnosis is based on nonspecific neurological signs indicating temporal lobe dysfunction and focal EEG abnormalities. MRI is the initial diagnostic imaging method because of its high sensitivity and anatomical resolution of limbic structures. However, when inconclusive, brain perfusion SPECT or FDG-PET may be diagnostic. Increased tracer accumulation in the medial and lateral portions of the temporal lobe is characteristic of herpes encephalitis, although extratemporal sites sometimes may be seen.

Primary and secondary brain tumors generally have increased metabolism that can be seen on FDG-PET imaging. Although blood flow usually follows metabolism and is increased with most tumors, ^{99m}Tc HM-PAO SPECT cerebral perfusion studies rarely show increased uptake with tumors. The reason is uncertain—perhaps a lack of receptors. Seizure foci have increased uptake on FDG-PET and brain perfusion SPECT during the ictal phase but have decreased uptake during the interictal phase.

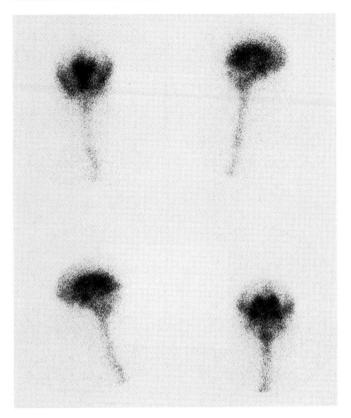

A 65-year-old man was referred for radionuclide cisternography. CT showed enlarged cerebrospinal spaces.

1. What is the radiopharmaceutical and route of administration?

2. Describe the findings on these images acquired at 24 hours after injection. *Top row:* anterior and right lateral. *Bottom row:* left lateral and posterior.

3. What is the diagnosis?

4. What are the patient's likely symptoms?

Central Nervous System: Normal-Pressure Hydrocephalus

1. [111]In DTPA administered intrathecally by lumbar puncture.

2. Ventricular reflux and convexity block with no flow over the cerebral hemispheres above the sylvian fissure.

3. Communicating hydrocephalus, in this case normal-pressure hydrocephalus.

4. Triad of dementia, ataxia, and incontinence.

Reference

Harbert JC: Radionuclide cisternography. In Harbert JC, Eckelman WC, Neumann RD, editors: *Nuclear medicine, diagnosis and therapy,* New York, 1996, Thieme Medical Publishers, pp 387-400.

Cross-Reference

Nuclear Medicine: THE REQUISITES, ed 2, pp 317-318.

Comment

Cerebrospinal fluid (CSF) is secreted by the choroid plexus of the ventricles, then drains from the lateral ventricles through the interventricular foramen of the third and fourth ventricles and diffuses into the subarachnoid space that surrounds the brain and spinal cord. It then is absorbed by the pacchionian granulations of the pia arachnoid villa and enters the superior sagittal sinus. When injected intrathecally into the lumbar space, ^{111}In DTPA, a small molecule, follows the flow of CSF. Normally it reaches the basal cisterns by 1 hour, the frontal poles and sylvian fissure by 6 hours, the cerebral convexities by 12 hours, and the sagittal sinus by 24 hours. It does not normally enter the ventricular system (except transiently in some normals) because physiological flow is in the opposite direction.

Normal-pressure hydrocephalus is a communicating hydrocephalus associated with dilation of the ventricular system but normal cerebrospinal pressure. The patterns of cerebral atrophy and normal-pressure hydrocephalus overlap on MRI. Surgical shunting (ventricular peritoneal, ventriculoatrial, or lumbar peritoneal shunting) can reverse the progressive dysfunction; however, not all patients improve with surgery. Radionuclide cisternography in combination with clinical findings, e.g., mental clearing after removal of cerebrospinal fluid, is used to confirm the clinical diagnosis and to predict response to shunting. The pattern of prolonged ventricular reflux is associated with improvement after ventricular shunting.

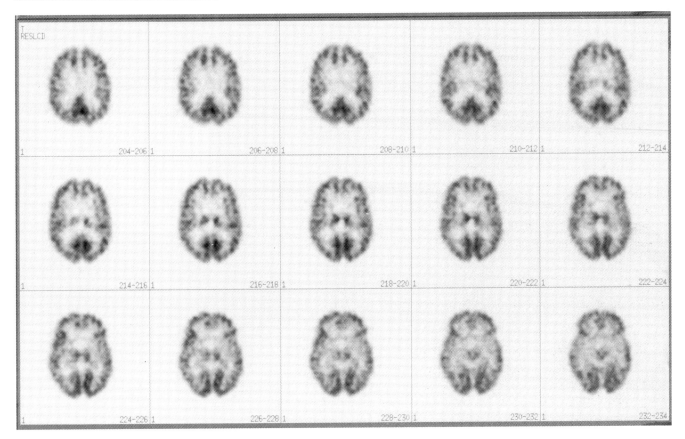

A 33-year-old man with neurological disorder was referred for a ^{18}F FDG-PET brain scan.

1. What is the FDG-PET scan abnormality?

2. What symptoms are likely?

3. What is the pathological condition?

4. What is the diagnosis?

Central Nervous System: Huntington's Disease

1. Hypometabolism of the basal ganglion.

2. Progressive motor abnormalities of involuntary choreiform movements and akinetic rigidity with progressive cognitive deterioration.

3. Neuronal degeneration in the striatum, with the caudate more involved than the putamen.

4. Huntington's disease.

References

Boecker H, Kuwert T, Langen KJ, et al: SPECT with HMPAO compared to PET with FDG in Huntington's disease, *J Comput Assist Tomogr* 18:524-528, 1994.

VanHeertum RL, Tikofsky RS, Rubens AB: Dementia. In VanHeertum RL, Tikofsky RS, editors: *Functional cerebral SPECT and PET imaging,* ed 3, New York, 2000, Lippincott Williams & Wilkins, pp 165-169.

Cross-Reference
Nuclear Medicine: THE REQUISITES, ed 2, p 314.

Comment

Huntington's disease is an autosomal dominant disorder of unknown origin that manifests in middle age. It is a progressive disease with symptoms and signs of involuntary choreiform movements and akinetic rigidity, behavioral changes, and dementia. CT and MRI scans often show no changes early in the course of the disease, although in later stages, atrophy of the head of the caudate and frontal cortex may be seen. PET studies show hypometabolism in the caudate and putamen nuclei, which as gray matter should have uptake similar to the cortex. These changes often precede atrophy seen on CT. Studies have found hypometabolism in the caudate nucleus of approximately one third of patients genetically at risk for the disease.

Parkinson's disease is another movement disorder, one that is caused by loss of the pigmented neurons in the substantia nigra and is characterized by bradykinesia, tremor, and rigidity. Dementia occurs in later stages in 20% to 30% of patients. No consistent characteristic SPECT or PET imaging pattern has been reported. However, patients with severe Parkinson's dementia late in the disease course may have scintigraphic findings indistinguishable from those of late Alzheimer's disease, i.e., bilateral hypoperfusion and hypometabolism of the posterior parietotemporal and frontal regions.

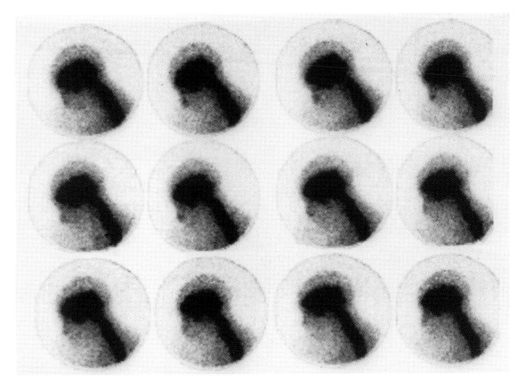

A 53-year-old woman has a history of head trauma, headache, and rhinorrhea. Left lateral views over 1 hour.

1. Name the appropriate radiopharmaceutical(s).

2. How is the radiopharmaceutical administered?

3. What is the imaging finding and interpretation?

4. How can the site of leakage be further defined?

Central Nervous System: CSF Leak

1. ^{111}In or ^{99m}Tc DTPA.

2. Intrathecal injection.

3. Activity in the region of the nose, indicating CSF leak, probably at the cribriform plate.

4. Anterior views. With the use of nasal pledgets placed in the superior, middle, and inferior nasal turbinates.

References

Harbert JC: Radionuclide cisternography. In Harbert JC, Eckelman WC, Neumann RD, editors: *Nuclear medicine, diagnosis and therapy,* New York, 1996, Thieme Publishers, pp 396-398.

Lawrence SK, Sandler MP, Partain CL, et al: Cerebrospinal fluid imaging. In Sandler MP, Coleman RE, Wackers FJTh, editors: *Diagnostic nuclear medicine,* ed 3, Baltimore, 1996, Williams & Wilkins, pp 1163-1176.

Cross-Reference
Nuclear Medicine: THE REQUISITES, ed 2, pp 318-320.

Comment

CSF rhinorrhea and otorrhea can be difficult diagnostic problems. Most leaks produce a small volume of fluid and leak intermittently. Some patients have repeated bouts of meningitis, and patient recognition of fluid drainage may be minimal or absent. Often imaging is required to confirm the CSF origin of rhinorrhea. Multiple modalities, e.g., CT with metrizamide and MRI, are also used for this purpose. The radionuclide method is an old, established technique and still useful in many cases.

Trauma and surgery are the most common causes for CSF rhinorrhea. Hydrocephalus and congenital defects are less common nontraumatic causes. CSF leak may occur at any site from the frontal sinuses to the temporal bone. The cribriform plate is the most susceptible to fracture. CSF otorrhea is a far less common cause of CSF leak. Perforation of the dura with communication through the petrous bone is the usual cause of otorrhea, although diversion through the eustachian tube also has been observed.

The study is performed with pledgets of cotton placed in the superior, middle, and inferior nasal turbinates bilaterally. The purpose is to differentiate frontal, ethmoidal, and sphenoidal sinus leakage. The pledgets are counted in a well counter rather than imaged and thus more sensitive for detection of leakage than imaging. Although lateral and anterior imaging is done for rhinorrhea, posterior imaging is performed for otorrhea.

A

B

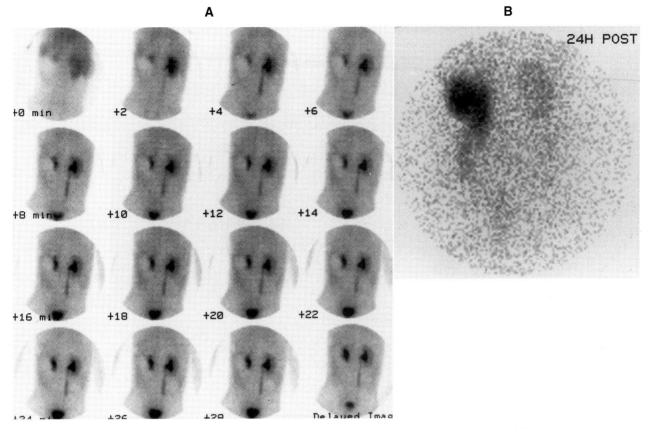

A 55-year-old woman with a history of renal stones is evaluated for recent onset of flank pain. ^{99m}Tc DTPA 30-minute dynamic radionuclide renogram *(A)* and 24-hour delayed image *(B)* are shown.

1. What are the scintigraphic findings?
2. Explain the changing imaging findings.
3. What is the diagnosis?
4. What is the likely cause?

Genitourinary System: Urinoma

1. A photopenic region, best seen on early images, involves most of the left renal fossa. Only the very upper pole is functioning. Urinary clearance into left renal pelvis appears displaced medially by the photopenic defect. The right pelvis and upper two thirds of the ureter fill. Poor clearance bilaterally. Delayed images show increased radiotracer uptake in the region of the initial cold defect and inferior to it.

2. The cold defect is a urinoma with an attenuating mass effect. Over time the radioactive urine enters this space and mixes with the nonradioactive urinoma. Activity in the region of the urinoma increases over time while the earlier seen kidney and background activity have cleared.

3. Active urinary leak and urinoma.

4. Urinary tract obstruction.

Reference

Talner LB: Urinary obstruction. In Pollack HM, McClennan BL, editors: *Clinical urography,* ed 2, Philadelphia, 2000, WB Saunders, pp 1944-1952.

Cross-Reference

Nuclear Medicine: THE REQUISITES, ed 2, pp 351-353.

Comment

Rupture of the weakest portion of the collecting system, the calyceal fornix, occurs when renal pelvic pressure exceeds a critical level. Less commonly the tear may affect the pelvis or ureter. This may occur during a bout of acute ureteral obstruction, retrograde pyelography, intravenous urography with abdominal compression, and massive vesicoureteral reflux. Spontaneous extravasation (not caused by trauma, instrumentation, or surgery) usually is caused by a ureteral calculus and almost always is benign and self-limited. Continued leakage of urine in the presence of obstruction may lead to the formation of an encapsulated retroperitoneal urine collection, a urinoma. In adults, spontaneous urinomas are confined to the perinephric space.

Urinomas generally do not result from small perforations unless the leak is accompanied by obstruction distal to the exit point. Until they become very large, urinomas often are clinically silent. Eventually a palpable tender mass may develop in conjunction with malaise, weight loss, nausea, and vague abdominal pain or back discomfort. The urinoma may worsen the obstruction because of its mass effect. Treatment consists of repair of the obstruction and excision and drainage of the urinoma.

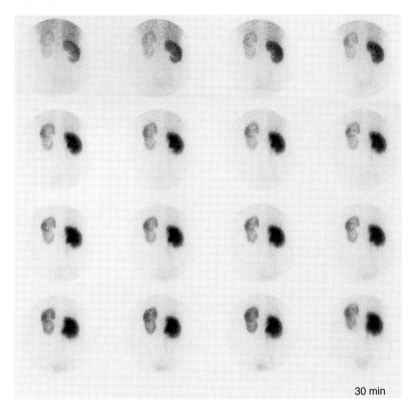

30 min

Furosemide

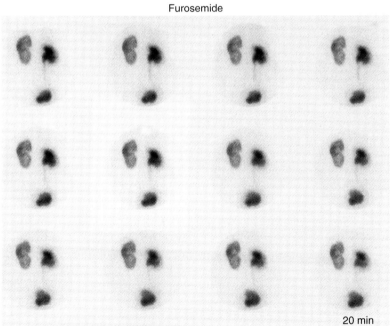

20 min

A 51-year-old woman with metastatic cervical cancer and new hydronephrosis on CT.

1. Describe the scintigraphic findings.
2. What is the diagnosis before and after the administration of diuretic (furosemide)?
3. What imaging finding should you see before administering furosemide?
4. How do you calculate differential renal function?

Genitourinary System: Diuretic Renography—Bilateral Obstruction

1. Left kidney: delayed and decreased cortical uptake, no clearance into the calyces or pelvis. Right kidney: prompt uptake and clearance into the collecting system, faint persistent visualization of the right ureter, and poor response to furosemide.

2. Before furosemide: high-grade obstruction on the left and hydronephrosis on the right, suspicious for obstruction. After furosemide: high-grade obstruction on the left and obstruction on the right.

3. Filling of the renal collecting system.

4. Percent radiopharmaceutical uptake by each kidney divided by total renal uptake between 1 and 3 minutes (before clearance into the calyces and pelvis).

References

Fine EJ: Diuretic renography and angiotensin-converting enzyme inhibitor renography, *Radiol Clin North Am* 39:979-995, 2001.

Taylor AL: Radionuclide renography: a personal approach, *Semin Nucl Med* 29:102-127, 1999.

Cross-Reference

Nuclear Medicine: THE REQUISITES, ed 2, pp 340-348.

Comment

The administration of a diuretic is not indicated in high-grade obstruction because there is no collecting system radiotracer to challenge. Diuretic renography is useful in patients with lower-grade obstructions, i.e., urinary excretion into the collecting system but retention in the renal pelvis. If the collecting system drains with diuretic, it is not obstructed, e.g., patients with congenital hydronephrosis or hydronephrosis caused by ureteropelvic reflux. Another group of patients in whom this technique is valuable are those who have had surgical correction for obstruction but have persistent dilation. Finally, patients with known partial obstruction, e.g., those with pelvic tumor compressing the ureters and new hydronephrosis noted on CT. The question is not whether an obstruction exists. Rather the question is whether urgent intervention is needed, e.g., stenting, to save the kidney and its renal function. Drainage after administration of a diuretic in these patients suggests that renal function will not deteriorate in the short term.

Many nuclear medicine clinics quantify the rate of radiotracer washout after furosemide. A common method is to calculate a half-time of emptying. As in all nuclear medicine, quantification must be interpreted in conjunction with image analysis. Normal values for the rate of emptying depend to some extent on the methodology used. In some clinics, diuretic is administered as soon as the renal pelvis has filled. Other clinics administer the diuretic at the end of the initial 25- to 30-minute study. Still others administer it before the study. The technique should be standardized for the particular method.

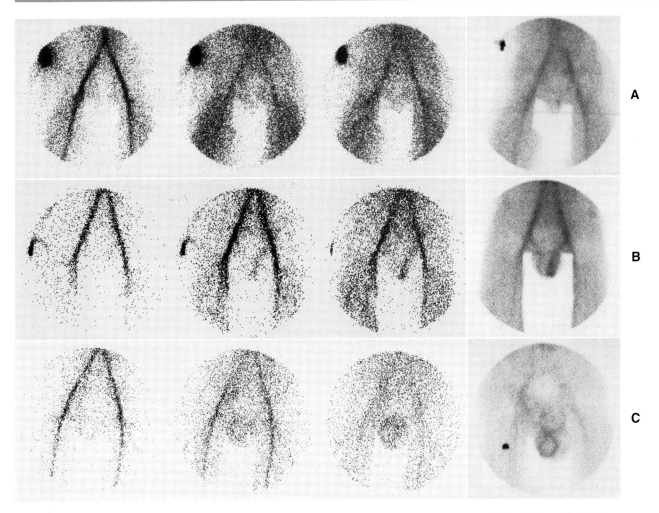

Three patients (*A, B,* and *C*) present with acute scrotal pain. All had testicular scans with blood flow *(left)* and post-flow static images *(right)*.

1. What are the scintigraphic findings in each case?
2. What is the most likely diagnosis in each patient?
3. What is the pathophysiological condition for patients *A, B,* and *C?*
4. What is the incidence of the most frequent final diagnoses in patients referred for acute scrotal pain?

Genitourinary System: Torsion of Testicular Appendage, Epididymitis, Delayed Torsion

1. *A,* Mildly increased flow and mild focal left upper scrotal uptake on the static image. *B,* Increased flow and increased distribution to the left hemiscrotum. *C,* Increased flow and delayed halo sign of the right hemiscrotum.

2. *A,* Torsion of a testicular appendage. *B,* Acute epididymitis/orchitis. *C,* Delayed testicular torsion.

3. *A,* Loss of blood supply to the appendage of the testicle. *B,* Infection, viral or bacterial. *C,* Infarction of the testicle caused by torsion more than 24 hours' duration.

4. Testicular torsion, 35%; torsion of the appendix testis, 35%; acute epididymitis, 25%, but varies with institution.

References

Melloul M, Paz A, Las D, et al: The pattern of radionuclide scrotal scan in torsion of testicular appendages, *Eur J Nucl Med* 23:967-997, 1996.

Siegel MJ: The acute scrotum, *Radiol Clin North Am* 35:959-976, 1997.

Cross-Reference
Nuclear Medicine: THE REQUISITES, ed 2, pp 357-362.

Comment

Torsion of the testicular appendage is treated medically. Affected patients (6 to 12 years of age) have acute pain localized to the superior pole of the testis. The classical physical examination finding is a small, firm paratesticular nodule exhibiting blue discoloration through overlying skin. Atrophy of the appendage and resolution of symptoms is the usual outcome. Scintigraphy may be normal, show focal uptake on delayed images as seen in this case, or have a more inflammatory appearance with increased flow, usually localized to the upper pole.

Acute epididymitis most commonly affects adolescent boys. It usually is caused by sexually transmitted organisms such as chlamydia and gonorrhea. This severe, acute inflammation is visualized on scintigraphy as increased flow and increased distribution to the inflamed side. It may be focal and localized to the epididymitis or more diffuse in orchitis.

Testicular torsion is the result of the testis and spermatic cord twisting one or more times, obstructing blood flow. A congenital predilection exists as a result of the bell-clapper deformity. Patients in whom acute torsion is suspected are taken immediately to surgery in an attempt to maintain testicular viability. The salvage rate is 100% at 6 hours, 70% from 6 to 12 hours, and 20% within 12 to 24 hours after the onset of pain. After 24 hours the testis rarely is salvageable. The increased flow seen on this study, *C,* is caused by the hyperemic dartos of the scrotum; the cold central region is nonviable testicle.

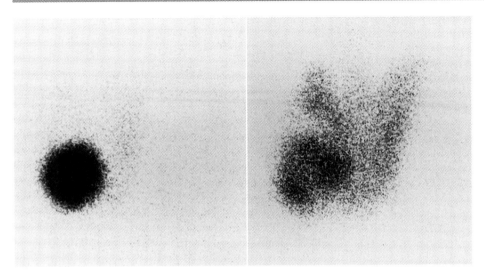

A 44-year-old woman had two ^{123}I thyroid scans performed 1 year apart.

1. What is the likely diagnosis in the first scan *(left)?* The patient is hyperthyroid.

2. What has happened in the intervening time?

3. What is the patient's thyroid function and diagnosis at the time of the second scan?

4. The patient has a suppressed thyroid-stimulating hormone (TSH) level but normal thyroxine (T$_4$) level. What is the diagnosis?

Endocrine System: Therapy of Toxic Nodule

1. Toxic autonomous thyroid adenoma in the right lobe.

2. The patient has been treated with radioactive iodine [131]I. The autonomous nodule is still hyperfunctional with cold areas, likely representing hemorrhage, necrosis, or both. However, it is no longer fully suppressing the remaining thyroid.

3. The patient may be euthyroid or possibly mildly hyperthyroid. The thyroid scan suggests partial suppression of the normal thyroid. Determination of the serum TSH level would answer the question.

4. Persistent hyperfunctioning autonomous adenoma (nodule), inadequately treated.

Reference

Becker DV, Hurley JR: Radioiodine treatment of hyperthyroidism. In Sandler MP, Coleman RE, Wackers FJTh, et al, editors: *Diagnostic nuclear medicine,* ed 3, Baltimore, 1996, Williams & Wilkins, pp 943-958.

Cross-Reference

Nuclear Medicine: THE REQUISITES, ed 2, pp 272-274.

Comment

This patient became clinically euthyroid after ^{131}I therapy after the first scan. She returned for a repeat thyroid scan because of a persistent right lower lobe thyroid nodule on examination and a suppressed serum TSH level. The second study shows that the palpable nodule is still hyperfunctioning but to a lesser extent than before therapy. The patient received additional radioiodine therapy. The effectiveness of radioactive iodine therapy for single autonomous nodules is quite high; however, occasionally a second therapy is needed. Effective therapy would have resulted in a totally cold (nonfunctioning) nodule.

Short- and long-term adverse effects from radioactive iodine are few. Radioactive iodine therapy has been given for hyperthyroidism for more than 50 years. It is safe and effective. The usual ^{131}I dose for autonomous nodule(s) is 20 to 30 mCi. This dose is typically greater than for patients with Graves' disease because thyroid nodules are more resistant to therapy. Many studies have sought to find adverse effects, e.g., second tumors, leukemia, infertility, abnormal offspring; however, no significant increase in these problems has been found in treated patients. Transient worsening of hyperthyroid symptoms and local pain may be noted in a minority of patients in the days after therapy. These are easily controlled with β-blocking and antiinflammatory drugs. [131]I therapy is contraindicated if the patient is pregnant. Iodine crosses the placenta. The fetal thyroid traps and organifies iodine after 10 weeks; therefore congenital hypothyroidism will result if ^{131}I is administered to the mother.

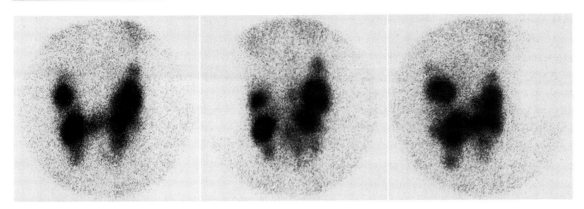

A 53-year-old woman was referred for recent enlargement of the right lower lobe of a known multinodular thyroid gland and a suppressed TSH level. The patient had radiation therapy for acne as a teenager.

1. Describe the scintigraphic findings of this ^{99m}Tc pertechnetate scan (*left to right:* anterior, left anterior oblique, right anterior oblique).

2. Give the likely diagnosis.

3. What are the therapeutic options?

4. What is the likelihood of thyroid cancer in this patient?

Endocrine System: Toxic Nodular Goiter and Thyroid Cancer

1. Multiple hot and cold regions throughout both lobes with apparent suppression of nonnodular gland.

2. Multinodular toxic goiter.

3. Biopsy. If benign, then ^{131}I therapy or surgery for multinodular goiter.

4. The likelihood of thyroid cancer is less than 5% in patients with a multinodular goiter. A dominant nodule increases the suspicion for cancer. A history of radiation therapy to the head and neck significantly increases this patient's risk of thyroid cancer.

Reference

Cases JA, Surks MI: The changing role of scintigraphy in the evaluation of thyroid nodules, *Semin Nucl Med* 30:81-87, 2000.

Cross-Reference

Nuclear Medicine: THE REQUISITES, ed 2, pp 369-374.

Comment

This patient not only had a toxic multinodular goiter with a radioactive iodine uptake (RAIU) of 36% but also had papillary follicular thyroid cancer. She subsequently had a near-total thyroidectomy and radioactive iodine therapy. The incidence of thyroid cancer approaches 30% in a patient with a history of radiation therapy to the neck and a nodular gland. Patients treated with radiation to the neck for acne, ringworm, and tonsillar enlargement often received a radiation dose of 10 to 50 rads to the thyroid. The scan has the appearance of a multinodular toxic goiter. This is a ^{99m}Tc pertechnetate scan. Note the salivary glands above the thyroid and the high background, neither of which is seen with ^{123}I. Normally thyroid uptake and salivary uptake are similar with ^{99m}Tc pertechnetate. The high thyroid uptake compared with salivary uptake here is consistent with hyperthyroidism. ^{131}I, 10 μCi, was administered orally, for the radioactive iodine uptake study. The RAIU was 38%. The usual administered dose for therapy of multinodular toxic goiter is 20 to 30 mCi. Toxic nodular goiter is more resistant to ^{131}I therapy than Graves' disease. Once the nodules are effectively treated, which may require 3 to 4 months, the function of the remaining suppressed gland will return. Hypothyroidism as a result of radioactive iodine therapy is uncommon because the suppressed gland does not take up the radioactive iodine. However, in this case the patient's biopsy showed cancer, so she received a thyroid cancer ablation dose after a near-total thyroidectomy.

A

ANT

B

POST

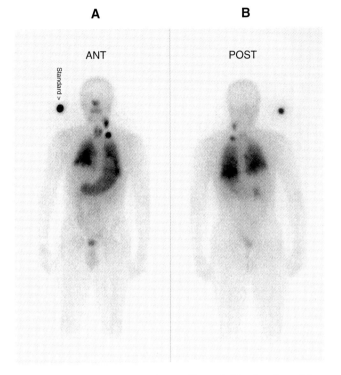

A 53-year-old woman with papillary-follicular thyroid cancer after near-total thyroidectomy.

1. What is the study? What is the radiopharmaceutical?

2. Describe the pattern of uptake and your interpretation.

3. What dose of ^{131}I is used for thyroid uptake and scan for a patient with suspected substernal goiter *(A)* and for a thyroid cancer patient *(B)* after thyroidectomy?

4. Explain why ^{131}I therapy but not ^{123}I is effective for Graves' hyperthyroidism, toxic nodules, and thyroid cancer.

Endocrine System: Thyroid Cancer Whole-Body Scan

1. [123]I whole-body thyroid cancer scan. [131]I is most commonly used, but the excellent image quality and similar biodistribution indicate this is [123]I.

2. Abnormal diffuse uptake in the lungs, uptake in the midline neck, left supraclavicular and lower cervical, all consistent with metastatic tumor

3. Uptake, 10 μCi; scan, 50 μCi; thyroid cancer scan, 2 to 4 mCi. Be careful to distinguish between millicuries (mCi) and microcuries (μCi).

4. The beta particle emissions of ^{131}I are taken up by thyroid follicular cells and are responsible for its therapeutic effect.

References

Freitas JE: Therapy of differentiated thyroid cancer. In Freeman LM, editor: *Nuclear Medicine Annual 1998,* Philadelphia, 1998, Lippincott-Raven.

Hurley JR, Becker DV: Treatment of thyroid cancer with radioiodine (131-I). In Sandler MP, Coleman RE, Wackers FJTh, et al, editors: *Diagnostic nuclear medicine,* ed 3, Baltimore, 1996, Williams & Wilkins, pp 959-989.

Cross-Reference

Nuclear Medicine: THE REQUISITES, ed 2, pp 379-380.

Comment

[131]I is most commonly used for whole-body thyroid cancer scintigraphy; however, there is a high total body radiation dose (0.5 rads/mCi) and the potential for thyroid stunning, i.e., decreased uptake of the subsequent therapeutic dose. Preliminary reports suggest that ^{123}I is now being used as an alternative to ^{131}I with similar diagnostic information. Disadvantages of ^{123}I are its short physical half-life (13 hours), which limits delayed imaging to 24 hours, and its higher expense. The administered dose for thyroid cancer scans is approximately 1.5 mCi, compared with 200 μCi for routine thyroid scans.

The only accepted clinical indication for a ^{131}I thyroid scan other than thyroid cancer is substernal goiter. The higher energy photopeak (364 keV) allows for better detectability compared with possible attenuation of [123]I (159 keV) by the sternum. The radiation dose to the normal thyroid from ^{131}I is high, 1 rad/μCi, resulting in approximately 50 rads to the thyroid. Most patients referred for this indication are elderly patients with goiter. Many clinics use ^{123}I first and reserve ^{131}I as a second-line evaluation for a substernal gland.

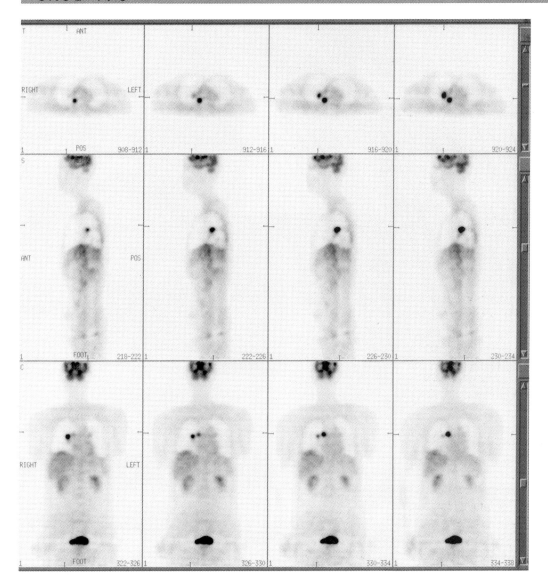

A patient has a history of papillary thyroid cancer and has undergone thyroidectomy. The patient received two ^{131}I treatments, 150 mCi each. The serum thyroglobulin level is elevated. Findings of a recent ^{131}I whole-body scan were negative.

1. What is the purpose of a serum thyroglobulin level determination?

2. What are the scintigraphic findings and interpretation of the FDG-PET study?

3. Why is there a discrepancy between the ^{131}I study and the ^{18}F FDG study?

4. Must the patient be withdrawn from thyroid replacement/suppression therapy before the FDG-PET study?

Endocrine System: FDG-PET and Thyroid Cancer

1. Serum thyroglobulin is used as a thyroid cancer serum marker. After gland ablation, detection indicates persistent tumor. It is increased with active disease.

2. Focal uptake in the right hilum and mediastinum consistent with tumor adenopathy.

3. The tumor has differentiated. Well-differentiated thyroid tumors usually have ^{131}I uptake. Poorly differentiated tumors are likely to be ^{131}I negative, FDG positive.

4. No. FDG uptake is not TSH-dependent; thus patients do not have to be withdrawn from suppression.

Reference

Wang W, Macapinlac H, Larson SM, et al: [^{18}F] FDG positron emission tomography localizes residual thyroid cancer in patients with negative diagnostic ^{131}I whole body scans and elevated serum thyroglobulin levels, *J Clin Endocrinol Metab* 84:2291-2302, 1999.

Cross-Reference

Nuclear Medicine: THE REQUISITES, ed 2, pp 376-378.

Comment

Approximately 85% of differentiated thyroid carcinomas take up [131]I. However, some uncommon thyroid cancers are known to have inconsistent ^{131}I uptake, e.g., Hürthle cell tumor, anaplastic thyroid cancer. The current clinical indication for FDG-PET in thyroid cancer is for patients with negative findings on ^{131}I whole-body scans but elevated serum thyroglobulin levels. FDG localization allows for possible tumor resection and serves as a baseline for evaluating response to therapy. Treatment of these patients with high-dose ^{131}I often produces a decline of the serum thyroglobulin level, although patients are rarely cured. Tumor response indicates tumor uptake, albeit very low (not seen on 2 mCi diagnostic scan, but seen on scan 7 to 10 days after high-dose therapy). [201]Tl and ^{99m}Tc sestamibi have been used for thyroid tumor localization; however, FDG-PET is considered superior. Thyroid metastases that trap ^{131}I often do not take up FDG, whereas FDG-avid metastases often have lost their ability to trap iodine. Dedifferentiated tumors lose their normal functional ability to concentrate iodine but tend to have increased glucose metabolism typical of higher-grade tumors. The sensitivity of FDG-PET for detecting metastases in all patients with differentiated thyroid cancer is only about 50%, but the combined use of FDG and ^{131}I scan has a 95% sensitivity. However, for patients with negative ^{131}I scans and elevated serum thyroglobulin levels, the sensitivity of FDG-PET is considerably higher (70% to 90%).

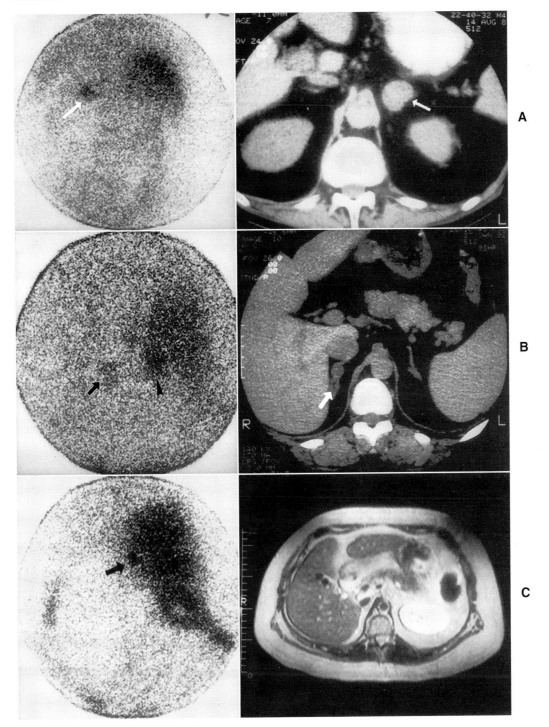

Three patients with Cushing's syndrome were referred for an ^{131}I iodocholesterol study (NP-59). CT and NP-59 *(posterior views)* studies are shown. Arrows are a bonus.

1. Patients *A* and *B* have a similar history of newly diagnosed hypercortisolism. Describe the findings and give interpretations.

2. Patient *C* had previous adrenalectomy for Cushing's syndrome but continues to have hypercortisolism. Describe the findings and give an interpretation.

3. What is the mechanism of uptake of the radiopharmaceutical?

4. What other diseases besides Cushing's syndrome can be diagnosed with NP-59?

Endocrine System: Adrenocortical Scintigraphy

1. *A,* Unilateral NP-59 uptake consistent with left adrenal adenoma; concordant with the CT study. *B,* Bilateral adrenal hyperplasia; discordant with CT study.

2. Uptake in the right adrenal bed region indicating adrenal remnant. Discordant with the negative CT.

3. Transport and receptors systems for serum cholesterol account for adrenal uptake. Cholesterol is required for the production of adrenal hormones.

4. Hyperaldosteronism (adrenal adenoma or hyperplasia) and hyperandrogenism.

References

Gross MD, Shulkin BL, Shapiro B, et al: Adrenal scintigraphy and therapy of neuroendocrine tumors with I-131 MIBG. In Sandler MP, Coleman RE, editors: *Diagnostic nuclear medicine,* ed 3, Baltimore, 1996, Williams & Wilkins, pp 1023-1045.

Yu KC, Alexander HR, Ziessman HA, et al: The role of preoperative iodocholesterol scintiscanning in patients undergoing adrenalectomy for Cushing's syndrome, *Surgery* 118: 981-987, 1995.

Cross-Reference

Nuclear Medicine: THE REQUISITES, ed 2, pp 380-383.

Comment

[131]I-6β-iodomethyl-19-iodocholesterol (NP-59, "new pharmaceutical," investigational number) is not approved by the FDA but available from the University of Michigan on an investigational new drug basis. It is an "orphan" drug. However, its clinical utility is proven. It can provide important functional information either not available or in contradiction to the findings suggested by the anatomical imaging study. When used to diagnose hyperaldosterolism or hyperadrenalism, the patient must be pretreated with dexamethasone to suppress adrenocorticotropic hormone (ACTH) secretion and inhibit adrenal uptake by the zona fasciculata and zona reticulosa. NP-59 is used to localize disease proved to be hyperfunctional by biochemical testing. It can determine whether the disease is unilateral or bilateral. The most common indication is Cushing's "syndrome," or hypercortisolism. Cushing's "disease" is caused by excess pituitary ACTH, the most common cause for Cushing's syndrome. In these patients bilateral uptake is seen. With autonomous cortisol production from an adrenal adenoma, unilateral uptake is seen. With adrenal cortical carcinoma, no uptake is seen. The tumor is hypofunctional and thus does not take up enough radiotracer in most cases to be detected scintigraphically. No uptake is seen on the contralateral normal side because it is suppressed.

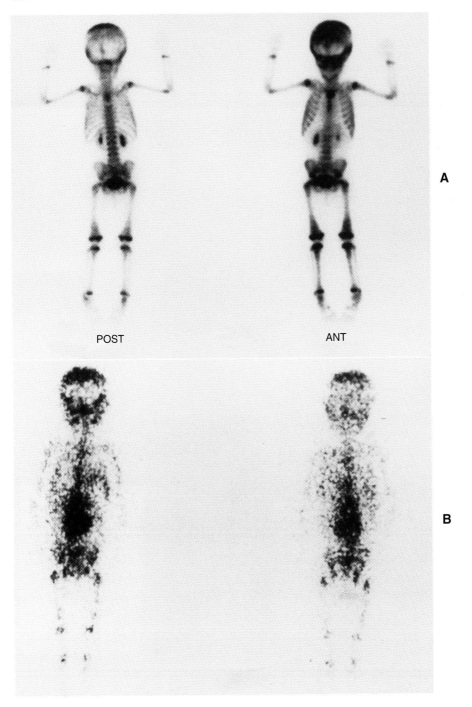

POST

ANT

A

B

A 3-year-old boy with a recently diagnosed retroperitoneal tumor.

1. Describe the imaging findings of the ^{99m}Tc MDP bone scan *(A)* and the ^{131}I MIBG study *(B)*.

2. What is your interpretation of the two studies?

3. What are the most common tumor causes for extraosseous uptake of bone-seeking radiopharmaceuticals in this age group?

4. What is the most sensitive imaging method for detection of bone metastases in this disease?

Endocrine System: Bone Scan and ^{131}I MIBG-Neuroblastoma

1. Bone scan shows uptake symmetrically in the distal femurs, cranial, and facial bones. [131]I MIBG study shows a large area of midline abdominal uptake. Inspection of the bone scan in the same area suggests a soft tissue left perirenal density, best seen in the anterior view. In addition, diffuse marrow/bone uptake is seen on the MIBG study.

2. The prominent midline uptake on the MIBG study is consistent with neuroblastoma. Subtle bone uptake is seen in that region. The symmetrical bone uptake in the distal femurs, cranial, and facial bones is very suggestive of tumor. The MIBG study confirms metastatic disease with extensive tumor in the marrow/bone from skull to feet.

3. First, primary neuroblastoma. Osteosarcoma metastatic to the lung is another. Metastases of various tumors occasionally are seen on bone scans, lung, colon, and breast.

4. Combination of ^{99m}Tc bone scan and ^{131}I MIBG.

References

Shulkin BL, Shapiro B: Current concepts on the diagnostic use of MIBG in children, *J Nucl Med* 39:667-688, 1998.

Gelfand MJ: Metaiodobenzylguanidine in children, *Semin Nucl Med* 23:231-242, 1993.

Cross-Reference

Nuclear Medicine: THE REQUISITES, ed 2, pp 383-384.

Comment

Neuroblastoma commonly manifests at an advanced stage and bone scans are used routinely for detection of metastatic lesions. Because the metastatic lesions of neuroblastoma originate in the bone marrow cavity, bone scans may underestimate the early stages of spread. The propensity of metastatic neuroblastoma to localize in metaphyseal regions adjacent to hot growth plates can also hinder early detection. The relatively subtle bone scan changes in this case contrast with the very abnormal MIBG study. Both studies are required for the highest detection rate of metastases.

[131]I MIBG is taken up and localized in presynaptic adrenergic nerves, adrenal medulla, and neuroblastic tumors. On scintigraphy, normal MIBG uptake is seen in the liver, soft tissue, and blood pool but not in normal bones or bone marrow. Normal uptake also may be seen in organs with adrenergic intervention, e.g., heart, salivary glands, spleen. Normal bilateral adrenal uptake is seen in 10% of patients. MIBG commonly is ordered for staging and monitoring the effectiveness of therapy. Response to therapy is seen on the MIBG study before the bone scan.

LBBB. *see* Left bundle branch block

Le Veen peritoneovenous shunt, 352

Left bundle branch block, 167-168

Left ventricular ejection fraction, 36, 169-170

Legg-Calve-Perthes disease, spontaneous osteonecrosis associated with, 142

Leiomyoma, small intestine bleeding associated with, 346

Leiomyosarcoma, small intestine bleeding associated with, 346

Leontiasis ossea, 24

Lesion
  on bone scan, 272
  malignant, in spine, 256
  photopenic, 254

Leukemia
  cold spine defect and, 148
  spontaneous osteonecrosis associated with, 142

Leukocyte
  labeling of, 310
  oxine, 186
  ^{99m}technetium studies of, 181-184

Leukocyte study, radiolabeled, 312

Lewy body disease, 232

Lingual thyroid, 246

Liver
  benign tumor in, 342
  bleeding in, 74
  cavernous hemangioma in, 72, 218
  colorectal cancer and, 196
  dysfunction of, 212
  ^{67}gallium uptake in, 190
  infection in, 310
  lesions in, 71
  leukocyte uptake in, 184
  malignancy in, 114
  metastases to, 142
  neuroblastoma in, 132
  ^{99m}technetium sulfur colloid scan of, 220, 343-344
  ^{99m}technetium sulfur colloid uptake in, causes of, 343-344
  tumor in, 72, 188
  uptake in, radiation therapy and, 150

Liver disease
  biliary atresia and, 216
  parenchymal, 212

Lobectomy, temporal, 230

Lung
  abnormal activity of, differential diagnosis of, 150
  cancer of, 132
    pulmonary embolism and, 42
  carcinoma of, superscan associated with, 130
  hyperparathyroidism and uptake in, 136
  lower, hypoperfusion of, 178
  metastatic, bone scan uptake and, 14
  metastatic calcification in, 150
  oligemia of, 48
  osteosarcoma in, 138

Lung—cont'd
  right-to-left shunt in, 306
  stripe sign in, 46
  uptake in, abnormal lung activity and, 150
  ventilation-perfusion scan of, 303
  ^{133}Xenon ventilation imaging of, 304

Lung cancer, 132
  detection of, 188
  ^{18}fluorine fluorodeoxyglucose positron emission tomography for evaluation of, 194
  fluorodeoxyglucose positron emission tomography for detection of, 193
  lung scan for diagnosis of, 42
  perfusion defect associated with, 304
  pulmonary embolism evaluation and, 300

Lung disease
  adenosine contraindicated by, 158
  diagnosis of, 46
  evaluation of, 186

Lung/myocardial activity, 40

Lung scan
  hot spots on, 44
  pulmonary embolism diagnosed with, 42

Lupus erythematosus, spontaneous osteonecrosis associated with, 142

LVEF. *see* Left ventricular ejection fraction

Lymph node
  breast cancer and, 18
  uptake in, 26

Lymphangiomatosis, soft tissue hypertrophy associated with, 24

Lymphedema, 18
  breast cancer and, 202
  description of, 276

Lymphocyte, labeling of, 310

Lymphoma
  brain, 326
  brain tumor and, 60
  detection of, 188
  ^{18}fluorine fluorodeoxyglucose positron emission tomography for detection of, 192
  intracranial, evaluation of, 200
  malignant, 293, 326
  malignant B-cell, 191
  non-Hodgkin's, 55, 56
  superscan associated with, 130

Lymphoscintigraphy
  breast, 201-202
  lower extremities evaluated with, 276
  melanoma evaluated with, 204

M

MAA. *see* Macroaggregated albumin study

Macroaggregated albumin study, 305-306

Macrodystrophia lipomatosa, soft tissue hypertrophy associated with, 24